Absolute Hospital Medicine Review

Kevin Conrad
Editor

Absolute Hospital Medicine Review

An Intensive Question and Answer Guide

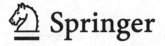 Springer

Editor
Kevin Conrad
Med. Dir. Comm. Aff. and Health Policy
Ochsner Health Systems Queensland
School of Medicine
New Orleans
Louisiana
USA

ISBN 978-3-319-23747-3   ISBN 978-3-319-23748-0   (eBook)
DOI 10.1007/978-3-319-23748-0

Library of Congress Control Number: 2015960185

Springer Cham Heidelberg New York Dordrecht London

Printed on acid-free paper

Springer International Publishing AG Switzerland is part of Springer Science+Business Media (www.springer.com)

Preface

Welcome to *Absolute Hospital Medicine Review: A Intensive Question and Answer Guide*

This book reflects the evolution of hospital medicine from its inception to its current rapidly expanding role in the delivery of healthcare. There is an emphasis in this book on the problems that hospitalists encounter daily. The goal of the book is to have an up-to-date referenced question-based learning text that encompasses all aspects of hospital care. It is divided into three sections: inpatient medicine, consultative and co-management, and hospital systems management. It is suitable for junior and senior clinicians, for those preparing for boards, and for those in training who would like to be exposed to the complexities of hospital medicine.

The content of this is book follows the framework set forth by the Society of Hospital Medicine. It relies heavily on the actual cases presenting to our facility and solutions that are based on available research.

These questions reflect the great variety of clinical, ethical, and administrative situations a hospitalist encounters. The definitive role of the hospitals has been somewhat of a moving target. I have been part of a program that began in the early days of hospital medicine. In the past 20 years since its formal inception, hospital medicine has grown to nearly 40,000 practitioners. No specialty has come so far so fast. The original intent of our own hospitalist program was to provide stability to our house staff teaching program. This has continued to be a major component, but we have also been called upon to co-manage surgical patients, provide cost-effective services, provide perioperative services, and lead a wide variety of quality initiatives.

As soon as the scope of our practice and our goals have been defined, they are changed. No doubt this trend will continue as hospitalists are viewed as the solution to many of the ever-increasing financial pressures on the healthcare system. As hospitalists, we have learned to be adaptable. Each week we face a new set expectations, requirements, and time constraints.

Our clinical future is uncertain as studies attempt to define which specialty provides the highest quality and most cost-effective care to the hospitalized patient. We need to understand the limitations of those studies, conduct our own research, and advocate for our clinical privileges. I believe the questions in this book will illustrate some of those issues.

Hospitalists often understand the acutely ill patient best. Their physical, emotional, and social needs can be rapidly assessed by our skill sets. We are often called upon to be the patient's advocate. With that comes the challenge of understanding the treatment options and proven efficacy of the options offered.

Now more so than ever, it is important that we define what we do, do it well, and communicate our value to the healthcare system. I hope that this question-based guide helps that process by demonstrating the issues that hospitalists are expert at solving and reveal those areas that need further research.

We hope to receive your feedback in improving future editions. Please share your thoughts on what topics should be added and how they should be presented.

New Orleans, LA, USA   Kevin Conrad, MD

Contents

Contributors

Editor in Chief

Kevin Conrad, MD, MBA Department of Hospital Medicine, Ochsner Health Systems, New Orleans, LA, USA

Tulane University School of Medicine, New Orleans, LA, USA

University of Queensland School of Medicine, New Orleans, LA, USA

Associate Editors

Laura E. Bateman, MD Internal Medicine Department, Ochsner Health Systems, New Orleans, LA, USA

Ashley Casey, Pharm.D, BCPS, MT, ASCP Department of Pharmacy, Ochsner Health Systems, New Orleans, LA, USA

Marianne Maumus, MD Department of Hospital Medicine, Ochsner Health Systems, New Orleans, LA, USA

Inpatient Medicine

Laura Bateman and Kevin Conrad

1. A 30-year-old female with systemic lupus erythematosus is recovering from a fracture of the right femur and right radius following a motor vehicle accident. She has been in the hospital for 5 days. She has a temperature spike of 39.0 °C (102.2 °F). Blood cultures are drawn which grow yeast, species to be identified. She does not appear ill or toxic. No obvious source of infection is found. The patient has an indwelling central catheter.

   In addition to changing the patient's central line, which of the following do you recommend?
   A) Continued observation.
   B) Computed tomography of the chest and abdomen.
   C) Start fluconazole.
   D) Start liposomal amphotericin B.
   E) Repeat blood cultures and treat if positive.

Answer: C
Candida is an increasingly common pathogen found due to line infections. It is currently the fourth leading bloodstream pathogen. In this particular case, despite the patient not appearing ill, treatment directed toward *Candida* should be initiated. The most common antifungal agents used for the treatment of candidemia are fluconazole and the echinocandins. These include caspofungin, micafungin, and anidulafungin. Amphotericin B is given less often due to the risk of nephrotoxicity. Both the echinocandins and the azoles are better tolerated than amphotericin B formulations. Candidemia requires treatment with antifungal agents. Catheter removal alone is not adequate therapy for candidemia. Several studies have noted the high mortality rates associated with candidemia. Furthermore, prompt initiation of therapy is crucial.

Reference
Manolakaki D, Velmahos G, Kourkoumpetis T, Chang Y, Alam HB, De Moya MM Mylonakis, E. Candida infection and colonization among trauma patients. Virulence. 2010;1(5):367–75.

2. A 41-year-old male presented to the emergency room with shortness of breath and chest pain. Imaging reveals a pulmonary embolus. He is started on enoxaparin 1 mg/kg SQ BID and warfarin 5 mg PO daily. Nursing staff reports to perform enoxaparin teaching in preparation for his discharge the following day; however, he reports that he is terrified of needles and feels as if twice daily injections will not be possible (weight = 77 kg, CrCl = 89 ml/min).

   Are there any other options to decrease the number of injections for this patient?
   A) Enoxaparin 1 mg/kg SQ daily
   B) Enoxaparin 0.5 mg/kg SQ daily
   C) Enoxaparin 1.5 mg/kg SQ daily
   D) Both A and C

Answer: C
Enoxaparin 1 mg/kg SQ daily would be used if a patient had a CrCl < 30 ml/min. Enoxaparin 0.5 mg/kg SQ is the indicated dose for infants >2 months and children </=18 years of age for thromboembolism prophylaxis and would be dosed BID, not daily. Enoxaparin 1.5 mg/kg SQ daily is an appropriate outpatient dosing regimen for patients with a CrCl > 30 ml/min for treatment.

Reference
Garcia DA, et al. CHEST guidelines – parenteral anticoagulants. Chest. 2012;141(2_suppl):e24S–43S.

L. Bateman, MD
Internal Medicine Department, Ochsner Clinic Foundation,
1521 Jefferson Hwy, New Orleans 70121, LA, USA
e-mail: lbateman@ochsner.org

K. Conrad, MBA, MD (✉)
Department of Hospital Medicine, Ochsner Medical Center,
1521 Jefferson Hwy, New Orleans 70121, LA, USA
e-mail: kconrad@ochsner.org

© Springer International Publishing Switzerland 2016
K. Conrad (ed.), *Absolute Hospital Medicine Review: An Intensive Question & Answer Guide*,
DOI 10.1007/978-3-319-23748-0_1

3. A 39-year-old female presents to the emergency room with progressive worsening of imbalance and vertigo accompanied by recent falls. She has a 5-year history of multiple sclerosis. Her last admit for a multiple sclerosis flair was 6 months ago. Medications are currently interferon beta-1a and gabapentin for neuropathic pain.

On physical examination, she is afebrile. Blood pressure is 120/66 mmHg. Heart rate is 60 bpm. Internuclear ophthalmoplegia is noted on the left. Gait testing shows imbalance when she walks, which is markedly worse from baseline. An MRI is scheduled for the morning.

Which of the following is the most appropriate first-line treatment?

A) Oral prednisone 60 mg daily
B) Intravenous methylprednisolone 1 g daily administration
C) Methylprednisolone 125 mg Q 6 h
D) Increase gabapentin dosage
E) Plasmapheresis
F) B and E

Answer: F

Intravenous methylprednisolone with a suggested dose of 1 g/day for 3–5 days has been the traditional treatment for acute exacerbations of multiple sclerosis. This patient is experiencing an acute exacerbation or relapse of her underlying multiple sclerosis. The data supports the use of high-dose intravenous corticosteroids. This treatment regimen has been demonstrated to speed the recovery from a multiple sclerosis attacks; however, it is uncertain whether this impacts long-term disability.

The 2011 American Academy of Neurology (AAN) Plasmapheresis Guideline Update states that plasmapheresis is effective and may be considered in fulminant demyelinating CNS disease as a first-line agent.

Plasmapheresis can also be considered in cases resistant to corticosteroid therapy, and clinical improvement should be followed closely. Previous clinical trials have demonstrated that oral prednisone is inferior to high-dose intravenous corticosteroids. A change in this patient's chronic disease-modifying therapy may be considered in consultation with a multiple sclerosis specialist, but would be of no benefit in the acute multiple sclerosis flair.

Reference

Rodriguez M, Karnes WE, Bartleson JD, Pineda AA. Plasmapheresis in acute episodes of fulminant CNS inflammatory demyelination. Neurology. 1993;43(6):1100–4.

4. A 65-year-old woman presents complaining of severe dizziness. Some mild nausea with eating is reported as well. She notes it especially occurs when she turns over in bed and immediately upon standing. She has had an episode of this before which resolved without medical care. She is currently unable to take care of herself at home and is admitted for further workup and intravenous fluids.

On physical exam, you ask the patient to sit on the bedside with her head turned approximately 45° to the right. You slowly lower the patient to the supine position and extend her head backward 20°. This maneuver immediately reproduces the patient's dizziness, and you note increased nystagmus.

What is the appropriate management in the evaluation and treatment of this patient?

A) MRI of her cerebellum
B) Methylprednisolone taper beginning at 60 mg daily
C) Repositioning (Epley) maneuvers
D) Rizatriptan 10 mg orally once
E) Valacyclovir 1000 mg three times daily for 10 days

Answer: C

The symptoms and physical examination of this patient are typical of benign paroxysmal positional vertigo (BPPV). Referral to ENT or physical therapy for repositioning maneuvers is the best treatment.

BPPV is a common cause of vertigo. Episodes of BPPV are typically brief, lasting no more than 1 min. They are brought about by changes in position. Typical reported movements that elicit vertigo are lying down, rolling over in bed, rising from bed, sitting up and tilting the head to look upward. Vertigo is often accompanied by nystagmus that beats upward and torsionally toward the affected ear. This can be elicited by the Dix–Hallpike maneuver which was performed on physical exam.

The history and physical examination are not consistent with a central cause of vertigo. An MRI can probably be avoided. Methylprednisolone is the primary treatment of acute vestibular neuritis. It is of benefit if used within the first 3 days of symptoms. Vestibular neuritis often presents with more prolonged and persistent symptoms. Most patients recover spontaneously, but when used early, methylprednisolone will decrease the duration of symptoms. Antiviral therapy is not indicated unless there is an obvious herpes zoster infection. Likewise, the symptoms are not consistent with migrainous vertigo, which would be persistent for hours and not be affected by positional changes.

Reference

Epley JM. The canalith repositioning procedure: for treatment of benign paroxysmal positional vertigo. Otolaryngol Head Neck Surg. 1992;107(3):399–404.

5. A 26-year-old woman presents to the emergency department with shortness of breath as her primary complaint, which has been progressively increasing for several days

since starting her menstrual period. She has also been experiencing increasing weakness during the past week as well. She notes a worsening of her symptoms at the end of the day, and she has noticed weakness while brushing her hair. Occasionally she reports blurry vision or difficulty with reading. On physical exam, no specific weakness is noted. She seems fatigued in general and has a depressed affect. Pulmonary exam is normal. All labs are within normal range.

Which of the following neuromuscular disorders is most likely the cause of this patient's symptoms?
A) Guillain–Barré syndrome
B) Bilateral diaphragmatic paralysis
C) Myasthenia gravis
D) Duchenne muscular dystrophy
E) Amyotrophic lateral sclerosis (ALS)

Answer: C

Multiple neuromuscular disorders may affect respiratory function. Guillain–Barré syndrome usually presents as an ascending paralysis with respiratory symptoms occurring later and rarely as a presenting symptom. Although bilateral diaphragmatic paralysis would explain this patient's shortness of breath, the proximal muscle weakness and ocular symptoms would remain unexplained. Duchenne muscular dystrophy is an X-linked disorder that exclusively affects males that presents by 12 years of age.

The majority of patients with ALS present clinically with progressive asymmetrical weakness, fasciculations, and prominent muscle atrophy. The distal musculature is primarily involved. Myasthenia gravis is an autoimmune disorder that interferes with the postsynaptic acetylcholine receptor. Patients usually present with intermittent symptoms that are usually worse at the end of the day. Respiratory symptoms may be the presenting symptom. The most common severe symptom of myasthenia gravis is respiratory failure. Exposure to bright sunlight, surgery, immunization, emotional stress, menstruation, infection and physical factors might trigger or worsen exacerbations.

Reference
Keesey JC. Clinical evaluation and management of myasthenia gravis. Muscle Nerve. 2004;29(4):484–505.

6. A 57-year-old white man is admitted with exertional shortness of breath. His symptom began several months ago and has gotten progressively worse over time. He reports occasional upper respiratory complaints, some fatigue, and a nonpainful, nonpruritic rash on his lower extremities. His medical history is significant only for diabetes.

On physical exam, you note a mildly erythematous, papular rash with a few nodules on his lower extremities.

His pulmonary examination is notable for bilateral crackles. Initial workup is unrevealing. A chest radiograph reveals interstitial abnormalities bilaterally. Urine dipstick testing reveals proteinuria and hematuria. A blood test for cytoplasmic antineutrophil cytoplasmic antibodies (c-ANCA) is pending. A subsequent biopsy reveals a necrotizing granulomatous vasculitis.

This patient's findings are most consistent with which of the following diagnoses?
A) Lymphomatoid granulomatosis
B) Systemic lupus erythematosus (SLE)
C) Granulomatosis with polyangiitis (GPA)
D) Churg-Strauss syndrome
E) Goodpasture disease

Answer: C

This patient has granulomatosis with polyangiitis (GPA), which was formerly known as Wegener's disease. It is associated with both distinctive and nonspecific mucocutaneous signs. Palpable purpura suggestive of vasculitis is one of the most common skin findings. A variety of other dermatologic conditions have been reported including ulcers, papules, and nodules. In addition to upper and lower pulmonary symptoms, nasal ulcerations and septal perforation should suggest the diagnosis. Biopsy is required. Diagnosis is made by the demonstration of a necrotizing granulomatous vasculitis in a patient with upper and lower respiratory tract disease and glomerulonephritis. C-ANCA autoantibodies make several autoimmune diseases less likely.

The absence of asthma makes the diagnosis of Churg-Strauss syndrome unlikely. Patients with lymphomatoid granulomatosis present with a predominance of pulmonary and nervous system manifestations, and tests for ANCA autoantibodies are usually negative.

Reference
Cartin-Ceba R, Peikert T, Specks U. Pathogenesis of ANCA-associated vasculitis. Curr Rheumatol Rep. 2012;14(6): 481–93.

7. A 68-year-old male was admitted to the hospital for pneumonia. He had a chest X-ray done that reveals a left lung infiltrate and pleural effusion. He underwent a thoracentesis that revealed an exudative effusion. With no resolution of the effusion, a repeat thoracentesis and chest tube was placed 2 days later. Three days later, he is spiking temperatures to 103 °F. Repeat chest X-ray reveals a worsening effusion on the left.

Which of the following is the best option in management at this time?
A) Expand antibiotic coverage
B) Repeat chest tube placement

C) Change antibiotics and continue with chest tube drainage
D) Perform video-assisted thoracic surgery (VATS)
E) No change required at this time

Answer: D

Patients with pneumonia and exudative effusion resistant to drainage should be considered for video-assisted thoracoscopic surgery (VATS).

Approximately 15–40% of patients with exudative effusion require surgical drainage of the infected pleural space. Chest tubes often become clogged or effusions become loculated. Patients should be considered for surgery if they have ongoing signs of sepsis in association with a persistent pleural collection. VATS is used as a first-line therapy in many hospitals if cardiothoracic surgery support is available. Open thoracic drainage remains a frequently used alternative technique.

Reference

Ferguson AD, Prescott RJ, Selkon JB, Watson D, Swinburn CR. The clinical course and management of thoracic empyema. QJM. 1996;89(4):285–9.

8. You are called to see a patient on the floor for acute obtundation. She has been admitted for chronic abdominal pain and possible pancreatitis. She has been in the hospital for 6 h and has received several doses of narcotics. Her last dose was 4 mg of hydromorphone 15 min ago. She has been on hydromorphone every 4 h. After you assess the patient, you administer a dose of naloxone. The patient has an immediate improvement of her symptoms. She is alert and oriented. One hour later, you are called again to see the patient, who has become somnolent again. The most likely cause of patient's worsening mental status is:
   A) Worsening CO_2 retention
   B) Diminishing effects of naloxone
   C) Further narcotic use
   D) Sepsis
   E) Delirium secondary to pancreatitis

Answer: B

Naloxone has an extremely rapid onset of action. The duration of naloxone is no greater than 1–2 h. This is of importance as patients who have received a one-time dose may have a return of intoxication symptoms. All opiates have a longer duration of action than naloxone. All patients with opiate overdose symptoms both in the emergency room and on the floor should be monitored for a return of symptoms after naloxone has been given.

Naloxone is most commonly injected intravenously for fastest action, which usually causes the drug to act within a minute. When IV access is not available, it can also be administered via intramuscular or subcutaneous injection. In emergency circumstances, it can be administered intranasally.

Reference

Orman JS, Keating GM. Buprenorphine/naloxone: a review of its use in the treatment of opioid dependence. Drugs. 2009;69(5):577–607.

9. A 55-year-old female presents with an the inability to close her left eye, mild numbness, and tingling of the left cheek. She has a history of hypertension. You are consulted by the emergency room to admit the patient for probable stroke.

   On physical examination, vital signs are normal. No lesions of the skin or mucous membranes are noted. Neurologic examination reveals a weakness of the left upper and lower facial muscles and an inability to close the left eye. Sensory examination reveals the facial sensation is normal bilaterally.

   CT scan is performed which reveals no significant abnormalities. Other labs are within normal limits.

   Which of the following is the most appropriate treatment?
   A) Acyclovir
   B) Intravenous methylprednisolone
   C) Aspirin
   D) Sumatriptan
   E) Prednisone

Answer: E

This patient has an acute onset of Bell's palsy. The current treatment of choice is prednisone. Mounting evidence suggests that Bell's palsy is due to human herpes virus 1. It is often is seen after a viral prodrome. Physical examination reveals paralysis of both the upper and lower facial motor neurons which distinguishes it from a cerebrovascular accident.

The patient may also report dry mouth, impaired taste, and pain and numbness in the ear. Abrupt onset of symptoms usually occurs over 1–2 days. The most appropriate treatment is oral prednisone 40 mg per day, started within the first 72 h. Antiviral agents have been used in the past. There is no evidence to date that anti-herpes virus agents, such as acyclovir, as monotherapy for Bell's palsy are of benefit. High-dose intravenous corticosteroids are not indicated for the treatment of Bell's palsy.

Reference

Baugh RF, Basura GJ, Ishii LE, Schwartz SR, Drumheller CM, Burkholder R, et al. Clinical practice guideline: Bell's Palsy executive summary. Otolaryngol Head Neck Surg. 2013;149(5):656–63.

10. A 23-year-old female is brought to the emergency room by her roommate with the chief complaint of increasing agitation, which began this morning. All history is obtained from the roommate who reports that the patient has been out for the past two days and has been acting strange and paranoid since returning home. Nothing is known about what the patient may have ingested.

    On physical exam, she is diaphoretic, alert, and agitated. She exhibits some unusual behaviors, such as picking at her legs. Her temperature is 38.3 °C (101.0 °F), heart rate is 120 bpm, and respirations are 26 per minute. Her blood pressure is 165/100 mmHg. On physical exam, it is noted that she has poor dentition. A few pustules and scabs are noted on the face. Cardiopulmonary and abdominal exams are normal. She is slightly hyperreflexic. Laboratory examination reveals normal liver enzymes and a normal basic metabolic profile.

    Which of the following substances is the most likely cause of the patient's clinical picture?
    A) Cocaine
    B) Benocyclidine
    C) Methamphetamine (Crystal Meth)
    D) MDMA (ecstasy)
    E) LSD

Answer: C
Methamphetamine, which has multiple street names including crystal or crystal meth, presents with hypertension, tachycardia, hyperthermia, and often with poor dentition and evidence of skin excoriations. Other common symptoms are paranoia and diaphoresis. Methamphetamine ingestion is commonly seen in both urban and rural settings. Ingestions often occur at extended late night events, concerts, and within group settings. Methamphetamine users and addicts may lose their teeth abnormally quickly. This may be due to several factors that lead to dry mouth as well as specific behaviors that are induced by the drug.
5–15 % of users may fail to recover completely after cessation of drug use. Antipsychotic medications may effectively resolve the symptoms of acute amphetamine psychosis.

Reference
Darke S, Kaye S, McKetin R, Duflou J. Major physical and psychological harms of methamphetamine use. Drug Alcohol Rev. 2011;27(3):253–62.

11. A 28-year-old white male presents to ED with a large swollen left arm and severe left arm pain and redness. He believes the only significant event that happened prior to the swelling was picking up a propane tank with his left arm. Of note, he is a construction worker who operates cranes and is seated for the majority of his workday. He works 6 days a week with Sunday being his only day off. He is eager to get back to work. After initial workup and imaging, a DVT is confirmed in the upper extremity.

    What would be an appropriate therapy to start?
    A) Rivaroxaban
    B) Warfarin plus Enoxaparin 1 mg/kg SQ BID x minimum 5 days
    C) Warfarin alone
    D) Enoxaparin 1 mg/kg for 2 weeks alone
    E) A or B

Answer: E
Rivaroxaban may be a great choice for this patient due to his age and work lifestyle. It can be started without the need for bridging therapy. Coumadin monitoring can be problematic and leads to a great deal of noncompliance.
If agreeable to the patient, warfarin plus enoxaparin is also an acceptable option. This dosing regimen is well established and validated.
Current guidelines recommend that patients with upper extremity DVTs require treatment similar to lower extremity DVT. Option C is incorrect because of the lack of bridging required initially for this disease state.

References
Ansel J, et al. Pharmacology and management of the vitamin K antagonists – ACCP evidence-based clinical practice guidelines (8th edition). Chest. 2008;133(6_suppl):160S–98S.
The EINSTEIN Investigators. Oral Rivaroxaban for treatment of VTE. N Engl J Med. 2010;363:2499–510.

12. A 38-year-old female patient with a history of end-stage renal disease on home peritoneal dialysis presents with a chief complaint of new onset abdominal pain. A peritoneal catheter was placed 6 months ago and since that time has had no complications.

    On physical exam, the abdomen is diffusely tender. She is afebrile. Serum WBC count is 15,000/μL.

    Initial therapy for treatment of suspected peritoneal dialysis-induced peritonitis would include which of the following?
    A) Ceftriaxone
    B) Vancomycin plus ceftriaxone
    C) Vancomycin, ceftriaxone, and diflucan
    D) Vancomycin
    E) Ceftriaxone and catheter removal

Answer: B
Peritonitis is a common complication seen in peritoneal dialysis patients. Unlike peritonitis seen in end-stage liver disease, the majority of infections are gram-positive bacteria. For this reason, vancomycin or other MRSA-covering antibiotic should be included in the initial

therapy. Antifungal therapy should be initiated only if the gram stain reveals yeast. Catheter removal should be considered in certain circumstances but is not necessarily indicated with every infection. Indications for removal of catheter include a repeat infection after 4 weeks of antibiotic therapy, infection not responding to antibiotics, fungal peritonitis, or other resistant causes of peritonitis.

Reference

Piraino B, Bailie GR, Bernardini J, et al. Peritoneal dialysis-related infections recommendations: 2005 update. Perit Dial Int. 2005;25(2):107–31.

13. A 65-year-old man with a history of hepatitis C and progressive liver disease presents to the hospital with increasing low-grade fever, abdominal pain, and distension. He is currently on furosemide, spironolactone, and nadolol.

    On physical examination, his temperature is 37.5 °C(99.5 °F), blood pressure is 100/50 mmHg. Abdominal examination reveals distended abdomen and marked ascites. The abdomen is mildly tender upon palpation. Creatinine is 0.8 mg/dl and total bilirubin is 2.1 mg/dl.

    Abdominal ultrasound is consistent with cirrhosis, splenomegaly, and large volume of ascites. Diagnostic paracentesis is scheduled.

    The most appropriate initial treatment is?
    A) Cefotaxime
    B) Cefotaxime and albumin
    C) Furosemide and spironolactone
    D) Large volume paracentesis

Answer: A

Spontaneous bacterial peritonitis (SBP) is a common complication of end-stage liver disease. Initial treatment consists of antibiotics that have coverage of gram-negative bacteria. Common isolates are *Escherichia coli* and *Klebsiella pneumonia*. There is no evidence that large volume paracentesis improves outcomes in patients with spontaneous bacterial peritonitis. Diagnostic paracentesis should be undertaken to confirm the diagnosis. SBP is confirmed when a WBC count of >250 per microliter is found. Additional paracentesis can be considered to determine the efficacy of treatment or to relieve symptoms.

Reference

Cholongitas E, Papatheodoridis GV, Lahanas A, Xanthaki A, Kontou-Kastellanou C, Archimandritis AJ. Increasing frequency of Gram-positive bacteria in spontaneous bacterial peritonitis. Liver Int. 2005;25(1):57–61.

14. A 45-year-old woman is being admitted for continued fever. Her symptoms started five weeks ago with the onset of low-grade daily fever. Over the past 2 weeks,

she has developed erythematous rash, fatigue, and weight loss. She has been seen twice by her primary care physician. Limited workup has been unrevealing. Her medical history is only significant for hypertension. She takes lisinopril.

    On physical exam, the patient's temperature is found to be 38.3 °C (101.0 °F), a 2/6 murmur is heard in the mitral area of the chest, and an erythematous rash is noted on both legs. A complete blood count shows anemia. The patient's erythrocyte sedimentation rate (ESR) is elevated at 80 mm/h. A transthoracic echocardiogram shows a 2 cm pedunculated mass in the left atrium.

    Which of the following is the most likely diagnosis?
    A) Metastatic colon adenocarcinoma
    B) Cardiac rhabdomyosarcoma
    C) Papillary fibroelastoma
    D) Cardiac myxoma
    E) Endocarditis

Answer: D

This patient has an atrial myxoma. Myxomas consist of benign scattered stellate cells embedded in a mucinous matrix. About 70 % of myxomas are in the left atrium. Myxomas often present clinically with mechanical hemodynamic effects, which often simulate mitral or tricuspid stenoses or regurgitation. Systemic symptoms include fatigue, fever, erythematous rash, myalgias, and weight loss, accompanied by anemia and an increased ESR. These symptoms may mimic endocarditis. About 10 % of myxomas are genetic. Surgery is the primary treatment.

Cardiac tumors are usually metastatic. Metastatic cardiac involvement occurs 20–40 times more frequently than primary tumors. Eighty percent of all primary cardiac tumors are benign. Myxomas account for more than half of these in adults.

Reference

Larsson S, Lepore V, Kennergren C. Atrial myxomas: results of 25 years' experience and review of the literature. Surgery. 1989;105(6):695–8

15. You are asked to admit a 40-year-old man with atypical chest pain. He reports the abrupt onset of an exertional type of pain. The emergency room staff is concerned that the pain may be angina. On further questioning by you, he reports a constant pain of 4 days duration. The pain is worse with inspiration and is positional. He also reports recent fever.

    On physical exam, he has diffuse mild chest wall tenderness but is primarily positional in nature. An ECG shows 2 mm elevation ST elevation in the precordial leads, without reciprocal changes and with PR segment depression in lead 2. An echocardiogram performed in the emergency room is normal. A CT angiogram of the chest is pending.

What is the most likely diagnosis and treatment for this patient?

A) Acute pericarditis; nonsteroidal anti-inflammatory drug (NSAID) are indicated
B) Acute pericarditis; start prednisone
C) Acute pericarditis; echocardiogram in 1 week to confirm diagnosis
D) Musculoskeletal strain; observation alone
E) Pulmonary embolism

Answer: A

The patient has acute pericarditis. The chest pain of acute pericarditis is sudden and severe. It is constant over the anterior chest. In acute pericarditis, the pain worsens with inspiration and is reliably positional. The absence of a significant effusion on echocardiography is not evidence against acute pericarditis. Salicylates or NSAIDs are the first-line agents for treatment. Corticosteroids should be reserved for severe cases that are unresponsive to initial therapy. Symptoms may recur after steroid withdrawal, making their use problematic. Low-grade fever and sinus tachycardia may be present.

If carefully auscultated, a pericardial friction rub can be detected in most patients when symptoms are acute. Electrocardiographic changes are common in infectious pericarditis and can occur with other etiologies as well. The characteristic change is an elevation in the ST segment in all leads. The absence of reciprocal ST segment depression distinguishes this characteristic pattern of acute pericarditis from acute myocardial infarction. Depression of the PR interval, which is not as obvious, is often the earliest electrocardiographic manifestation.

Reference

Maisch B, Seferovic PM, Ristic AD, Erbel R, Rienmüller R, Adler Y, et al. Guidelines on the diagnosis and management of pericardial diseases executive summary; the Task force on the diagnosis and management of pericardial diseases of the European society of cardiology. Eur Heart J. 2004;25(7):587–610.

16. A 45-year-old-man is brought to the emergency department by his family for lethargy, altered mental status, and abdominal discomfort. His past medical history includes combined diastolic and systolic heart disease with EF of 30 %, diabetes mellitus 2 with a HgA1c of 11 %, and a baseline creatinine of 1.8 units/L checked last week in clinic. However, the patient is not currently taking any medications for diabetic management. His glucose on admission was 450 mg/dL with negative serum ketones. A diagnosis of hyperosmolar nonketotic

acidosis was made. The patient was treated with an intensive insulin drip and fluids with resolution of symptoms. A successful transition to basal-prandial insulin regimen is made the next day.

What is the best diabetic regimen to discharge your patient home on?

A) Metformin BID plus lantus 10U SQ nightly
B) Levemir SQ nightly with prandial novolog with meals
C) Glyburide 5 mg daily and insulin sliding scale
D) Dual oral therapy with metformin and rosiglitazone

Answer: B

The patient presented with hyperosmolar nonketotic acidosis and a hemoglobin A1c of 11 % meeting requirements to begin a basal-prandial insulin regimen. In patients with consistent extreme hyperglycemia greater than 300 mg/dl, hgbA1c greater than 10 %, insulin should be started immediately.

Metformin is contraindicated in men with a creatinine >1.5 mg/dL and women with creatinine >1.4 mg/dL. The glitazones are typically not recommended for diabetics in the setting of severe uncontrolled hyperglycemia.

Reference

American Diabetes Association. Standards of Medical Care in Diabetes-2015: Abridged for Primary Care Providers. Clinical Diabetes. 2015. 33(2)

17. A 27-year-old male is brought to the emergency room after being found down in the parking lot of a grocery store. While in the emergency room, he awakens and reports chest pain. An ECG reveals a 4 mm ST segment elevation in leads II, III, and aVF. Rapid drug screen is positive for cocaine. The emergency room staff administers aspirin, Ativan, and sublingual nitroglycerin. You are consulted for admission. His heart rate is 120 beats per minute. After 5 min, chest pain is not alleviated by nitroglycerin.

Which of the following is the most appropriate treatment?

A) Enoxaparin
B) Repeat lorazepam
C) IV metoprolol
D) Nitroprusside
E) Urgent coronary arteriography

Answer: E

Cocaine often induces vascular syndromes due to increased platelet aggregation and endothelial dysfunction. In this particular case, the patient is suffering an acute myocardial infarction due to cocaine. Urgent coronary arteriography, if available, is recommended. Avoidance of beta-blockers acutely after cocaine use is currently a part of the American Heart Association guidelines. This is due to the possibility that beta-blockers may lead to unopposed alpha-adrenergic stimulation with subsequent worsening coronary vasospasm. There have been no controlled trials on this issue yet. It is important to recognize that cocaine can induce myocardial infarctions and other thrombotic events in a low-incidence population such as the case here.

Reference
Hiestand BC, Smith SW. Cocaine chest pain: between a (crack) rock and a hard place. Acad Emerg Med. 2011;18(1):68–71.

18. A 65-year-old man with acute respiratory distress is transferred to the intensive care unit. He has just been intubated and placed on mechanical ventilation for respiratory failure secondary to aspiration pneumonia. Before intubation, his oxygen saturation was 81 % breathing 100 % oxygen with a nonrebreather mask.

On physical examination, temperature is 37.0 °C (98.6 °F), blood pressure is 145/85 mmHg, and pulse rate is 110 bpm. His height is 150 cm (59 in) and his weight is 78.0 kg (154.3 lb). Ideal body weight is calculated to be 50.0 kg (114.6 lb). Central venous pressure is 9 cm H_2O. Cardiac examination reveals normal heart sounds, no murmurs, and no rubs. Crackles are auscultated in the right and left lung fields. The patient is sedated. Neurologic examination is nonfocal.

Mechanical ventilation is set on the assist/control mode at a rate of 16/min. Positive end-expiratory pressure is 8 cm H_2O, and FIO_2 is 1.0.

Which of the following is the correct tidal volume?
A) 300 mL
B) 450 mL
C) 700 mL
D) 840 mL

Answer: A
This patient's presentation is consistent with acute respiratory distress syndrome (ARDS). The most appropriate tidal volume is 300 mL. Survival in ARDS is improved when patients are ventilated with a tidal volume of 6 mL/kg of ideal body weight (IBW). A low tidal volume mechanical ventilation strategy is now the standard of care for ARDS.
Lung injury is presumed to arise from repetitive opening and closing of alveoli. Barotrauma may be limited by low tidal volumes. This can be achieved by delivering limited size tidal volumes, minimizing plateau pressure, optimizing PEEP, and reducing FIO_2 to less than 0.6. Ideal body weight rather than actual body weight should be used. Use caution in patients who are overweight or edematous. Calculating actual body weight will typically result in inappropriately large tidal volumes.

Reference
The Acute Respiratory Distress Syndrome Network. Ventilation with lower tidal volumes as compared with traditional tidal volumes for acute lung injury and the acute respiratory distress syndrome. N Engl J Med. 2000;342(18):1301–8.

19. A 75 year old Vietnamese male presents with a one month history of bilateral hand swelling and recurrent ulcerations. Over that time period he has been treated with several course of oral antibiotics for presumed cellulitis with no improvement. The family reports that he has had several ulcerations on his fingers develop in the past month that have resolved. He is an active gardener and spends several hours per day tending to his plants. He has no other past medical history.

On physical exam one 3x 3cm superative ulceration is noted distally on his right fifth finger. Some erythema around the ulceration is noted. Both hands are markedly swollen. He is admitted and started on IV vancomycin. After three days no improvement is seen. No fever or elevation in WBC is noted.

On day three, one new lesion similar to the previous lesion develops on the dorsum of his hand. On day four another lesion develops proximally on the forearm.

Which of the following is the most likely diagnosis?
A) Rheumatoid arthritis
B) Cutaneous Sporotrichosis
C) Mycobacterium Marinum
D) Hypersensitivity Reaction
E) Small Vessel Vasculitis

Answer: B
A non healing cellulitis with ulceration is suugestive of an atypical bacterial or fungal infection. In this patient with significant environmental exposure and classic lymphatic spread, Sporotrichosis is the likely diagnosis. Sporotrichosis is a subacute infection caused by the saprophytic dimorphic fungus *Sporothrix schenckii*.
The characteristic infection involves ulcerative subcutaneous nodules that progress proximally along lymphatic channels. The primary lesion develops at the site of cutaneous inoculation, typically in the distal upper extremities. After several weeks, new lesions appear along the lymphatic tracts. Patients are typically afebrile and not systemically ill. The lesions usually cause minimal pain. Many affected patients have received one or more courses of antibacterial therapy without benefit.
Sporotrichosis may involve other organs, including the eye, prostate oral mucosa, paranasal sinuses, larynx and joints. In such patients, the clinical manifestations depend on the organs involved.

Soil, plants, moss and other organic material are common sources. The rose bush thorn has been described as the classic source.

Sporotrichosis occurs worldwide, with focal areas of hyper-endemicity, such as Peru and China.

Treatment can be lengthy. One recent guideline recommends oral itraconazole 200 mg/d until 2-4 weeks after all lesions have resolved, usually for a total of 3-6 months.

Reference

Barros MB, de Almeida Paes R, Schubach AO. Sporothrix schenckii and Sporotrichosis. Clin Micro Rev. Oct/2011. 24:633–654.

20. A 24 year-old presents with rash, hypotension, and fever. One week ago she was involved in a biking accident, where she sustained a laceration to the leg. It did not require sutures. She has had no recent travel, gardening exposure, or exposure to pets. She is up-to-date on all of her vaccinations. She does not use IV drugs.

    On examination her heart rate is 120 bpm, blood pressure is 87/58. The leg laceration looks clean with a well-granulated base and no erythema, warmth, or pustular discharge. She does have diffuse erythema that is prominent on her palms, conjunctiva, and oral mucosa. There is some mild desquamation noted on her fingertips.

    Laboratory results are notable for a creatinine of 3.0 mg/dL, aspartate aminotransferase of 289 U/L, alanine aminotransferase of 372 U/L, total bilirubin of 2.8 mg/dL, INR of 1.5, and platelets at 82,000/μL. She is started on broad-spectrum antibiotics and IV fluids.

    What is the most likely diagnosis?
    A) Sepsis
    B) Leptospirosis
    C) Staphylococcal toxic shock syndrome
    D) Streptococcal toxic shock syndrome
    E) Drug reaction

Answer: C

She has toxic shock syndrome. The characteristic diffuse rash and systemic symptoms make *Staphylococcus* the most likely inciting agent. Antibiotic treatment should cover both the leading causes, *S. pyogenes* and *S. aureus*. This may include a combination of cephalosporins, vancomycin, or drugs effective against MRSA. The addition of clindamycin may reduce toxin production and mortality. Toxic shock usually has a prominent primary site of infection or source. Staphylococcal toxic shock can be associated with immunosuppression, surgical wounds, or retained tampons. *Staphylococcus aureus* colonization can incite toxic shock. In certain circumstances and loca-

tion, it has been suggested that Rocky Mountain spotted fever and leptospirosis which can have a similar presentation be ruled out serologically to confirm the diagnosis. This patient is at very low risk for these diagnoses.

References

Lappin E, Ferguson AJ. Gram-positive toxic shock syndromes. Lancet Infect Dis. 2009 May. 9(5):281–90.

Schlievert PM, Kelly JA. Clindamycin-induced suppression of toxic-shock syndrome-associated exotoxin production. J Infect Dis. 1984;149(3):471.

21. What is the appropriate rivaroxaban dose for an indication of pulmonary embolism (weight=77 kg, CrCl=89 ml/min)?
    A) 15 mg PO BID×3 weeks, then 20 mg PO daily
    B) 20 mg PO daily
    C) 15 mg PO daily
    D) 10 mg PO BID×3 weeks, then 5 mg PO daily

Answer: A

Per package labeling by the pharmaceutical manufacturer, for patients with a CrCl>30 ml/min and for the treatment of DVT/PE, take 15 mg PO BID×3 weeks, and then 20 mg PO daily. 15 mg PO daily is a renally adjusted regimen for atrial fibrillation. A 10 mg daily dose is indicated for postoperative VTE prophylaxis.

Reference

Garcia DA, et al. CHEST guidelines – parenteral anticoagulants. Chest. 2012;141(2_suppl):e24S–43S.

22. An 18-year-old male is admitted for a 2-day history of fever, abdominal pain, and left knee pain. In the past year, he has had three similar episodes, each lasting 2 days. He feels well between episodes. He takes no medications and reports no other medical history. He is sexually active with one partner.

    On physical examination, the temperature is 38.2 °C (100.8 °F), blood pressure is 144/86 mmHg, heart rate is 90/min, and respiration rate is 18/min. There is diffuse abdominal tenderness without rebound. There is no evidence of hepatosplenomegaly. No lymph nodes are palpable. The left knee has a small effusion. Flexion of the knee is limited to 90°. A well-demarcated, raised, erythematous rash is noted on the right lower extremity overlying the shin. It is tender to touch.

    Laboratory studies reveal an elevated erythrocyte sedimentation rate of 56 mm/h. Screening antinuclear antibody test results are negative. Urinalysis reveals 1+ protein with no cells or casts.

Which of the following is the most likely diagnosis?
A) Adult-onset Still disease
B) Crohn's disease
C) Familial Mediterranean fever
D) Reactive arthritis
E) Gonococcal arthritis

Answer: C

Familial Mediterranean fever (FMF) also known as recurrent polyserositis presents with monoarticular arthritis and systemic complaints. It is episodic and recurrent which suggests an autoimmune disease. The symptoms presented here are most compatible with familial Mediterranean fever (FMF). It is an autosomal recessive disorder characterized by recurrent 12–72 h episodes of fever with serositis, synovitis, most often monoarticular. Ten percent of patients experience their first episode in early adulthood. FMF is most prevalent in persons of Mediterranean ethnicity. Laboratory studies are consistent with acute inflammation. Serology results are negative for autoimmune disease. Proteinuria may occur from renal amyloidosis. Colchicine is the standard therapy. It reduces both acute attacks and amyloidosis.

Adult-onset Still disease (AOSD) which may have a similar presentation is characterized by fever, rash, joint pain, and serositis. Pleuritis or pericarditis may occur. Fever associated with AOSD is quotidian, lasting less than 4 h, and often peaks in the early evening. The characteristic rash is evanescent, salmon-colored, and not painful. Abdominal pain is rare. Finally, a markedly elevated serum ferritin level occurs in most patients with AOSD.

Reference

Kuky O, Livneh A, Ben-David A, et al. Familial Mediterranean Fever (FMF) with proteinuria: clinical features, histology, predictors, and prognosis in a cohort of 25 patients. J Rheumatol. 2013;40:2083–7.

23. Which of the following is NOT consistent with self-induced infection or factitious fever?
A) Tachycardia with fever
B) Polymicrobic bacteremia
C) Recurrent soft tissue infections
D) Self inoculation with body fluids
E) Healthcare background

Answer: A

Factitious fever and self-induced infections are encountered in the hospital with some frequency. The literature suggests an increase in all forms of factitious illness. In factitious fever, high temperatures are often not associated with tachycardia or skin warmth. Many creative methods have been described in the literature to induce an elevated temperature. A high index of suspicion will usually reveal some unusual patterns.

Self-induced infection generally occurs by self-injection of body fluids, pyretic substances, or other contaminated materials. This includes various substances including materials contaminated with feces, pure microbiological cultures, coliform bacilli, and foreign proteins. Patients may have serial episodes of unexplained polymicrobial bacteremia or recurrent soft tissue infections. The underlying disorder for factitious fever may be the Munchausen syndrome and the Munchausen syndrome by proxy.

Reference

Aduan RP, Fauci AS, Dale DC, et al. Factitious fever and self-induced infection: a report of 32 cases and review of the literature. Ann Intern Med. 1979;90(2):230–42.

24. A 35-year-old male intravenous drug user is admitted for a febrile illness. Endocarditis is suspected but ruled out by blood cultures and echocardiography. He tested negative for HIV 8 months ago. He describes a one week onset of a cold, characterized by subjective fever, fatigue, and aching joints. In the hospital, he develops a morbilliform rash. You are now concerned that the patient may have an acute infection with HIV.

What test or tests should be ordered in diagnosing this patient?
A) Enzyme-linked immunosorbent assay (ELISA) for HIV antibody
B) CD4+ T cell count
C) Complete blood count for lymphopenia and thrombocytopenia
D) p24 antigen test of HIV RNA
E) HIV ELISA antibody test and a test for p24 antigen of HIV

Answer: E

After acquiring HIV, infected persons may develop a nonspecific febrile illness. The incubation period is 7–14 days after acquiring HIV. The symptoms are similar to influenza or mononucleosis in character. Laboratory testing often reveals lymphopenia and thrombocytopenia, but these findings are not diagnostic. Results of HIV ELISA antibody testing are usually negative because it typically takes 22–27 days for the HIV antibody to become positive. The CD4+ T cell count is usually normal at time of seroconversion.

The plasma p24 antigen test is highly specific for HIV infection but is not as sensitive as the HIV RNA assay. Patients typically have a high level of viremia. They are highly infectious at this stage. Plasma HIV RNA level of several million HIV RNA copies per milliliter of plasma are usually seen. The combination of a positive HIV RNA test and a negative screening HIV antibody test result confirms the diagnosis of acute HIV infection.

Reference

Delaney KP, Branson BM, Uniyal A, Phillips S, Candal D, Owen SM, et al. Evaluation of the performance characteristics of 6 rapid HIV antibody tests. Clin Infect Dis. 2011 Jan 15. 52(2):257–63.

25. A 22-year-old female is admitted with the acute onset of fever, severe throat pain, and inability to handle her oral secretions.

    On physical examinations, she has an erythematous oropharynx and cervical lymphadenopathy. The patient has no known history of drug allergy. She is started on an empirical regimen of amoxicillin for streptococcal pharyngitis.

    The next day she developed an erythematous maculopapular rash on several areas. The mono spot test comes back positive.

    Which of the following statements regarding this patient's exanthematous drug eruption is true?
    A) Fever is common in viral-related exanthematous eruptions.
    B) Systemic corticosteroids are required to treat this drug eruption.
    C) In the future she will be able to tolerate all β-lactam antibiotics, including ampicillin.
    D) The mechanism of exanthematous eruption caused by ampicillin is mast cell degranulation.
    E) This patient's rash can be expected to be severe.

Answer: C

This patient has ampicillin- or amoxicillin-related exanthematous eruption that can frequently occur with mononucleosis. This does not appear to be IgE mediated and is not a penicillin allergy. Patients may receive penicillins in the future. The etiology of the ampicillin rash that occurs in association with a viral infection is unknown.

Fever is not associated with simple exanthematous eruptions. These eruptions usually occur within 1 week after the beginning of therapy and generally resolve within 7–14 days. Scaling or desquamation may follow resolution. The treatment of exanthematous eruptions is generally supportive. Oral antihistamines used in conjunction with soothing baths may help relieve pruritus. Topical corticosteroids are indicated when antihistamines do not provide relief. Systemic corticosteroids are used only in severe cases. Discontinuance of ampicillin is recommended.

Reference

Kagan B. Ampicillin rash. West J Med. 1977;126(4):333–5.

26. A 44-year-old male is admitted for acute psychosis. He has a history of schizophrenia and has been on various antipsychotics, lithium, and paroxetine. His agitation in the hospital has been difficult to control and has required escalating doses of haloperidol. On the third day of his hospitalization, he develops temperature of 39.6 °C (103.3 °F). Blood pressure is 110/65. Other medications include lithium and valproic acid.

    On physical examination, he has generalized tremors, rigidity, agitation, and diaphoresis. These symptoms have increased since admission. Laboratory studies are significant for a creatinine kinase level of 1480 mg/dL.

    Which of the following is the most likely diagnosis?
    A) Lithium toxicity
    B) Malignant hyperthermia
    C) Neuroleptic malignant syndrome
    D) Serotonin syndrome
    E) Sepsis

Answer: C

This patient's symptoms of fever, tremor, agitation, and rigidity are consistent with the neuroleptic malignant syndrome. This is a potential life-threatening condition. It is characterized by hyperthermia that is accompanied by autonomic dysfunction, as seen in this patient. This syndrome presents as a reaction to new antipsychotic neuroleptic medications or an increase in neuroleptic medications, as is the case here. The most common offending agents are the older antipsychotics such as haloperidol and fluphenazine. Neuroleptic malignant syndrome rapidly develops over a 24-h period and peaks within 72 h.

References

Gurrera RJ, Caroff SN, Cohen A, et al. An international consensus study of neuroleptic malignant syndrome diagnostic criteria using the Delphi method. J Clin Psychiatry. 2011;72(9):1222–8

Trollor JN, Chen X, Sachdev PS. Neuroleptic malignant syndrome associated with atypical antipsychotic drugs. CNS Drugs. 2009;23(6):477–92.

27. A 27-year-old male is admitted with severe agitation, psychosis, and violent behavior. He was brought to the emergency room 2 h ago by police. Despite 3 mg of lorazepam given 2 h prior, he remains agitated and difficult to control.

    On physical examination, he is diaphoretic and is unable to answer questions. He has a heart rate of 170 bpm, blood pressure of 200/110 mmHg, and a marked vertical nystagmus. He is a known user of cannabis, but no other illicit drug history is known.

Which of the following is the most likely drug ingested?
A) Cocaine
B) Phencyclidine (PCP)
C) Lysergic acid diethylamide (LSD)
D) Heroin
E) Methylenedioxymethamphetamine (MDMA).

Answer: B

Phencyclidine, or PCP, often presents with severe agitation, psychosis, and violent behavior. Often, multiple people are required to restrain the patient. Vertical or rotatory nystagmus is a unique finding characteristic of PCP intoxication. Management of phencyclidine intoxication mostly consists of supportive care. Benzodiazepines have been used for agitation and for the treatment of seizures that can occur with PCP ingestion.

Cocaine intoxication may present with similar symptoms but is not reported to cause nystagmus. Lysergic acid diethylamide (LSD) is a typical hallucinogen, but no significant amount of violent behavior is reported. MDMA and ecstasy are both hallucinogenic and a stimulant. Violent behavior is not usually seen. Heroin causes a typical opioid symptom profile consisting of constricted pupils, sedation, and respiratory depression.

Since its peak use in urban areas, the 1970s PCP use has declined.

Reference

Zukin SR, Sloboda Z, Javitt DC. Phencyclidine PCP. In: Lowinson JH, Ruiz P, Millman RB, et al., editors. Substance abuse: a comprehensive textbook, 4th ed. Philadelphia: Lippincott Williams & Wilkins; 2005.

28. A 43-year-old white male presents to the emergency room for intractable nausea and vomiting. During inpatient admission paperwork, you complete his VTE risk assessment and realize he is a high VTE risk. What would you choose for DVT prophylaxis (BMI=45, CrCl=75 ml/min)?
A) Early ambulation
B) Lovenox 40 mg SQ daily
C) Lovenox 40 mg SQ BID
D) Sequential compression device

Answer: C

For thromboprophylaxis with fixed-dose enoxaparin, there is a strong negative correlation between total body weight and anti-Xa levels in obese patients. Several prospective trials have examined this issue in patients undergoing bariatric surgery, with inconclusive findings. However, guidelines have stated that increasing the prophylactic dose of enoxaparin in morbidly obese patients (body mass index >/=40 kg/m²) is appropriate. The most common dosing recommendation for this scenario is 40 mg SQ BID. However, other indications, such as bariatric surgery, have recommended 60 mg SQ BID if BMI>/= 50 kg/m². Early ambulation and sequential compression devices alone would not be appropriate DVT prophylaxis for a high VTE risk.

References

Frederiksen SG, Hedenbro JL, Norgren L. Enoxaparin effect depends on body-weight and current doses may be inadequate in obese patients. Br J Surg. 2003;90:547–8.
Garcia DA, et al. CHEST guidelines – parenteral anticoagulants. Chest 2012;141(2_suppl):e24S–43S.
Nutescu EA, Spinler SA, Wittkowsky A, Dager WE. Low-molecular-weight heparins in renal impairment and obesity: available evidence and clinical practice recommendations across medical and surgical settings. Ann Pharmacother. 2009;43:1064–83.

29. A 35-year-old woman with Crohn's disease presents with a flare of her disease consisting of fever, right lower quadrant pain, guaiac-positive diarrhea, and macrocytic anemia. She states she has lost 20 lbs from her usual weight of 101 lbs. She is still able to tolerate solid food and liquids. Previously, her disease has been limited to the small intestine and terminal ileum.

On physical exam, she has a temperature of 37.9 °C (100.3 °F), active bowel sounds are heard, and she has right lower quadrant tenderness.

Which of the following statements is true for this patient?
A) The anemia is probably caused by folate deficiency.
B) Sulfasalazine is the first-line therapy.
C) An aminosalicylate (5-ASA) will be required to control this flare.
D) Corticosteroids will be necessary to control her symptoms.
E) She should be hospitalized and given infliximab.

Answer: D

This patient has moderate to severe Crohn's disease. This is based on her symptoms of fever, weight loss, abdominal pain without obstruction, and ability to continue oral intake. For the treatment of moderate to severe Crohn's disease, the current recommendations include the "top-down" approach. This differs from the conventional step-up approach in that more potent agents are administered initially. For symptoms of this severity, corticosteroids will be necessary. The use of 5-ASA for the treatment of Crohn's disease is limited. In studies, only a small subset of patients have benefitted from this agent.

Infliximab may be used in patients who are not responsive to salicylates, antibiotics, or steroids. Unless the small bowel mucosal disease is very extensive, the macrocytic anemia is most likely caused by a deficiency of vitamin B12, which is absorbed in the terminal ileum.

Reference

Ford AC, Bernstein CN, Khan KJ, Abreu MT, Marshall JK, Talley NJ, et al. Glucocorticosteroid therapy in inflammatory bowel disease: systematic review and meta-analysis. Am J Gastroenterol. 2011;106(4):590–9.

30. A 65-year-old female with a history recently diagnosed small cell lung cancer presents with a chief complaint of fatigue, dizziness, and imbalance. Her sodium level on admission is 112 meq/L. She was noted to have a sodium of 142 mmol/L approximately 1 month ago. Her family reports no change in her dietary habits or excessive water intoxication.

On physical exam she appears to be euvolemic.

The most appropriate initial therapy includes:

A) Slow correction of her sodium with normal saline
B) Free water restriction
C) 3 % saline administration with close monitoring
D) Demeclocycline
E) Dexamethasone

Answer: C

In a setting of significant hyponatremia with neurologic symptoms, consideration must be given to administering hypertonic saline. This patient's condition is almost certainly due to syndrome of inappropriate antidiuretic hormone (SIADH) due to her small cell lung cancer. Isotonic normal saline would probably worsen the hyponatremia by the mechanism of water retention and sodium excretion. When hypertonic saline is administered, careful monitoring of her sodium levels should be done to prevent central pontine myelinolysis, which can occur with rapid correction. In less severe cases with no neurologic findings, water restriction would be the first line of treatment.

Reference

Zenenberg RD, Carluccio AL, Merlin MA. Hyponatremia: evaluation and management. Hosp Pract. 2010;38(1):89–96.

31. A 65-year-old male with a recent hospitalization for total knee replacement presents with the chief complaint of eight bowel movements per day. He reports a fever as high as 37.8 °C.

On physical exam, mild abdominal distention is noted, and he appears in no apparent distress. WBC is 16, 000 cells/μl.

Initial therapy for suspected *Clostridium difficile* disease would include the following:

A) Oral metronidazole 500 mg q 8
B) Oral vancomycin 125 mg q 6
C) IV metronidazole 500 mg q 6
D) Oral vancomycin 125 g q 6

Answer: D

The treatment for *Clostridium difficile* infections is changing as new protocols and therapies are developed. The patient in this question is characterized as having moderate *Clostridium difficile* infection. First-line treatment is based on the severity of illness and initial clinical response. Symptoms of moderate disease include 6–12 bowel movements per day, fever of 37.5–38.5 °C, a WBC count between 15,000 and 25,000 cells/μl, or visible GI bleeding. Oral vancomycin is the treatment of choice for moderate disease. For severe disease, oral vancomycin 125 mg q 6 and IV metronidazole 500 mg q 6 is the treatment of choice. For mild disease, oral Flagyl can be used alone, 500 mg q 8. New treatment modalities, such as fidaxomicin as well as stool replacement therapy, have shown promising results and are currently undergoing trials.

Reference

Ananthakrishnan AN. Clostridium difficile infection: epidemiology, risk factors and management. Nat Rev Gastroenterol Hepatol. 2011;8(1):17–26.

32. A 54-year-old man is admitted with abdominal pain. He had a similar episode 6 months ago for which he was seen in the emergency room several days after the onset of pain and was discharged home without a definitive diagnosis. He has a history of poorly controlled diabetes mellitus. He has pain for the past 3 days. He denies any alcohol use, which is confirmed by family members.

On physical exam, he is tachycardic and has diminished bowel sounds and epigastric tenderness. He has a papular rash on his knees.

Initial laboratory studies are significant for the following: leukocytes, 16,000 cells/mm³; blood glucose level of 400 mg/dl. An amylase level is normal.

Which of the following is the most likely diagnosis for this patient?

A) Acute or chronic idiopathic pancreatitis
B) Gallstone pancreatitis
C) Alcoholic pancreatitis
D) Pancreatitis secondary to hypertriglyceridemia
E) Malignancy-induced pancreatitis

Answer: D

This patient has triglyceride induced pancreatitis. The serum amylase level may be normal in some patients with acute pancreatitis associated with high triglycerides as marked elevations in the triglyceride level can interfere with the laboratory assay for amylase. The presence of a papular rash on this patient is consistent with eruptive xanthomas due to hypertriglyceridemia.

In the acute phase, the initial treatment of hypertriglyceridemia-induced acute pancreatitis focuses on good hydration and analgesia and is similar to the management of acute pancreatitis due to any etiology. The triglyceride levels usually rapidly decrease within 48 h of the onset of acute pancreatitis.

Gallstones and alcohol abuse combined account for 70–80 % of all cases of acute pancreatitis. Other etiologies include sphincter of Oddi dysfunction, strictures of the pancreatic duct, congenital anatomic abnormalities and genetic disorders, drugs, toxins, trauma, infections, and metabolic causes. Some cases are idiopathic. Metabolic causes of acute pancreatitis include not only hypertriglyceridemia but hypercalcemias well. Serum triglycerides generally need to be in excess of 1,000 mg/dl to produce acute pancreatitis. This is most commonly seen in type V hyperlipoproteinemia and is usually associated with diabetes mellitus. Acute pancreatitis can itself raise triglyceride levels, but not to this degree.

References

Suang W, Navaneethan U, Ruiz L, et al. Hypertriglyceridemic pancreatitis: presentation and management. Am J Gastroenterol. 2009;104:984–91.

Toskes PP. Hyperlipidemic pancreatitis. Gastroenterol Clin North Am. 1990;19:783–91.

33. An 80-year-old man has been admitted with a urinary tract infection. On the third day from his admission, he develops the acute onset of chest pain of 30 min duration. He has a history of an inferior myocardial infarction 3 years ago. His medical history is remarkable for hypertension and an ischemic stroke 8 years ago. Current medications include atenolol and aspirin.

    On physical exam, the patient is afebrile, his blood pressure is 170/100 mmHg, his pulse is 90 beats/min, and his respiratory rate is 20 breaths/min. He is diaphoretic and in apparent pain. ECG reveals 0.2 mm elevations in leads V2–V6.

    Which of the following features, in this case, would be an absolute contraindication to thrombolytic therapy?
    A) Failure to meet ECG criteria.
    B) Age greater than 75 years.
    C) History of stroke.
    D) Elevated blood pressure.
    E) There are no absolute contraindications.

Answer: E

In this case, there are no absolute contraindications to thrombolytic therapy.

The patient meets ECG criteria for the administration of thrombolytic therapy. This includes ST segment elevation greater than 0.1 mm in two contiguous leads.

Age greater than 75 years is not a contraindication to thrombolysis. In patients older than 75 years, there is an increased risk of hemorrhagic stroke. Overall mortality is reduced in such patients without other contraindications. A prior history of hemorrhagic stroke is an absolute contraindication to thrombolytic. A history of an ischemic stroke less than 1 year is an absolute contraindication. A stroke more than 1 year before presentation is a relative contraindication. Blood pressure >180/110 mmHg is a relative contraindication to thrombolytic therapy.

Reference

O'Gara PT, Kushner FG, Ascheim DD et al. 2013 ACCF/AHA guideline for the management of ST-elevation myocardial infarction: a report of the American College of Cardiology Foundation/American Heart Association Task Force on Practice Guidelines. Circulation. 2013;127:e362–452.

34. A 65-year-old male presents with progressive shortness of breath over the past month. He has a 40 pack-year history of smoking. CT scan of the chest reveals a right middle lobe mass for which he subsequently undergoes biopsy, which reveals adenocarcinoma. Magnetic resonance imaging of the brain reveals a 1 cm tumor in the left cerebral cortex, which is consistent with metastatic disease. The patient has no history of seizures or syncope. The patient is referred to outpatient therapy in the hematology/oncology service as well as follow-up with radiation oncology. The patient is ready for discharge.

    Which of the following would be the most appropriate therapy for primary seizure prevention?
    A) Seizure prophylaxis is not indicated.
    B) Valproate.
    C) Phenytoin.
    D) Phenobarbital.
    E) Oral prednisone 40 mg daily.

Answer: A

There is no indication for antiepileptic therapy for primary prevention in patients who have brain metastasis who have not undergone resection. Past studies have revealed no difference in seizure rates between placebo and antiepileptic therapy in patients who have brain tumors. Antiepileptic therapy has high rates of adverse reactions and caution should be used in their use.

Reference

Sirven JI, Wingerchuk DM, Drazkowski JF, Lyons MK, Zimmerman RS. Seizure prophylaxis in patients with brain tumors: a meta-analysis. Mayo Clin Proc. 2004;79(12):1489–94.

35. A 52-year-old male presents with new onset hemoptysis and shortness of breath. He is recovering from an ankle fracture. CT angiography reveals an intraluminal defect in the left lower lobar pulmonary artery and right upper lobe subsegment.

What additional measurements from CT angiography have been shown to have prognostic significance?
A) Clot burden (e.g., amount of clot seen)
B) Clot location
C) Right versus left ventricular volume
D) Clot size
E) Collateral flow

Answer: C

Risk stratification for pulmonary embolism is the goal of many current studies. A reliable method is currently being developed. In patients who are hemodynamically stable, a number of tests have been examined in this effort. Clot size and location are not good at predicting mortality or right ventricular strain.

Examination of ventricular volumes comparing right to left may be the best measurement for predicting outcomes. A ratio >1.2 that is suggestive of right ventricular strain has utility in predicting adverse outcome and death. Echocardiograms may look for right heart strain as well. Other tools that are being considered include biomarkers such as troponin and pro-brain natriuretic peptide (proBNP) levels, and clinical models such as PESI (Pulmonary Embolism Severity Index) and PREP (prognostic factors for PE).

References

Aujesky D, et al. Derivation and validation of a prognostic model for pulmonary embolism. Am J Respir Crit Care Med. 2005;172:1041–6.

Becattini C, et al. Acute pulmonary embolism: external validation of an integrated risk stratification model. Chest. 2013. doi:10.1378/chest.12-2938.

Sanchez O, et al. Prognostic factors for pulmonary embolism: the PREP study, a prospective multicenter cohort study. Am J Respir Crit Care Med. 2010;181:168–73.

36. A 68-year-old male with a history COPD presents with a 3-day history of worsening shortness of breath and fever. On the day prior to presentation, he developed abdominal pain and diarrhea. He is employed as an air conditioner repair technician.

On physical exam, his temperature is 39.5 °C (103.1 °F), pulse is 72, and respiratory rate is 30. He is in moderate respiratory distress. Oxygen saturation is 95 % on 2 l of oxygen. He has moderate abdominal pain.

Laboratory data is significant for mild elevation of his transaminases and a sodium of 128. Chest radiograph reveals bilateral infiltrates.

The most appropriate antibiotics and treatment are:
A) Vancomycin 1 g q12 and piperacillin/sulbactam 4.gms q 8
B) Ceftriaxone 1 g q 12 and azithromycin 500 mg q8
C) Vancomycin 1 g q12/gentamicin
D) Ceftriaxone 1 g q12/Prednisone 40 mg QD
E) Bactrim

Answer: B

This patient has legionella pneumonia, which should be treated with a quinolone or macrolide antibiotic. Legionella pneumonia presents with the common symptoms of fever, chills, and cough. Distinguishing features are loss of appetite, loss of coordination, and occasionally diarrhea and vomiting. Relative bradycardia has traditionally been considered a symptom. Laboratory tests may show significant changes in renal functions, liver functions, and electrolytes. This can include marked hyponatremia. Chest X-rays often show bi-basal consolidation. It is difficult to distinguish Legionnaires' disease from other types of pneumonia by symptoms alone. Serology is often required for diagnosis. Many hospitals utilize the urinary antigen test for initial detection when legionella pneumonia is suspected.

It is not spread from person to person, but rather often through exposure to aerosolized cool water, such is the case here.

It acquired its name after a July 1976 outbreak of a then unrecognized disease, which afflicted 221 persons, resulting in 34 deaths. The outbreak was first noticed among people attending a convention the American Legion.

References

Fraser DW, Tsai T, Orenstein W, et al. Legionnaires' disease: description of an epidemic of pneumonia. N Engl J Med. 1977;297:1186–96.

Woo AH, Goetz A, Yu VL. Transmission of Legionella by respiratory equipment and aerosol generating devices. Chest. 1992;102(5):1586–90.

37. You are called to the floor to see a 77-year-old man who has recently passed a large amount of red and maroon blood per rectum. He was admitted 2 days ago for a urinary tract infection. After this episode, the patient feels dizzy but is conscious and able to converse.

On physical exam, his blood pressure is 100/60 mmHg and the pulse rate is 110/min. He has no abdominal pain, nausea, vomiting, fever, or weight loss. He had a colonoscopy 1 year ago that showed a benign polyp and extensive diverticulosis. He has a single 22 g IV access.

Stat laboratory studies reveal a hemoglobin of 7.5 g/dL. The leukocyte count is 5600/μL. Prothrombin time and activated partial thromboplastin times are normal.

Which of the following is the most appropriate next step in the management of this patient?
A) Colonoscopy
B) Esophagogastroduodenoscopy
C) Increased intravenous access
D) Placement of a nasogastric tube with lavage
E) Technetium-labeled red blood cell scan

Answer: C

This patient is volume depleted and not hemodynamically stable. Survival may be dependent upon the correct management sequence. Two large-bore peripheral catheters or a central line for volume repletion is urgently required. Fluid resuscitation should be started as well as an urgent type and match for blood transfusion. Although rapid diagnosis may be of benefit, early resuscitation measures should not be delayed by diagnostic workup.

A nasogastric tube may be considered after volume resuscitation, if an upper source of gastrointestinal bleeding is likely. Regardless of the source of bleeding at this point in the management, the first rule is to achieve hemodynamic stability.

Although a colonoscopy is the diagnostic test of choice to evaluate for sources of lower gastrointestinal bleeding, this should not occur before volume resuscitation. A bleeding scan may be indicated if an endoscopic evaluation is not immediately possible or if an endoscopic evaluation has been non-revealing. Diverticular bleed is certainly a possibility in this case. If a bleeding diverticulum is detected on colonoscopy, it can be treated with thermal coagulation or epinephrine injection. Up to 90 % of diverticular bleeding resolves without intervention.

References
Laine L, Shah A. Randomized trial of urgent vs. elective colonoscopy in patients hospitalized with lower GI bleeding. Am J Gastroenterol. 2010;105(12):2636–41.
Scottish Intercollegiate Guidelines Network (SIGN). Management of acute upper and lower gastrointestinal bleeding. A national clinical guideline. SIGN publication; no. 105. Edinburgh (Scotland): Scottish Intercollegiate Guidelines Network (SIGN); 2008.

38. An 81-year-old female who is admitted to the hospital with a diagnosis of healthcare-associated pneumonia (HCAP). She is empirically started on vancomycin, ciprofloxacin, and piperacillin/tazobactam.

In treating this patient, what is the vancomycin trough goal for HCAP?
A) 10–15 ug/ml
B) 15–20 ug/ml
C) 25–30 ug/ml
D) 28–32 ug/ml

Answer: B
Healthcare-associated pneumonia (HCAP) treatment with vancomycin requires higher trough levels of 15–20 mcg/ml.

References
ATS Board of Directors and IDSA Guideline Committee. Guidelines of the management of adults with hospital-acquired, ventilator-associated, and healthcare-associated pneumonia. Am J Respir Crit Care Med. 2005;171:388–416.
Ryback M et al. Therapeutic monitoring of vancomycin in adult patients. Am J Health-Syst Pharm. 2009;66:82–98.

39. A 40-year-old male is admitted to the hospital for new-onset fever and chills. He denies any other symptoms. He was recently diagnosed with non-Hodgkin's lymphoma, for which he received his first cycle of chemotherapy 10 days ago. He currently does not have an indwelling venous catheter.

On physical examination, the temperature is 39.0 °C (102.2 °F). Blood pressure is 120/75 mmHg. There is no evidence of mucositis. Chest exam is normal. Heart examination is normal as well. Abdominal exam reveals normal bowel sounds and is nontender. Laboratory data shows a hemoglobin of 10.8 g/dL and leukocyte count of 600/mcL. The differential is 10 % neutrophils and 90 % lymphocytes. Chest X-ray is normal. Blood and urine cultures are pending.

Which is the most appropriate treatment course?
A) Begin vancomycin.
B) Await blood cultures and urine cultures.
C) Begin vancomycin, amphotericin, and acyclovir.
D) Begin piperacillin/tazobactam.
E) Begin vancomycin, amphotericin, acyclovir, and diflucan.

Answer: D
This patient is neutropenic and febrile and warrants rapid initiation of antibiotics. A stepwise and logical approach is needed for the selection of antibiotics. Febrile neutropenia is a medical emergency. Patients may not present with overt signs of infection. However, septic shock and death can occur within hours of presentation.
Initial antibiotic choices may include a third-generation cephalosporin, penicillin with beta-lactamase inhibitor, or cefepime. Endogenous flora from the gastrointestinal

tract is the probable cause for most cases of febrile neutropenia. Vancomycin may be considered but alone would not be sufficient coverage for this patient. Empiric antifungal therapy is usually reserved for patients who are febrile after the source of infection is not found following 4–7 days of broad-spectrum antimicrobial therapy. Viral infections are not common, and empiric therapy with antiviral agents such as acyclovir is not warranted.

Reference

Hughes WT, Armstrong D, Bodey GP, et al. 2002 guidelines for the use of antimicrobial agents in neutropenic patients with cancer. Clin Infect Dis. 2002;34(6):730–51.

40. An 82-year-old female presents to the emergency department complaining nausea and vomiting. She is admitted for dehydration due to probable viral gastroenteritis. On admission her serum creatinine is noted to be 3.0 mg/dL, her baseline is 1.2 mg/dl.

    After transfer to the floor, she acutely develops dizziness with a heart rate of 34/min. 12-lead ECG shows marked sinus bradycardia without any ST segment changes. Stat glucose is 95 mg/dl.

    Home medications include atenolol 100 mg daily and hydrochlorothiazide 25 mg daily. Blood pressure is 85/68 mmHg.

    Which of the following medications is the most appropriate to administer next?
    A) Intravenous 50 % dextrose solution and insulin
    B) Intravenous glucagon
    C) Intravenous calcium gluconate
    D) Intravenous magnesium sulfate
    E) Intravenous atropine
    F) B or E

Answer: F

This patient has bradycardia and hypotension from betablocker toxicity. This is caused by a reduced clearance of atenolol, which is renally excreted and impaired because of her prerenal kidney failure. Glucagon is used to reverse beta-blocker toxicity and is often used as a first-line agent when beta-blocker toxicity is the confirmed issue. Atropine may be used according protocols as well.

She should also receive fluid resuscitation with intravenous normal saline solution. If she does not improve with glucagon and IV fluids, external pacemaker or transvenous pacemaker can also be used.

Reference

Hoot NR, Benitez JG, Palm KH. Hemodynamically unstable: accidental atenolol toxicity?. J Emerg Med. 2013;45(3):355–7.

41. A homeless man is found unconscious by police. He is admitted for hypothermia and possible cellulitis of his left foot. His past medical history is unknown.

    On examination, the foot appears atypical for cellulitis. It has hemorrhagic vesicles distributed throughout the foot distal to the ankle. The left foot is cool and has no sensation to pain or temperature. The right foot is hyperemic but does not have vesicles and has normal sensation. The remainders of the physical examination findings are normal. He is started on antibiotics, and further therapy is considered.

    Which of the following statements regarding the management of his foot is true?
    A) Rewarming should not be attempted.
    B) Heparin has been shown to improve outcomes.
    C) Surgical consultation and debridement are indicated.
    D) Normal sensation is likely to return with rewarming.
    E) Antibiotics improves limb survival.
    F) During the period of rewarming, intense pain will occur.

Answer: F

This patient presents with frostbite of the left foot. One of the common presenting symptoms of this is sensory changes that affect both pain and temperature reception. Hemorrhagic vesicles are caused by injury to the vasculature. The prognosis is more favorable when the presenting area has a rapid return to normal temperature and color returns as well. Treatment of extremities is with rapid rewarming, which usually is accomplished with a 37–40 °C (98.6–104 °F) water bath.

The period of rewarming can be intensely painful for the patient, and often narcotic analgesia is warranted and should be anticipated to improve compliance. If the pain is intolerable, the temperature of the water bath may be lowered slightly. Compartment syndrome can develop. Rewarming should be closely followed. No medications have been shown to improve outcomes. This includes heparin, steroids, calcium channel blockers, and hyperbaric oxygen. Emergent surgical decisions about the need for debridement should be deferred until the boundaries of the tissue injury are determined. Neuronal injury often occurs with abnormal sympathetic tone in the extremity. This may be permanent or resolve over the course of several months.

References

McCauley RL, Hing DN, Robson MC, Heggers JP. Frostbite injuries: a rational approach based on the pathophysiology. J Trauma. 1983;23(2):143–7.

Twomey JA, Peltier GL, Zera RT. An open-label study to evaluate the safety and efficacy of tissue plasminogen activator in treatment of severe frostbite. J Trauma. 2005;59(6):1350–4; discussion 1354–5.

42. An 18-year-old female is admitted for observation after sustaining a head-to-head blow during a high school soccer game. She briefly lost consciousness on the field but was able to walk on the sidelines without assistance. She was immediately brought to the emergency room and subsequently admitted to the hospital medicine service.

After an overnight stay in the observation unit, she appears back to her usual baseline mental status. Physical examination in the morning is within normal range. Neurologic examination is within normal limits as well.

Which of the following is the most appropriate next step in management?

A) CT of the head and return to competition if normal
B) Observation for 24 more hours
C) Exclusion from competition for 1 week
D) Clearance for return to competition
E) Funduscopic examination

Answer: C

This patient has a grade 3 concussion. A concussion is defined as trauma-induced alteration in mental status that may be associated with transient loss of consciousness. Neither a grade 1 nor a grade 2 concussion involves a loss of consciousness. A grade I concussion, or mild bruising of brain tissue, is the most common form of head injury. The athlete may briefly appear or act confused; however, he or she is able to remember all events following the impact. The difference between a grade II and a grade I concussion is the presence of post-traumatic amnesia. A grade 3 concussion, such as is seen in this patient, is defined by a brief or prolonged loss of consciousness. Current recommendations state that a grade 1 concussion are permitted to return to the contest on the same day as the injury. The athlete should be removed from competition for at least 20 min and examined every 5 min.

Those with grade 2 or grade 3 concussions are prohibited from returning that day. Grade 3 concussions are prohibited from returning to competition until the athlete is asymptomatic for 1 week. Hospitalization is indicated in the presence of traumatic findings, abnormal neuroimaging studies, or with persistent abnormalities seen on physical examination.

Reference

Giza CC, Kutcher JS, Ashwal S, Barth J, Getchius TS, Gioia GA, et al. Summary of evidence-based guideline update: evaluation and management of concussion in sports: report of the Guideline Development Subcommittee of the American Academy of Neurology. Neurology. 2013;80(24):2250–7.

43. A 77-year-old male presents to the emergency room with a chief complaint of syncope while getting out of bed to go to the bathroom at 2:00 AM. He has no recollection of the event. He was found by his wife on the floor confused. He has no prior history of syncope and denies chest pain.

On physical examination, the patient is alert and oriented to person, place, time, and event. Temperature is 36.6 °C (97.9 °F). Pulse rate is 60 per minute. Respirations are 16 per minute. Blood pressure is 110/40. Cardiopulmonary and neurologic exams are normal. A small laceration to the chin is noted, but otherwise, there is no evidence of trauma to the head.

Which of the following diagnostic test has the highest yield for determining this patient's cause of syncope?

A) Measurement of postural blood pressure
B) Cardiac enzymes
C) Ultrasonography of the carotid arteries
D) Computed tomography
E) Electroencephalography

Answer: A

Syncope is a common admission to the hospital. The majority of cases are vasovagal in origin and warrant limited and focused workup. History and physical examination are the most specific and sensitive ways of evaluating syncope. These measures, along with 12-lead electrocardiography (ECG), are the only current level A recommendations listed in the 2007 American College of Emergency Physicians (ACEP) Clinical Policy on Syncope.

Several tests commonly ordered have little yield. Cardiac enzymes determine the etiology of syncope in only 0.5 % of patients. Carotid ultrasonography determines the etiology of syncope in 0.8 % of patients. Computed tomography of the brain determines the etiology of syncope in 0.5 % of patients. Electroencephalography determines the etiology of syncope in only 0.8 % of patients. The use of these tests is warranted only when there is evidence to suggest that vasovagal syncope is not the cause.

A common scenario is for vasovagal syncope to occur in the middle of the night while going to the bathroom, as is the case here. Confusion is often present and does not necessarily point toward a postictal state. Reassurance and lifestyle modifications are the best treatment. This includes methods to reduce nighttime bathroom use, which is common cause of syncope and injury inducing falls.

Measurement of postural blood pressure may confirm the diagnosis and is often a cost-effective test in determining the cause of syncope.

Reference

Huff JS, Decker WW, Quinn JV, et al. Clinical policy: critical issues in the evaluation and management of adult patients presenting to the emergency department with syncope. Ann Emerg Med. 2007;49(4):431–44.

44. A 50-year-old male is admitted with complaints of moderate mid-epigastric pain in his upper abdomen for a few weeks. He reports moderate heartburn for the past 2 months. He also complains of weight loss of 10 lbs in the last 2 months as well. He does not take any medications except occasional ibuprofen for back pain.

    On physical exam he has moderate tenderness in the epigastric area. The patient's amylase and lipase are normal. CT scan of the abdomen is normal.

    What is the next appropriate step in the management of this patient?
    A) Start PPI.
    B) H. pylori treatment.
    C) Stop ibuprofen.
    D) Manometry studies.
    E) Upper endoscopy.

Answer: E

Many patients with gastroesophageal reflux disease are appropriately treated with empiric therapy. Endoscopy is reserved for those with chronic symptoms who are at risk for Barrett's esophagus and those with alarm symptoms.

Alarm symptoms include dysphagia, odynophagia, gastrointestinal bleeding or anemia, weight loss, and chest pain. Other alarm features are age greater than 55 years and family history of gastric cancer. This patient's weight loss would warrant endoscopic evaluation.

Reference

DeVault KR, Castell DO. Updated guidelines for the diagnosis and treatment of gastroesophageal reflux disease. Am J Gastroenterol. 1999;94:1434–42.

45. An EEG showing triphasic waves is most suggestive of which of the following clinical disorders?
    A) Brain abscess
    B) Herpes simplex encephalitis
    C) Locked-in syndrome
    D) Metabolic encephalopathy
    E) Nonconvulsive status epilepticus

Answer: D

Triphasic waves have been associated with a wide range of toxic, metabolic, and structural abnormalities. They were first described in a patient with hepatic encephalopathy.

The EEG can often provide clinically useful information in comatose patients. Certain EEG patterns may help in determining diagnosis and prognosis. The EEG becomes slower as consciousness is depressed, regardless of the underlying cause. The EEG is usually normal in patients with locked-in syndrome and helps in distinguishing this disorder from the comatose state. Epileptiform activity characterized by bursts of abnormal discharges containing spikes or sharp waves may be useful to diagnose and treat unrecognized nonconvulsive status in a presumed comatose patient. Patients with herpes simplex encephalitis may show a characteristic pattern of focal, often in the temporal regions or lateralized periodic slow-wave complexes.

Yang SS, Wu CH, Chiang TR, et al. Somatosensory evoked potentials in subclinical portosystemic encephalopathy: a comparison with psychometric tests. Hepatology. 1998;27:357–9.

46. Blood cultures should be obtained in which patients admitted for cellulitis?
    A) Presence of lymphedema
    B) Liver cirrhosis
    C) Presence of ipsilateral orthopedic implant
    D) Leukocytosis of $<13.5 \times 106 \, \mu L$
    E) A, B, and C
    F) All of the above

Answer: E

Blood cultures are not beneficial for many patients admitted with uncomplicated cellulitis. They should be limited to certain high-risk populations. Any form of immunosuppression or underlying structural damage would increase the risk of bacteremia, and thus a blood culture should be performed and may be of benefit.

Reference

Phoenix G, Das S, Joshi M. Diagnosis and management of cellulitis. BMJ (Clinical Research ed.). 2012;345:e4955.

47. A 31-year-old woman presented to the emergency room with a history of low-grade intermittent fever and reported joint pain, swelling, and rapid onset of decreased mental status over the past 2 days. Per family, the joint pains have developed gradually over the past 4 months. In the past 36 h, she first developed profound personality changes that included agitation and mild visual hallucinations. Increasing lethargy followed this.

    On physical exam she appears obtunded. Joint tenderness is difficult to assess due to decreased mental status. Mild swelling is noted in several joints.

A CT scan of the brain reveals possible diffuse mild cerebral edema.

Magnetic resonance imaging reveals diffuse microinfarcts. Hemoglobin, WBC, and platelet counts are within normal range. The CSF report 110 lymphocytes and an elevated protein.

The most likely diagnoses is?

A) Herpes encephalitis
B) Lupus cerebritis
C) Endocarditis
D) Lyme disease
E) Drug injection

Answer: B

Lupus cerebritis can pose as a major diagnostic challenge, as many lupus patients have underlying neuropsychiatric symptoms. The case here has some classical findings, but many cases are elusive. Patients may present with acute confusion, lethargy, coma, chronic dementia, depression, mania, affective disturbances, or psychosis.

Prompt identification can be extremely difficult, mainly because there is no single laboratory or radiological confirmatory test. Inflammatory markers can be variable. Lupus cerebritis should be included as a possible diagnosis in any young female patient who presents with complicated neurologic manifestations and no alternative diagnosis.

Reference
Calabrese LV, Stern TA. Neuropsychiatric manifestations of systemic lupus erythematosus. Psychosomatics. 1995;36:344–8.
Greenberg BM. The neurologic manifestations of systemic lupus erythematosus. Neurologist. 2009 May. 15(3):115–21

48. Which of the following regimens are most appropriate for the treatment of *Clostridium difficile* infections?

A) Moderate to severe initial episode: vancomycin 125 mg QID for a total of 10–14 days
B) Severe initial episode complicated with shock and megacolon: vancomycin 125 mg po QID plus metronidazole 500 mg Q8 h IV.
C) Severe initial episode but with a complete ileus: consider rectal instillation of vancomycin
D) None of the above
E) All of the above

Answer: E

The following are 2010 guidelines for the treatment of the first episode of *Clostridium difficile* colitis:

First episode with mild or moderate leukocytosis with a white blood cell count of 15,000 cells/mL or lower and a serum creatinine level less than 1.5 times the premorbid level – metronidazole 500 mg 3 times per day by mouth for 10–14 days

First episode, severe and leukocytosis with a white blood cell count of 15,000 cells/mL or higher or a serum creatinine level greater than or equal to 1.5 times the premorbid level – vancomycin 125 mg 4 times per day by mouth for 10–14 days

First episode, severe and complicated by hypotension or shock, ileus, megacolon – vancomycin 500 mg 4 times per day by mouth or by nasogastric tube, plus metronidazole 500 mg every 8 h intravenously

If complete ileus, consider adding rectal instillation of vancomycin.

Reference
Cohen SH, Gerding DN, Johnson S, Kelly CP, Loo VG, McDonald LC, Pepin J, Wilcox MH. Clinical Practice Guidelines for Clostridium difficile Infection in Adults: 2010 Update by the Society for Healthcare Epidemiology of America (SHEA) and the Infectious Diseases Society of America (IDSA). Infect Control Hosp Epidemiol. 2010;3:431–55.

49. A 52-year-old man is evaluated in the emergency department for a 2-week history of fatigue and nonspecific arthralgia. He reports some increasing shortness of breath over the past few days and now has some pleuritic chest pain. He has a history of coronary artery disease and hypertension. His medications include diltiazem, hydralazine, aspirin, and isosorbide dinitrate.

On physical examination, his temperature is 37.2 °C (99 °F), blood pressure is 145/90 mmHg, pulse rate is 80 bpm, and respiration rate is 24/min. Cardiac examination is normal. Pulmonary examination reveals a mild left pleural friction rub. There are small bilateral knee effusions. A nonblanching purpuric rash is noted over the distal upper and lower extremities.

Laboratory studies show hemoglobin of 7.9 g/dL, leukocyte count 2,200/µL, platelet count 124,000/µL, and erythrocyte sedimentation rate 88 mm/h. Urinalysis reveals 1+ protein, 2–5 erythrocytes/hpf, and 5–10 leukocytes/hpf.

Chest radiograph reveals small bilateral effusions.

Which of the following is the most appropriate diagnostic test to perform next?

A) Serum and urine electrophoresis
B) Bone marrow aspiration and biopsy
C) CT of the chest, abdomen, and pelvis
D) Rheumatoid factor and anti-cyclic citrullinated peptide antibody
E) Antinuclear antibody and anti-double-strand DNA antibody assay

Answer: E

This patient has drug-induced lupus erythematosus (DILE). The most common drugs that cause DILE are hydralazine, procainamide, quinidine, isoniazid, diltiazem, and minocycline.

He has new-onset fever, arthralgia, myalgia, nonblanching purpuric rash, pleuritis, pancytopenia, and proteinuria with active urine sediment.

Testing for antinuclear antibodies (ANA), as well as anti-double-stranded DNA antibodies and complement levels, is indicated. This multiorgan pattern is suggestive of an autoimmune disorder, in particular of systemic lupus erythematosus (SLE). No specific criteria establish the diagnosis of DILE. Excluding other underlying autoimmune diseases must first be done. SLE is typically ruled out first.

Drugs that cause DILE may take months to years before the associated symptoms occur. In addition similar drugs can also induce flairs of SLE.

References

Fritzler MJ. Drugs recently associated with lupus syndromes. Lupus. 1994;3(6):455–9.

Lowe G, Henderson CL, Grau RH, Hansen CB, Sontheimer RD. A systematic review of drug-induced subacute cutaneous lupus erythematosus. Br J Dermatol. 2011;164(3):465–72.

50. A 28-year-old woman was admitted due to severe head trauma after a motor vehicle accident. Three weeks after admission, there has been no change in her mental status. All vital signs are normal as well as laboratory values.

    She is noted to have spontaneous eye opening and is able to track an object visually at times. She does not speak or follow any commands. She in intubated but is fed through a gastrostomy tube. She moves extremities spontaneously but without purposeful movement.

    What term best describes this patient's condition?

    A) Coma
    B) Locked-in
    C) Minimally conscious state
    D) Persistent vegetative state
    E) Vegetative state

Answer: E

A vegetative state "of wakefulness without awareness" was first described in 1972. In the vegetative state, patients may open their eyelids occasionally and demonstrate sleep-wake cycles, but completely lack cognitive function, communication, or purposeful movement. In addition, extensive neurologic and medical test must be made to rule out treatable causes.

In the minimally conscious state, unlike the vegetative state, there is evidence that patients are aware of themselves and/or their environment.

Traditionally, per informal US guidelines, a vegetative state that lasts greater than 1 month is considered to be a persistent vegetative state. A diagnosis of persistent vegetative state does not absolutely imply permanent disability because in very rare cases patients can improve, reaching a minimally conscious state or a higher level of consciousness.

Reference

Ashwal S. The Multi-Society Task Force On Pvs. Medical aspects of the persistent vegetative state – second of two parts 1994. N Engl J Med. 330(22):1572–9.

51. An 87-year-old female was admitted to the hospital for a heart failure exacerbation. At baseline, she could ambulate, but needed help with some activities of daily living. She has ischemic cardiomyopathy, coronary artery disease, hypertension, and hyperlipidemia. Current medications are furosemide, lisinopril, metoprolol, aspirin, atorvastatin, and heparin given subcutaneously twice daily for deep venous thrombosis prophylaxis.

    Since admission, the patient has expressed her concern about receiving heparin injections. She has had a moderate amount of bruising on her abdomen, which is painful. She has asked her nurse several times if she really needs "those shots," and the nurse has relayed her concerns to you.

    On physical examination, heart rate is 82 beats per minute and blood pressure is 120/65 mmHg. Crackles are still heard a third the way up in both lung fields. Ecchymosis are seen on the abdomen. There is edema (1+) extending to the knees. She can walk slowly but safely with a walker or assistance.

    What is the best treatment?

    A) Continue the heparin, and explain its necessity to the patient.
    B) Stop the heparin, and start enoxaparin daily.
    C) Stop the heparin, and start venous foot pumps.
    D) Start Coumadin.
    E) Stop the heparin and encourage the patient to walk with her family.

Answer: E

The current guidelines recommend that adults older than age 40 who are hospitalized for medical reasons and are expected to be less mobile for 3 days or more be given some form of deep venous thrombosis (DVT) prophylaxis. This is based on several randomized controlled trials.

However, whether these recommendations should apply to older adults is less uncertain. A systematic review and meta-analysis examined the evidence for harm and efficacy of pharmacologic prophylaxis of DVT in older adults. For the most part older adults with comorbidities have been excluded from studies. The majority of events prevented in studies are asymptomatic DVTs. There is no consistent reduction in fatal pulmonary embolism or mortality. When data from the three trials with patients older than age 75 are pooled, a similar reduction in endpoints to other trials is seen. However, two-thirds of these events are asymptomatic DVTs. In the general population, the absolute bleeding risk is generally increased by 2 % in the heparin treatment group. Older age with its comorbidities may increase this risk.

The current data suggest that this patient would gain a very small absolute risk reduction for symptomatic DVTs and an even smaller risk for pulmonary embolism. Given her wishes, it is reasonable to stop heparin and encourage ambulation.

References

Greig MF, Rochow SB, Crilly MA, Mangoni AA. Routine pharmacological venous thromboembolism prophylaxis in frail older hospitalized patients: where is the evidence? Age Ageing. 2013;42:428–34.

Wakefield TW, Proctor MC. Current status of pulmonary embolism and venous thrombosis prophylaxis. Semin Vasc Surg. 2000;13(3):171–81.

52. A 26-year-old female presents with cellulitis of her left forearm. The patient has a history of IV heroin abuse but denies any recent heroin use. Current medications are lorazepam and methadone.

   On presentation, her temperature is 35.8 °C (96.4 °C), respirations are 10 per minute, and blood pressure is 124/72 mmHg. Electrocardiogram reveals wide complex variable focus tachycardia. Toxicology screen is positive for cannabis, alcohol, and opiates.

   Which of the following medications is the most likely cause of this patient's arrhythmia?
   A) Cannabis
   B) Benzodiazepines
   C) Alcohol
   D) Methadone
   E) Oxycodone

Answer: D

Cardiac arrhythmias in methadone users have been reported for several decades. The most serious have been wide complex tachycardias. Risk factors include female sex, hypokalemia, high-dose methadone, drug interactions, underlying cardiac conditions, and unrecognized congenital long Q-T interval syndrome.

In methadone patients, an ECG should be obtained on admission. QT prolongation may predict subsequent malignant arrhythmias and possible need to alter methadone treatment. Methadone has been used to treat heroin addicts for nearly 50 years, but little is known about its long-term side effects.

Reference

Justo D, Gal-Oz A, Paran Y et al. Methadone-associated torsades de pointes (polymorphic ventricular tachycardia) in opioid-dependent patients. Addiction. 2006;101:1333–8.

53. A 38-year-old man is admitted with atypical chest pain of 3 h duration. While waiting to be seen, his pain resolves. He reports that he has been smoking marijuana extensively and denies any other ingestions or substances.

   He reports no past medical history and is not on any meds. He is not sure but may have chest pain prior to this admission.

   On physical exam, his heart rate is 110, temperature is 37 °C (98.6 °F), and blood pressure is 180/90. He is 96 % on room air. He is agitated, tachycardic, and diaphoretic. His electrocardiogram reveals slight ST depressions in leads V3 through V5. Initial troponin level is 0.1 mg/mL. Toxicology screen is pending.

   Initial therapy should include the following:
   A) Tissue plasminogen activator (TPA)
   B) Percutaneous transluminal coronary angioplasty (PTCA)
   C) Aspirin
   D) Abciximab
   E) Metoprolol

Answer: C

This patient is exhibiting a sympathomimetic presentation probably due to crack cocaine ingestion. This should be considered as an additive in someone with a history of smoking marijuana. His possible myocardial ischemia is due to endothelial dysfunction as well as aggregation of platelets. In this particular scenario, there is no evidence of segment elevation myocardial infarction, so PTCA, tPA, and GP IIb/IIIa are not indicated. A reasonable approach would be an aspirin with further cardiovascular workup considered.

Beta-blockers are relatively contraindicated in cocaine-induced chest pain as there is a possible risk of increased peripheral vascular resistance. This has not been well tested.

References

Hobbs WE, Moore EE, Penkala RA, Bolgiano DD, López JA. Cocaine and specific cocaine metabolites induce von Willebrand factor release from endothelial cells in a tissue-specific manner. Arterioscler Thromb Vasc Bio. 2013;33:1230–7.

2014 AHA/ACC Guideline for the Management of Patients With Non-ST-Elevation Acute Coronary Syndromes: A Report of the American College of Cardiology/American Heart Association Task Force on Practice Guidelines. Circulation. 2014;130:e344–e426.

54. A 75-year-old male with Parkinson's disease is admitted for worsening tremor and confusion. On his first night of hospitalization, he is noted to be markedly agitated. Which of the following drugs should not be used for treatment?
    A) Haloperidol
    B) Olanzapine
    C) Risperidone
    D) All of the above

Answer: D

Delirium and psychosis occur in about one-third of patients with Parkinson's disease. There have been no conclusive studies on the best approach in the treatment of delirium in patients with Parkinson's disease.

There is a strong contraindication for haloperidol, olanzapine, and risperidone because of potential exacerbation of extrapyramidal symptoms. There is also a lack of efficacy reported with olanzapine. Other atypical antipsychotics such as quetiapine have been commonly used with caution and slow titration. Most studies suggest that quetiapine is safe in Parkinson's disease. Some reports suggest that there is an increased risk of adverse motor effects in these patients, predominantly in demented subjects.

Reference

David A. Quetiapine in the treatment of psychosis in Parkinson's disease. Ther Adv Neurol Disord. 2010; 3(6):339–50.

55. Which of the following options are appropriate prophylaxis of venous thromboembolism for hospitalized medical patients with a moderate risk of bleeding undergoing dialysis three times per week?
    A) Aspirin
    B) Warfarin to maintain INR between 1.5 and 2.5
    C) Heparin 5000U SQ TID
    D) Lovenox 40 mg SQ daily
    E) Lovenox 30 mg SQ daily

Answer: C

Venous thromboembolism, which includes pulmonary embolism and deep venous thrombosis, continues to be a common clinical problem. The American College of Physicians recommends pharmacologic prophylaxis with heparin or a related drug for venous thromboembolism in medical patients unless the assessed risk for bleeding outweighs the likely benefits. Aspirin and mechanical prophylaxis with graduated compression stockings have been shown to provide inferior coverage in comparison but in some circumstances may be the best option. Heparin 5000U SQ TID is recommended for patients with end-stage renal disease undergoing dialysis. Lovenox is cleared by hemodialysis in an irregular manner and is contraindicated in patients undergoing dialysis.

Reference

Qaseem A, et al. Venous thromboembolism prophylaxis in hospitalized patients: a clinical practice guideline from the American College of Physicians. Ann InternMed. 2011;155(9):625–32.

56. A 66-year-old man with history of diabetes, hypertension, and coronary artery disease is admitted with sepsis. Blood cultures drawn on day 1 started growing enterococci on day 3. He was also diagnosed with an infective endocarditis and was started on gentamicin and aqueous penicillin G.

His labs at the time of admission showed a BUN of 32 mg/dL and serum creatinine of 0.8 mg/dL. He started complaining of worsening shortness of breath on the next day, and a CT angiogram of the chest was obtained and pulmonary embolism was ruled out. His BUN on day 7 was 53 mg/dL with a serum creatinine of 2.8 mg/dL. Urine output dropped to 600 cc in 24 h. His vital signs and urinalysis were normal.

What is the reason for this acute renal failure?
    A) Aminoglycoside toxicity
    B) Drug-induced interstitial nephritis
    C) Acute glomerulonephritis
    D) Diabetic nephropathy
    E) Contrast-induced nephropathy

Answer: E

This patient has developed acute renal failure secondary to contrast-induced nephropathy. Several causes of renal failure are possible. They include interstitial nephritis secondary to penicillin and infective endocarditis. Aminoglycoside toxicity should also be considered.

Normal complement levels (C2,3,4) and rapid onset point toward contrast-induced nephropathy. Aminoglycoside toxicity usually happens 4–5 days after the therapy.

Reference

Murphy SW, Barrett BJ, Parfrey PS. Contrast nephropathy. J Am Soc Nephrol. 2000;11(1):177–82.

57. A 75-year-old female was admitted to the hospital 3 days prior for community-acquired pneumonia. She has a history of hypertension, hyperlipidemia, and peripheral vascular disease. Medications on admission are lisinopril, metoprolol, hydrochlorothiazide, pravastatin, and aspirin. On admission, Zosyn and vancomycin were initiated. She underwent a CT angiogram to rule out pulmonary embolism. She is now afebrile. Her blood pressure is 110/55 mmHg. She has no evidence of orthostasis. Since admission, her respiratory status has improved and her creatinine level has increased from a baseline of 1.5–3.2 mg/dL. Laboratory studies reveal a urine sodium of 44 mEq. Her fractional excretion of sodium is 2 %, and her fractional excretion of urea is 50 %.

Which of the following is the most likely cause of this patient's acute renal injury?
A) Cholesterol emboli
B) Acute interstitial nephritis
C) Prerenal azotemia
D) Normotensive ischemic acute kidney injury
E) Contrast dye-induced kidney injury

Answer: D

This patient has normotensive ischemic kidney injury. The findings of elevated fractional excretion of sodium, fractional excretion of urea, and granular casts seen on urinalysis are all consistent with this diagnosis.

The patient's medical history reveals evidence of an underlying chronic kidney disease possibly due to vascular disease. This places the patient at increased risk for normotensive ischemic injury. The patient's lower blood pressure during hospitalization may be the result of a variety of factors, including infection, better medicine compliance, and the low-salt diet typically seen during a hospitalization.

Acute interstitial nephritis, which is often caused by a hypersensitive reaction to medication, is a possibility. However, the patient's lack of fever, rash, and leukocytes on her urinalysis argues against this diagnosis. Prerenal azotemia is common in the consideration of this patient's differential diagnosis. The patient's fractional excretion of sodium of 2 % and fractional excretion of urea of 50 % argues against this. The fractional excretion of urea is a more sensitive test for patients on diuretics.

Reference

Abuelo JG. Normotensive ischemic acute kidney injury. N Engl J Med. 2007;357(8):797–805.

58. A 72-year-old female was admitted with an ankle fracture. One hour after receiving a dose of morphine, she developed the acute onset of diffuse abdominal pain. She has a history of known cardiovascular disease and hepatitis C. Her current medications are atenolol, aspirin, and lisinopril.

On physical examination, her temperature is 36.7 °C(98.0 °F), blood pressure is 84/60 mmHg. Abdominal examination reveals diffuse abdominal tenderness upon palpation. No guarding or rebound is noted. No ascites is noted.

CT scan reveals small bowel wall thickening and intestinal pneumatosis. Her WBC count is 14,000 μm/l, and an elevated serum lactate is noted. The most likely diagnosis is:
A) Pancreatitis
B) Crohn's disease
C) Acute mesenteric ischemia
D) Spontaneous bacterial peritonitis
E) Infectious ileitis

Answer: C

Acute mesenteric ischemia (AMI) is a syndrome caused by inadequate blood flow through the mesenteric vessels from a combination of preexisting vascular disease, emboli, and hypotension. This results in ischemia and eventual gangrene of the bowel wall. It is a potentially life-threatening condition. This patient's drop in blood pressure due to morphine triggered the ischemic event.

AMI may be classified as either arterial or venous. CT scan and laboratory values in this case are consistent with an acute event. CT scan may reveal bowel wall thickening or, in some instances, intestinal pneumatosis as in this case. Treatment options for acute thrombosis can be surgical, stenting, or thrombolytics. Early and aggressive diagnostic imaging and early surgical consultation are warranted. Angiography is the test of choice for both diagnosis and possible therapeutic vasodilation and stenting.

Because of the high mortality and the difficulty of diagnosis, mesenteric ischemia has traditionally been considered a diagnostic challenge.

Reference

Boley SJ, Brandt LJ, Sammartano RJ. History of mesenteric ischemia. The evolution of a diagnosis and management. Surg Clin North Am. 1997 Apr. 77(2):275–88.

59. A 91-year-old African American female was admitted from her nursing home for altered mental status and foul-smelling urine.

UA is positive with 3+ leukocytes and many bacteria. The admitting physician empirically started moxifloxacin 400 mg IV daily. You are assuming care the following day. Her vital signs are stable, and she seems in no distress.

What would be the next best step?

A) Continue current regimen.
B) Discontinue moxifloxacin and start ceftriaxone.
C) Continue moxifloxacin but change to PO.
D) None of the above.

Answer: B

Moxifloxacin is a quinolone antibiotic that does not achieve adequate concentration in the urine, thereby eliminating its use in the treatment of urinary tract infections. It does not matter whether moxifloxacin is given either oral or IV – the bioavailability of the oral is 100 % and the IV formulation has no ability to concentrate in urine.

Reference

Gupta K, Hooton TM, Naber KG et al. International clinical practice guidelines for the treatment of acute uncomplicated cystitis pyelonephritis in women: a 2010 Update by the Infectious Disease Society of America and the European Society of Microbiology and Infectious Disease. Clin Inf Dis. 2011;52:e103–20.

60. You are called in consultation to see a 35-year-old male who was in a motor vehicle accident and underwent surgical repair of a right femur fracture. Postoperatively, the patient has received acetaminophen and scheduled doses of oral morphine. He has become acutely agitated and is oriented only to person. The only admission labs were a complete blood count and a basic metabolic panel, which are normal. His past medical history is not known.

On physical examination, his temperature is 39.0 °C (102.1°), pulse rate is 110 beats per minute, and respirations are 18 per minute. Blood pressure is 180/90 mmHg. The lungs are clear upon auscultation. There are no signs of infection noted. The patient seems agitated with a mild tremor. He is diaphoretic.

Which of the following is the most likely diagnosis?

A) Drug-induced delirium from morphine
B) Fat emboli
C) Alcohol withdrawal
D) Pneumonia
E) Deep wound infection

Answer: C

Alcohol use disorders are common and can complicate postoperative recovery. In this particular case, the fever, tachycardia, hypertension, and tremor are suggestive of alcohol withdrawal. The alcohol level in trauma patients should be checked on admission, as withdrawal is a common source of delirium in this population.

About 9 % of US adults meet the criteria for an alcohol use disorder. Less than 50 % of alcohol-dependent persons

develop any significant withdrawal symptoms that require pharmacologic treatment upon cessation of alcohol intake. Minor withdrawal occurs within 6–24 h following the patient's last drink and is characterized by tremor, anxiety, nausea, vomiting, and insomnia. Major withdrawal occurs 10–72 h after the last drink. The signs and symptoms include visual and auditory hallucinations, whole body tremor, vomiting, diaphoresis, and hypertension.

The most objective and best-validated tool to assess the severity of alcohol withdrawal is the Clinical Institute Withdrawal Assessment for Alcohol.

Reference

Mayo-Smith MF, Beecher LH, Fischer TL, et al. Management of alcohol withdrawal delirium. An evidence-based practice guideline. Arch Intern Med. 2004 Jul 12. 164(13): 1405–12.

61. A 57-year-old man is admitted for recent onset of fatigue and weakness. He has been seen twice in the past 2 months as an outpatient for similar symptoms with no diagnoses made. The family states that he is currently unable to take care of himself. The patient further reports nocturia, polyuria, and weight loss over the past 3 months. He has COPD and a 58-pack-year smoking history.

On physical examination, the temperature is 36.4 °C (97.5 °F), blood pressure is 178/97 mmHg, pulse rate is 86/min, and respiration rate is 24/min. Proximal muscle weakness is noted in the upper and lower extremities. Hyperpigmented mucous membranes are noted.

Laboratory studies are as follows: creatinine is 1.4 mg/dL, sodium is 149 mEq/L, glucose is 273, urine cortisol is 472ug per 24 h, and ACTH is 257 pg/ml.

Chest radiographs show hyperinflated lung fields but no masses.

Which of the following is the most likely cause of this patient's findings?

A) Adrenal adenoma
B) Adrenal carcinoma
C) Ectopic ACTH secretion
D) Pituitary adenoma
E) New onset diabetes

Answer: C

This patient has Cushing syndrome due to excessive ACTH production. This is almost certainly due to underlying malignancy such as lung cancer which is the case here. Approximately half of all cases of ectopic ACTH secretion are due to small cell lung cancer, which has a long list of paraneoplastic syndromes associated with it.

Adrenal adenomas can be associated with hypercortisolism, but the features tend to cause a mild Cushing syndrome.

Adrenal adenomas are associated with suppressed ACTH levels. Hyperpigmentation suggests excessive ACTH production.

A chest radiograph does not rule out the possibility of a lung malignancy and computed topography of the chest is needed.

Reference

Iias I, Torpy DJ, Pacak K, Mullen N, Wesley RA, Nieman LK. Cushing's syndrome due to ectopic corticotropin secretion: twenty years' experience at the National Institutes of Health. J Clin Endocrinol Metab. 2005;90(8):4955–62.

62. A 67-year-old female is admitted to the hospital service with an unexpected syncopal episode. There are no factors to suggest a vasovagal episode. She reports worsening shortness of breath with exertion over the past 3 months. Otherwise, she has enjoyed good health.

    Physical exam is pertinent for a 3/6 systolic crescendo-decrescendo murmur at the left sternal border with radiation to the carotids. You suspect aortic stenosis as the cause of the syncope and order a 2D cardiac echo with color flow Doppler. Results of the 2D echo indicate aortic stenosis.

    Which of the following are indications to refer your patient for evaluation for aortic valve replacement?
    A) Exertional dyspnea
    B) Aortic valve mean pressure gradient of 40 mmHg or higher
    C) Aortic stenosis in the setting of LVEF less than 50 %
    D) All of the above
    E) A and B

Answer: D

Aortic valve replacement is recommended for symptomatic patients with severe aortic stenosis. Severe aortic stenosis is defined as an aortic velocity 4.0 m per second or greater or by a mean pressure gradient 40 mmHg or higher. Symptoms of heart failure, syncope, exertional dyspnea, angina, or presyncope by history or on exercise testing are also indications.

Reference

Nishimura R, et al. 2014 AHA/ACC guidelines for the Management of patients with Valvular Heart Disease. A Report of the American College of Cardiology/American Heart Association Task Force on Practice Guidelines. J Am Coll Cardiol. 2014;63:57–185.

63. A 71-year-old woman is admitted from a nursing home with confusion, fever, and flank pain. She has a presumed urinary tract infection.

    On physical exam, temperature is 38.8 °C (101.8 °F), blood pressure is 86/50 mmHg, pulse rate is 125/min, and respiration rate is 24/min. Mucous membranes are dry, and there is costovertebral angle tenderness, poor skin turgor, and no edema.

    Hemoglobin concentration is 10.5 g/dL, leukocyte count is 15,600/μL, and urinalysis reveals 50–75 leukocytes/hpf and many bacteria/hpf. The patient has an increase anion gap metabolic acidosis. The patient is admitted to the intensive care unit and antibiotic therapy is started.

    Which of the following in the next goal of therapy?
    A) Aggressive fluid resuscitation
    B) Hemodynamic monitoring with a pulmonary artery catheter
    C) Maintaining hemoglobin concentration above 12 g/dL (120 g/L)
    D) Maintaining PCO_2 below 50 mmHg
    E) Vasopressor therapy

Answer: A

The patient has severe sepsis from pyelonephritis. Aggressive fluid resuscitation is indicated. Resolution of lactic acidosis within 6 h will have a beneficial effect on this patient's survival. Resuscitation of the circulation should target a central venous oxygen saturation or mixed venous oxygen saturation of at least 70 %. Other goals include a central venous pressure of 8–12 mmHg, a mean arterial pressure of at least 65 mmHg, and a urine output of at least 0.5 mL/kg/h.

Fluid requirements are often as much as 5–6 L of fluid. Early goal-directed therapy sees the most benefits within the first 6 h. End points that improve survival include maintaining a $SCVO_2$ of greater than 70 % and resolution of lactic acidosis.

Blood transfusion may be part of resuscitation for anemic patients in shock. In stable patients who have not had major blood loss or further blood loss is anticipated, a transfusion threshold of 7 g/dL is an acceptable approach. There are no data to support that maintaining a lower PCO_2 is of any benefit. In addition placement of a pulmonary artery catheter would help to increase survival in this patient.

Reference

Rivers E, Nguyen B, Havstad S, Ressler J, et al. Early goal-directed therapy in the treatment of severe sepsis and septic shock. N Engl J Med. 2001;345(19):1368–77.

64. A 52-year-old woman is admitted for a syncopal event while having her blood drawn. She has no past medical history and takes no medications. She experiences a brief loss of consciousness for about 20 s. She had no seizure-like activity and immediately returns to her usual level of functioning. You diagnose her with vasovagal syncope, and discharge the next day with no follow-up testing.

Which of the following statements regarding neurally mediated syncope is TRUE?

A) Neurally mediated syncope occurs when there are abnormalities of the autonomic nervous system.
B) Myoclonus does not occur during neurally mediated syncope.
C) The final pathway of neurally mediated syncope results in a surge of the sympathetic nervous system with inhibition of the parasympathetic nervous system.
D) The usual finding with cardiovascular monitoring is hypotension and tachycardia.
E) The primary therapy for neurally mediated syncope is reassurance, avoidance of triggers, and plasma volume expansion.

Answer: E

Syncope accounts for 3 % of all emergency department visits and 1 % of all hospitalizations. Additionally, it is estimated that 35 % of all individuals will experience at least one syncopal event in their lifetime. Currently, no specific testing has sufficient power to be recommended for evaluation of syncope.

Syncope occurs when blood flow to the brain suddenly drops. Vasovagal syncope is one category without a clearly defined mechanism but can occur with intense emotions, strong odors, or orthostatic factors. Neurally mediated syncope can be brought about by specific mechanical events such as cough, micturition, swallowing, or carotid sensitivity. Reassurance and avoidance of triggers are the primary treatments. Liberal intake of fluids and salt and prevention of dehydration are protective against all forms of syncopal events.

In randomized controlled trials, isometric counterpressure maneuvers are also protective. In patients with refractory syncope, fludrocortisone, beta-blockers, and other vasoconstricting agents have been used with limited success. However, there are no clinical trial data to support their use.

References

Moya A, Sutton R, Ammirati F, et al. Guidelines for the diagnosis and management of syncope (version 2009): the Task Force for the Diagnosis and Management of Syncope of the European Society of Cardiology (ESC). Eur Heart J. 2009;30(21):2631–71.

Tan MP, Parry SW. Vasovagal syncope in the older patient. J Am Coll Cardiol. 2008;51(6):599–606.

65. A 56-year-old woman who is listed for liver transplantation due to hepatitis C and portal hypertension is admitted for worsening ascites. She has had required one uncomplicated, large-volume paracentesis during the past 5 months. Her current medications are furosemide 40 mg daily and spironolactone 100 mg daily. She adheres to a daily diet containing less than 2000 mg of sodium and 2 L of free water.

On physical exam, her blood pressure is 115/78 mmHg. She has mild muscle wasting. A prominent second heart sound is noted on cardiac auscultation. The abdomen is protuberant with moderate ascites. No tenderness is noted. No lower extremity edema is evident, and the patient exhibits no confusion or asterixis.

Her sodium is 132 mmol/L, creatinine is 1.4 mg/dl.

Which of the following is the correct approach to treat this patients worsening ascites?

A) Adjust fluid restriction to 1.5 L daily
B) Antibiotics for possible bacterial peritonitis
C) Continue serial paracenteses with albumin infusions
D) Refer for transjugular intrahepatic portosystemic shunt
E) Increase furosemide and spironolactone

Answer: E

It would be reasonable to try an increased diuretic dose in this patient. The recommended initial regimen is furosemide 40 mg plus spironolactone 100 mg daily. This patient is not at the maximum diuretic dose. Diuretics can be increased every 3–5 days, while maintaining the 40:100 mg ratio. In ascites due to end-stage liver disease, the maximum dose for furosemide is 160 mg daily and for spironolactone it is 400 mg daily. At the higher doses, decreasing efficacy will be seen. As the total diuretic dose is increased, it can be given once daily or divided as twice daily dosing.

Serum electrolytes and renal function tests should be carefully monitored as dose adjustments are made. The patient should discontinue diuretic therapy if the serum sodium decreases to less than 120 mmol/L, uncontrolled or recurrent encephalopathy develops, or the serum creatinine exceeds 2.0 mg/dL.

Reference

Runyon BA, AASLD Practice Guidelines Committee. Management of adult patients with ascites due to cirrhosis: an update. Hepatology. 2009;49:2087–107.

66. A 76-year-old female is admitted for respiratory failure. She has a history of prior dementia. On her previous admissions, she has had episodes of delirium, which have resulted in prolonged hospitalization. On admission she is on no sedatives or antipsychotic meds. The family is concerned about the possibility of hospital-induced delirium and would like efforts be made to prevent this.

In an effort to reduce the incidence of delirium in this patient, which of the following should you undertake?

A) Nighttime use of melatonin
B) Mobilizing patient to the chair early
C) Prophylactic use of rivastigmine
D) Maintaining lights on for visual stimulation

Answer: B

Delirium is a common problem in the hospitalized patient, especially with a history of underlying dementia or psychiatric disease. So far, only simple interventions focused on maintaining normal environmental issues have been proven to be of any benefit. These include promoting sleep by decreasing nighttime stimuli, use of hearing aids and eyeglasses, and minimizing restraints. One study showed a reduction of sound during the night by using earplugs in patients in the ICU setting resulted in a decreased risk of delirium by 53 %.

Family can play a role in decreasing delirium. They can assist in orienting and reassuring the patient. Support from a familiar nurse and staff should also be encouraged.

There are no definitive studies that demonstrate the use of any prophylactic medicines, such as haloperidol or risperidone, provides any benefit. The use of these and other sedatives should be minimized. Pain can contribute to delirium as well as the excessive use of narcotics. Rivastigmine has been shown to worsen delirium in the hospitalized patient. Melatonin has had no clear clinical benefit in reduction of delirium. Early physical and occupational therapy may also be of some benefit.

Reference

Inouye SK, Bogardus ST, Charpentier PA, et al. A multicomponent intervention to prevent delirium in hospitalized older patients. N Engl J Med. 4 1999;340(9):669–76

67. A 62-year-old male has been admitted for diabetic foot ulcer and associated cellulitis for the past 4 weeks. He has chronic diabetic kidney disease, hypertension, and type 1 diabetes mellitus. Medications are metformin, insulin, and lisinopril.

   He is started on vancomycin and ciprofloxacin.

   On physical examination, blood pressure is 145/90 mmHg. An area of erythema extends about 3 cm around a 3×3 cm ulcer on the right great toe. The area involved is tender warm and fluctuant.

   Laboratory studies reveal an albumin of 2.9 g/dL, and a serum creatinine of 4.1 mg/dL. For acute renal failure, complement levels are checked and they are low. Urine studies show a urine sodium of 15 mEq/L. Urinalysis reveals 25 erythrocytes per HPF and 1–2 erythrocyte casts.

Which of the following is the most likely cause of this patient's acute kidney injury?

A) Diabetic nephropathy
B) IgA nephropathy
C) Post-infectious glomerulonephritis
D) Membranous glomerulonephritis
E) Drug-induced acute renal failure

Answer: C

This patient has post-infectious glomerulonephritis (PIGN). PIGN presents as an acute nephritic syndrome characterized by rapid onset of edema, hypertension, oliguria, and erythrocyte casts seen in the urine sediment. Low complement levels further suggest the exudative proliferative glomerulonephritis patterns can be seen by light microscopy on biopsy specimens.

Diabetic nephropathy does not explain the onset of this patient's acute kidney injury. The decline of the glomerular filtration is predictable and usually no greater than 12–16 mL/min/1.73 m^2 per year. Patients with IgA nephropathy may present with an episode of acute renal injury precipitated by infection. Gross hematuria is often seen. Adult patients with primary membranous glomerulonephritis frequently present with a nephritic picture. In these patients, the urine sediment can be active and reveal granular casts. Erythrocyte casts are not seen. In addition, complement levels are normal.

It has been suggested that PIGN was the cause of death of the composer Wolfgang Amadeus Mozart.

References

Rodriguez-Iturbe B, Musser JM. The current state of post streptococcal glomerulonephritis. J Am Soc Nephrol. 2008;19(10):1855–64.

Zegers RH, Weigl A. Steptoe A death of Wolfgang Amadeus Mozart: an epidemiologic perspective. Ann Intern Med. 2009;151(4):274–8, W96-7 (ISSN: 1539–3704).

68. A 60-year-old male with end-stage liver disease was admitted for shortness of breath. He reports progressive ascites over the past few weeks and a low-grade temperature.

   On physical exam, his lungs are clear upon auscultation. The abdomen is tender and distended. Oxygenation is 84 % by pulse oximetry, which improves slightly to 87 % with 5 l of oxygen. Chest X-ray reveals lung fields without infiltrate or pleural effusions. Computed tomography reveals no evidence of pulmonary embolism.

   Paracentesis is performed which reveals a white blood cell count of 1,500 WBCs, of which 58 are neutrophils. The patient is started on antibiotics. Two days later, the patient continues with shortness of breath and marked hypoxia. Pulse oximetry is 93 % when supine but decreases to 84 % when sitting.

Which of the following studies is most likely to confirm patient's cause of hypoxia?

A) Ventilation perfusion scan of the lungs
B) High contrast CT scan of the chest
C) Pulmonary arteriography
D) Lung biopsies
E) Echocardiography with saline bubble contrast

Answer: E

This patient has hepatopulmonary syndrome. In these cases, contrast- or bubble-enhanced echocardiography will reveal a intrapulmonary shunt. Hepatopulmonary syndrome is associated with platypnea, which is increased dyspnea in the upright position, and orthodeoxia, which is increased hypoxia when transitioning from the lying to the standing position. Hypoxemia, in this case due to intrapulmonary shunt, is not significantly affected by an increase in inhaled O_2 concentration. This syndrome may resolve with liver transplantation and does not exclude the patient from being considered for transplant.

Reference
Rodriguez-Roisin R, Krowka MJ. Hepatopulmonary syndrome – a liver-induced lung vascular disorder. N Engl J Med. 2008;358:2378–87.

69. You have just admitted a 28-year-old man with a witnessed seizure. He has a prior history of seizure disorder. The event was witnessed by family members. His family describes movement of his right hand that spread to involve the entire arm. He did not lose consciousness.

On physical examination, sensation is intact in the affected limb, but his strength is 0 out of 5 in the musculature of the right hand. . His electrolytes and complete blood count are within normal limits. A toxicology screen is normal. A noncontrast CT scan of his head is unremarkable.

What is the best course of action at this time?

A) Cerebral angiogram
B) Magnetic resonance angiogram
C) Reassess in a few hours
D) Psychiatric evaluation
E) Lumbar puncture

Answer: C

The patient has Todd's paralysis, which may take minutes to many hours to return to normal. The abnormal motor movements that begin in a restricted area and then progress to involve a larger area are termed Jacksonian march. If his symptoms were to persist beyond several hours, it would be reasonable to investigate a different etiology of his hand weakness with imaging studies. The symptoms are too lim-

ited to suggest conversion disorder. Magnetic resonance angiogram or cerebral angiogram may be useful to evaluate for cerebrovascular disorders, if symptoms persist.

Reference
Gallmetzer P, Leutmezer F, Serles W, Assem-Hilger E, Spatt J, Baumgartner C. Postictal paresis in focal epilepsies–incidence, duration, and causes: a video-EEG monitoring study. Neurology. 2004;62(12):2160–4.

70. A 22-year-old woman is admitted with fatigue of 1 week's duration. She reports that she had a febrile illness 3 weeks ago, during which she experienced a transient rash and joint pain. She was treated for a possible urinary tract infection with ciprofloxacin. She works in a day care facility, where there has been an outbreak of a febrile illness with a rash during the past few weeks. The patient has a history of hereditary spherocytosis. On physical examination, she is pale, somewhat lethargic, but otherwise there are no significant findings.

Her laboratory tests show a hematocrit of 22 %, the reticulocyte count is 0.5 %.

Which of the following is the most likely diagnosis for this patient?

A) Acute leukemia
B) Glucose-6-phosphate dehydrogenase (G6PD) deficiency
C) Systemic lupus erythematosus
D) Hereditary spherocytosis in hemolytic crisis
E) Aplastic crisis caused by parvovirus B19

Answer: E

This patient has a parvovirus B19 infection. This is the virus that causes the common childhood disease known as erythema infectiosum or fifth disease. It can cause aplastic crises in persons with hemolytic disorders, chronic anemia in immunocompromised hosts, and fetal loss in pregnant women.

The rash of erythema infectiosum usually appears without prodromal symptoms after an incubation period of 4–14 days. The rash starts as a fiery-red rash on both cheeks. It then extends as an erythematous maculopapular eruption on the proximal extremities and trunk in a reticular pattern. The rash may wax and wane for several weeks. Arthralgia and arthritis are seen in up to 80 % of infected adults.

Parvovirus B19 can cause an aplastic crises in patients who have sickle cell anemia, hereditary spherocytosis, thalassemia, and various other hemolytic anemias. These aplastic crises are abrupt in onset and are associated with giant pronormoblasts in the bone marrow. They generally resolve spontaneously after 1 or 2 weeks. In immunocompromised patients, acute infection may lead to viral persistence and chronic bone marrow suppression. In this patient, the anemia with a low reticulocyte count suggests a transient aplastic process and not a hemolytic crisis.

Reference

Servey JT, Reamy BV, Hodge J. Clinical presentations of parvovirus B19 infection. Am Fam Physician. 2007;75(3):373–6.

71. A 55-year-old woman is admitted with epigastric abdominal pain. Initial clinical exam and laboratory findings are consistent with acute pancreatitis. She is admitted for aggressive hydration and observation. Lipase and amylase have decreased. Four days later she is doing better but pain and nausea still persist. A CT scan with contrast reveals necrotizing pancreatitis. The patient is hemodynamically stable, afebrile, with WBC of 11,000.

      What should be done next?
   A) CT-guided aspiration for culture and gram stain
   B) Repeat CT scan in 48 h
   C) Immediate initiation of broad-spectrum antibiotics
   D) Referral to general surgery for immediate debridement
   E) Continued observation and hydration

Answer: E

The current recommendations do not support the use of prophylactic antibiotics to prevent pancreatic infection among patients with necrotizing pancreatitis. Some studies suggest that the use of potent antibiotics may lead to a superimposed fungal infection. The current guidelines recommend medical management during the first 2–3 weeks. After 3 weeks, if symptoms persist or clinical condition deteriorates, a surgical debridement should be considered. If symptoms worsen or fail to improve, repeat imaging or biopsy can be considered.

References

Telem DA, Bowman K, Hwang J, Chin EH, Nguyen SQ, Divino CM. Selective management of patients with acute biliary pancreatitis. J Gastrointest Surg. 2009;13(12):2183–8.

Tenner S, Baillie J, Dewitt J, et al. American College of Gastroenterology guidelines: management of acute pancreatitis. Am J Gastroenterol. 2013;108(9):1400–15.

72. You are asked to admit a 49-year-old female with the acute onset of fever and severe headache. Her past medical history is significant for renal transplant due to diabetes mellitus type 1. While in the emergency room, she develops chills, photophobia, and stiffness of her neck.

      On physical exam, temperature is 38.6 °C (101.2 °F), heart rate is 90, and blood pressure is 120/68 mmHg

      You have significant concern for meningitis.

Which of the following is NOT an appropriate next step in the patient's management?
   A) Draw stat blood cultures while placing the orders for empiric antibiotics.
   B) Perform stat lumbar puncture while waiting for MRI.
   C) Check CT scan of brain without contrast before lumbar puncture.
   D) Give dexamethasone with first dose of antibiotics.
   E) A than D

Answer: E

It is important to recognize the treatment sequence in the management of suspected bacterial meningitis. Imaging and lumbar puncture should not delay empiric antibiotic coverage and steroids. The necessity of a CT scan prior to a lumbar puncture in all instances has been debated. The management algorithm for adults with suspected bacterial meningitis per Infectious Disease Society of America (IDSA) guidelines is as follows:

1. Blood cultures STAT.
2. Begin dexamethasone + empiric antimicrobial therapy.
3. Check CT scan of the head before performing lumbar puncture.

Reference

Tunkel AR, Hartman BJ, Kaplan SL, Kaufman BA, Roos KL, Scheld WM, Whitley RJ. Practice Guidelines for the management of bacterial meningitis. IDSA. Clin Infect Dis. 2004;39:1267–84.

73. A 68-year-old female with metastatic breast cancer involving the lungs is admitted for increasing agitation. She has been enrolled in home hospice for the past 4 weeks. She has diffuse back pain, which is moderately well controlled with transdermal fentanyl and oral hydromorphone.

      On physical exam, the patient is frail and cachectic. Tachycardia is noted. She is neurologically intact as well as alert and oriented. Her daughter tells you that she produces a small amount of concentrated urine a few times daily and that she eats occasional small meals but is often nauseated. Her daughter notes that she becomes agitated just before dawn if she is still awake. The daughter would like to take the patient home if the behavior can be controlled.

      Which of the following should you do to decrease this patient's agitation?
   A) Prescribe lorazepam on an as-needed basis.
   B) Prescribe zolpidem at bedtime.
   C) Prescribe an evening dose of quetiapine.
   D) Request that the hospice social worker meets with the patient to address her fears and worries.
   E) Admit to inpatient hospice.

Answer: C

Quetiapine can be used for agitation in critically ill patients. In a prospective, randomized, double-blind, placebo-controlled study conducted on 36 adult critically ill patients with delirium, quetiapine in escalating doses was shown to be effective in palliating agitation.

The use of lorazepam may worsen her agitation in her medically fragile state. The use of zolpidem will address this patient's disrupted sleep but may increase her agitation. Supporting the family with rapid control of behavior issues is needed. While inclusion of psychosocial support is helpful, this patient is rapidly declining and medication can provide immediate benefit.

References

Devlin JW, Roberts RJ, Fong JJ, et al. Efficacy and safety of quetiapine in critically ill patients with delirium: a prospective, multicenter, randomized, double-blind, placebo-controlled pilot study. Crit Care Med. 2010;38(2):419–27.

Larson AM, Polson J, Fontana RJ, Davern TJ, Lalani E, Hynan LS, Reisch JS, Schiødt FV, Ostapowicz G, Shakil AO, Lee WM, Acute Liver Failure Study Group. Acetaminophen-induced acute liver failure: results of a United States multicenter, prospective study. Hepatology. 2005;42(6):1364–72.

74. A 34-year-old female is admitted with a 2-day history of right eye redness and pain, photophobia, and decreased visual acuity. She has a 2-year history of recurrent oral ulcerations and tender nodules on her shins. She has had mild rotating joint tenderness for the past 4 months. Her only medication is ibuprofen. She has been treated for genital herpes in the past.

    On physical examination, the temperature is 37.4 °C (99.3 °F), blood pressure is 130/80 mmHg, pulse rate is 110/min, and respiration rate is 16/min. Oral ulcerations are noted on the inner cheek, palate, and tongue. The lungs are clear. The abdomen is nontender. No bruits are noted. The right knee and right ankle are swollen. Peripheral pulses are normal. An ophthalmology consultation reveals anterior and posterior uveitis.

    Complete blood count and the basic metabolic panel and INR are within normal limits. Chest X-ray reveals a prominent right pulmonary artery. CT of the chest demonstrates an aneurysm of the right pulmonary artery.

    Which of the following is the most likely diagnosis?
    A) Behçet disease
    B) Granulomatosis with polyangiitis
    C) Polyarteritis nodosa
    D) Gonococcal arthritis
    E) Reiter's syndrome

Answer: A

This patient has Behçet disease. Behçet disease is characterized by the triad of recurrent oral aphthous ulcers, genital ulcers, and uveitis.

Behçet disease is a systemic disorder characterized by vasculitis and multiple organ involvement. The diagnostic clues are intermittent mucous membrane ulcerations and ocular involvement. Gastrointestinal, pulmonary, musculoskeletal, and neurologic manifestations may be present. This patient has a 2-year history of recurrent oral ulcerations. The skin lesions are erythema nodosum. She now presents with panuveitis. Pulmonary artery aneurysm also strongly suggests Behçet disease.

Exposure to an infectious agent may trigger a cross-reactive immune response. Proposed infectious agents have included herpes simplex virus, *Streptococcus* species, *Staphylococcus* species, and *Escherichia coli*. There may be relationship to flora of the mouth.

The treatment approach depends on the severity of the disease and major organ involvement. This may include systemic corticosteroids, azathioprine, pentoxifylline, dapsone, interferon-alfa, colchicine, and thalidomide.

References

Hatemi G, Silman A, Bang D, et al. EULAR recommendations for the management of Behçet disease. Ann Rheum Dis. 2008;67(12):1656–62.

Study Group for Behçet's Disease. Criteria for diagnosis of Behçet's disease. International Study Group for Behçet's Disease. Lancet. 1990;335(8697):1078–80.

75. A 58-year-old female is admitted for nausea, vomiting, and a diffuse rash. Four days before admission, she was bitten on her hand by her neighbor's dog. The patient reports no other symptoms. Ten years ago, she underwent splenectomy following a motor vehicle collision. On physical exam, temperature is 36.8 °C (98.2 °F), pulse rate is 90 per minute, respirations are 16 per minute, and blood pressure is 120/76 mmHg. The patient appears alert and cooperative. The neck is supple. The lungs are clear. Two deep lesions are noted on the dorsum of the left hand. Faint purple, macular lesions are seen on the trunk and extremities. The lesions are not compressible, painful, or pruritic.

    The leukocyte count is 17,000/μL with 15 % band forms. Despite rapid administration of intravenous fluids, vancomycin, piperacillin/tazobactam, and clindamycin, the patient's blood pressure drops and is transferred to the ICU for vasopressor support.

    Which of the following organisms is the most likely cause of the findings in this patient?
    A) *Pasteurella multocida*
    B) *Neisseria meningitidis*
    C) *Streptococcus pneumoniae*
    D) *Capnocytophaga canimorsus*

Answer: D

This patient has disseminated *C. canimorsus* infection due to a dog bite and asplenia. *C. canimorsus* is a normal colonizing bacterium of dog and cat saliva. Canimorsus is Latin for "dog bite."

Clinical symptoms usually begin 5–6 days after the dog bite, scratch, or other exposure. Patients typically present with signs of sepsis including fever, vomiting, and abdominal pain. There is progressive cutaneous hemorrhage with infarction that leads to extensive skin necrosis.

Several other organisms can produce purpura fulminans including endotoxin-producing *Neisseria meningitidis* and encapsulated *Streptococcus pneumoniae* and *Haemophilus influenzae*.

References

Pers C, Gahrn-Hansen B, Frederiksen W. Capnocytophaga canimorsus septicemia in Denmark, 1982–1995: review of 39 cases. Clin Infect Dis. 1996;23(1):71–5.

Eefting M, Paardenkooper T. Capnocytophaga canimorsus sepsis. Blood. 2010;116(9):1396.

76. A 28-year-old male is admitted with acute agitation. He was brought to the hospital by emergency medical services, which was called by his neighbor. He was found on the roof of his house. Little is known of his past medical history.

    On physical exam, he is actively hallucinating, diaphoretic, and is nonresponsive to painful stimuli. In addition to emergency room staff, he requires four security guards to restrain. Drug screen is negative. Computed tomography of his head is not possible due to agitation. Over the course of next 2 days, he requires large doses of benzodiazepines and haloperidol for management and sedation. In addition he requires physical restraints. He gradually returns to his usual functional status in 5 days with little recollection of the event.

    The most likely ingested substance was:
    A) Synthetic cathinones "bath salts"
    B) Hallucinogenic mushrooms
    C) Heroin
    D) Cocaine
    E) Ecstasy

Answer: A

Synthetic cathinones, drugs known as "bath salts," were first described in the United States in 2010. Users of bath salts experience vivid disturbing hallucinations, agitation, paranoia, and extreme pain intolerance. They are more potent as compared to other hallucinogens. Episodes of intoxication are unpredictable and are often prolonged lasting several days. Large dose of sedatives are often required as well as careful use of physical restraints. Decreased pain sensation makes physical restraint difficult and reports of injury during sedation are common.

Reference

Coppola M, Mondola R. Synthetic cathinones: Chemistry, pharmacology and toxicology of a new class of designer drugs of abuse marketed as "bath salts" or "plant food". Toxicol Lett. 2012;211(2):144–9. doi:10.1016/j.toxlet.2012.03.009. PMID 22459606.

77. A 22-year-old male college student is admitted for having a witnessed generalized tonic-clonic seizure. This occurred in the morning as witnessed by his roommate.

    The patient reports that he was out late the night before and drank more than usual over the course of the evening. He reports having sudden jerks of his arms this morning before the generalized seizure was witnessed. He has had similar muscular jerks in the previous mornings. This has particularly occurred on days when he has little sleep. He reports no history of excessive alcohol use or illicit substance abuse. He takes no medications.

    Neurologic examination is normal. He is oriented and feeling well the day after admission.

    Results of laboratory studies are normal. A CT scan of the head shows no abnormalities.

    Which of the following is the most likely diagnosis?
    A) Alcohol withdrawal seizure
    B) Benign rolandic epilepsy
    C) Illicit drug-induced seizure
    D) Temporal lobe epilepsy
    E) Juvenile myoclonic epilepsy

Answer: E

This patient has juvenile myoclonic epilepsy. A history of rapid, unprovoked jerks and generalized tonic-clonic seizures on awakening is a common presentation. Onset is usually in adolescence, but may occur in an early adulthood.

Juvenile myoclonic epilepsy may affect 5–10 % of all patients with epilepsy. Seizures are often provoked by sleep deprivation, alcohol, video games, or exposure to flickering lights.

Recognizing the specific epilepsy syndrome affecting a patient is important in selecting the appropriate therapy.

Alcohol withdrawal seizures develop in chronic users of alcohol. It is generally seen in combination with other signs and symptoms of alcohol withdrawal, such as delirium, tremor, tachycardia, and diaphoresis.

Benign rolandic epilepsy is a syndrome seen in younger children who have seizures, usually during sleep. Temporal lobe epilepsy is the most common of the localization-related epilepsies. This often is due to a specific brain malformation, such as trauma, infarct, or congenital. The most common seizure occurring with temporal lobe epilepsy is complex partial seizure. Patients with complex partial seizures are awake but exhibit altered awareness, such as unresponsiveness or staring.

References

Prasad A, Kuzniecky RI, Knowlton RC, et al. Evolving anti-epileptic drug treatment in juvenile myoclonic epilepsy. Arch Neurol. 2003;60(8):1100–5

Proposal for revised classification of epilepsies and epileptic syndromes. Commission on Classification and Terminology of the International League Against Epilepsy. Epilepsia. 1989;30(4):389–99.

78. A 38-year-old female is admitted to the hospital for a 2-day history of fever and abdominal pain. Her medical history is notable for cirrhosis due to chronic hepatitis C, esophageal varices, and ascites. Her medications are furosemide, spironolactone, nadolol, and lactulose.

    On physical examination, the temperature is 36.5 °C (97.7 °F), blood pressure is 110/60 mmHg, pulse rate is 90/min, and respiration rate is 20/min. Abdominal examination discloses distention. The abdomen is mildly tender upon palpation.

    Laboratory studies show hemoglobin of 9 g/dL, leukocyte count 3,700/µL platelet count 82,000/µL, INR 1.6, albumin 2.3 g/dL, alkaline phosphatase 162 units/L, alanine aminotransferase 27 units/L, aspartate aminotransferase 32 units/L, total bilirubin 3.8 mg/dL, and creatinine 2.4 mg/dL. Abdominal ultrasound reveals cirrhosis, splenomegaly, and ascites. Diagnostic paracentesis discloses a cell count of 1,700/µL with 20 % neutrophils, a total protein level of 1.2 g/dL, and an albumin level of 0.7 g/dL.

    Which of the following is the most appropriate treatment?

    A) Cefotaxime
    B) Cefotaxime and albumin
    C) Furosemide and spironolactone
    D) Large-volume paracentesis
    E) Vancomycin and cefotaxime
    F) Ciprofloxacin

Answer: B

This patient has spontaneous bacterial peritonitis and acute kidney injury . The diagnosis of spontaneous bacterial peritonitis (SBP) is made in the setting of an elevated ascitic fluid absolute polymorphonuclear (PMN) cell count of greater than 250/µl without evidence of secondary causes of peritonitis. A positive bacterial culture of the ascitic fluid is not needed. Intravenous cefotaxime or a similar third-generation cephalosporin is the treatment of choice for SBP. However per Cochrane review, this class has not been shown to be superior to other classes of antibiotics. Most common isolates are *Escherichia coli*, *Klebsiella pneumoniae*, and pneumococci. Vancomycin is not needed for initial treatment. Oral fluoroquinolone treatment may be indicated in mild cases treated as an outpatient.

Several strategies may be employed to improve renal vascular flow in the setting of SBP. Intravenous albumin is the most widely used.

The use of cefotaxime plus intravenous albumin at 1.5 g/kg on day 3 has been shown to decrease in-hospital mortality by 20 % in patients with serum creatinine values of 1.5 mg/dL or greater. There is no evidence that large-volume paracentesis improves outcomes in patients with SBP and should be done with caution. Excessive fluid shifts may worsen kidney function.

References

Chavez-Tapia NC, Soares-Weiser K, Brezis M, Leibovici L. Antibiotics for spontaneous bacterial peritonitis in cirrhotic patients. Cochrane Database Syst Rev. 2009;1:CD002232.

Sort P, Navasa M, Arroyo V, et al. Effect of intravenous albumin on renal impairment and mortality in patients with cirrhosis and spontaneous bacterial peritonitis. N Engl J Med. 1999;341(6):403–9.

79. A 55-year-old female presents to the emergency department 5 h after the onset of left hemiplegia and right gaze deviation. CT scan reveals an early large infarct. Her airway appears to be intact and she is arousable. She responds to voice commands appropriately. She is admitted to the hospitalist service with a neurology consult.

    Ten hours later, the patient becomes somnolent. On repeat examination, she is no longer responsive to voice and has minimal withdrawal to pain. The right pupil is large, irregular, and unresponsive. Repeat CT scan of the head reveals a 10 mm midline shift as well as the evolution of a well-demarcated right middle cerebral artery infarction.

    Which of the following is the most appropriate next step in her treatment and management?

    A) Neurosurgical consultation for possible hemicraniectomy
    B) Dexamethasone intravenously
    C) Transfer to the intensive care unit for intracranial pressure monitoring
    D) Aspirin
    E) Bedside intubation

Answer: A

Patients who have a large territory infarcts are at risk for herniation and should have frequent neurologic checks to follow for signs of deterioration. Early repeat imaging and neurosurgical consult is warranted with significant clinical decline. Three separate European studies reveal that hemicraniectomy reduces mortality and severe disability in patients with malignant middle cerebral artery infarction. This benefit is greatest if performed within the first 48 h after stroke and optimally before clinical herniation has occurred. This patient has evidence of elevated clinical intracranial pressure, and urgent neurosurgical consultation is needed as well as repeat imaging. The neurosurgical consult should come first while arranging for imaging, intensive care unit transfer, and further supportive measures.

Reference

Gupta R, Connolly ES, Mayer S, Elkind MSV. Hemicraniectomy for massive middle cerebral artery territory infarction: a systematic review. Stroke. 2004;35:539–43.

80. A 54-year-old male is admitted for observation after suffering a concussion in a syncopal episode and suffering a laceration of the head. This occurred while getting up at night to go to the bathroom. On presentation he continues to feel slightly dizzy and is noted to be dehydrated.

    He has no past medical history and no meds. He also reports increased thirst and urination for the past month. Urinalysis reveals 2+ glucose. His blood sugar is 305 mg/dl. His hemoglobin A1C is 11 %. He is started on intravenous fluids in the emergency room.

    What is an appropriate initial diabetic regimen for this patient?
    A) Metformin 500 mg PO BID
    B) Insulin
    C) Januvia 100 mg PO daily
    D) Metformin 500 mg PO BID and glipizide 5 mg PO daily

Answer: B

Initial diabetic therapy is guided by hemoglobin A1C and symptoms. According to the American Diabetes Association (ADA), the recommended goal A1C for this patient is less than 7 %. Metformin as monotherapy, if not contraindicated, may be first-line therapy. However, in newly diagnosed type 2 diabetics with marked symptoms and/or highly elevated blood glucose or A1C, insulin therapy is indicated.

The American Association of Clinical Endocrinology has more specific guidelines with respect to initiating therapy. Specifically, when the entry level A1C is greater than 9 % and/or the patient is symptomatic (urinalysis 2+ glucose, polydipsia, polyuria), insulin plus or minus other agents is recommended. Monotherapy is recommended when the entry A1C is less than 7.5 %. Similarly, dual therapy is recommended when the entry level A1C is greater than or equal to 7.5 %, but less than 9 %. Additionally, the oral agents will drop the A1C by approximately 1–2 % (not all oral agents); therefore, this would not be an adequate decrease for a patient with an A1C of 9 % or greater.

References

ADA Professional Practice Committee. Clinical practice recommendations. Diabetes Care 2014;37: S1–155.
American Association of Clinical Endocrinology. Comprehensive diabetes management algorithm 2013. Endocr Pract. 2013;19:1–48.

81. A 50-year-old male is admitted due to observation for chest pain and the possibility of myocardial ischemia. On presentation, he reported a brief episode of burning chest pain that occurred with maximal exertion. The pain lasted less than a minute.

    Since admission, he has had no further chest pain. He has a positive family history for coronary artery disease. He is currently a 1-pack/day smoker. On the first day of admission, blood pressure is noted to be 180/100.

    Which of the following is the most appropriate medicine for the treatment of his hypertension?
    A) Nifedipine
    B) Labetalol
    C) Clonidine
    D) Enalapril
    E) Hydrochlorothiazide

Answer: B

Beta-blockers are the best initial antihypertensive agent to use when the possibility of cardiac ischemia is present. This would be a reasonable first-line choice until the possibility of coronary artery disease is explored.

Reference

Marik PE, Varon J. Hypertensive crises: challenges and management. Chest. 2007;131(6):1949–62.

82. A-65-year-old male with a past medical history of hypertension is admitted with the diagnosis of a pulmonary embolism and is started on intravenous heparin.

    After being transported to his room, his heart rate increases to 130 bmp with a blood pressure of 100/60 mmHg. An ECG reveals atrial fibrillation with rapid ventricular response. Rate control is attempted with three doses of IV 5 mg Lopressor, but failed to decrease heart rate. A Cardizem drip is started.

    While at the bedside the patient's heart rate increases to 150 bpm and he begins to complain of chest pain. A repeat blood pressure is checked and noted to be 80/40.

You begin a 500 cc bolus of normal saline but the patient experiences a syncopal episode while sitting in bed. Pulses are faintly palpable and respirations remain intact. A cardiac code is called.

What is the most appropriate next step in acute management after activating the emergency response team?

A) Place the patient in reverse Trendelenburg.
B) Begin chest compressions at a rate of 30:2.
C) Push Lopressor 5 mg IV × 1 dose.
D) Immediate R-wave synchronized direct-current cardioversion.

Answer: D

When a rapid ventricular response does not respond promptly to pharmacologic measures for patients with atrial fibrillation with ongoing myocardial ischemia, symptomatic hypotension, angina, or heart failure, immediate R-wave synchronized direct-current cardioversion is recommended.

Reference

Anderson J et al. Management of patients with atrial fibrillation (compilation of 2006 ACCF/AHA/ESC and 2011 ACCF/AHA/HRS recommendations): a report of the American College of Cardiology/American Heart Association Task Force on Practice Guidelines. Circulation. 2013;127:1916–26.

83. A 75-year-old man was admitted to the hospital for diarrhea and hypotension. During the past year, he has had four prior admissions because of similar problems. Polymerase chain reaction assay comes back positive for *Clostridium difficile* infection. This is his third confirmed *Clostridium difficile* infection documented by stool polymerase chain reaction assay.

On physical exam, the patient's blood pressure is 80/40 mmHg. The abdomen has diffuse tenderness without peritoneal signs. Computed tomography scan of the abdomen did not show any bowel dilation. He is started on oral vancomycin and IV Flagyl.

Since admission, his hemodynamic profile has rapidly stabilized with additional fluid administration.

Which of the following should be considered now?

A) Rifaximin
B) Neomycin enema
C) Assessment for presence of vancomycin-resistant enterococci
D) Fecal microbiota transplantation
E) Probiotics

Answer: D

Recurrent *Clostridium difficile* infection can be life threatening. In this patient, the diagnosis is established, and colo-noscopy is unlikely to yield additional results of value. Fecal microbiota transplantation should be considered. Initial experience with a fecal transplant is promising, and certainly in a case of multiple recurrences such as this, it should be considered.

Both initial and sustained responses to fecal microbiota transplant for the treatment of refractory *C. difficile* infection remain high out to 18 months follow-up.

References

Bakken JS. Fecal bacteriotherapy for recurrent Clostridium difficile infection. Anaerobe 2009; 15:285–289.

Crooks NH, Snaith C, Webster D, et al. Clinical review: probiotics in critical care. Crit Care. 2012;16:237.

84. A 65-year-old male with end-stage liver disease secondary to alcohol presents with a chief complaint of worsening ascites.

On physical examination, minimal ascites is noted. Blood pressure is 90/50. Chemistries reveal a creatinine of 5.3 mg/dL and a BUN of 42 mg/d/L. Urine sodium is noted to be 5 mEq/L. Urine volume in the first 24 h of admission is 120 mL/day. No red blood cells are noted on initial exam.

Initial treatment includes which of the following?

A) Supportive care and IV hydration
B) Furosemide 80 mg IV push with albumin
C) Volume expansion with albumin 25 %, 1 g/kg
D) Intravenous albumin, midodrine, and octreotide
E) Large volume paracentesis

Answer: D

This patient's diagnosis is consistent with hepatorenal syndrome (HRS) . Most individuals with cirrhosis who develop HRS have nonspecific symptoms, such as fatigue or malaise. Diagnosis of HRS is based on the presence of acute renal failures in the absence of other causes in patients with chronic liver disease.

Clues to diagnosis include suddenly worsening renal function, a urine sodium <10 mEq/L, decreased urine output, and a relatively inactive urine sediment. Urinary indices are not considered reliable as they may be variable in HRS.

Intravenous albumin, midodrine, and octreotide have been shown to increase renal function and decrease mortality in hepatorenal syndrome. These medicines should be started as well as achieving an increase of 15 mmHg in mean arterial pressure.

Reference

Moreau R, Lebrec D. Diagnosis and treatment of acute renal failure in patients with cirrhosis. Best Pract Res Clin Gastroenterol. 2007;21(1):111–23.

85. A 57-year-old male patient is scheduled for urgent coronary angiography. His estimated glomerular filtration rate is 30 mL/min per 1.68 m² He has poorly controlled diabetes and hypertension.

On physical exam, his blood pressure is 137/75 mm/Hg. His renal function is at baseline. The procedure is due to begin in 2 h, and you would like to prevent or reduce the risk of contrast nephropathy.

Which agent will best reduce the risk of contrast nephropathy?
A) Dopamine
B) Fenoldopam
C) Indomethacin
D) N-acetylcysteine
E) Sodium bicarbonate

Answer: E

Of the other measures mentioned here, only sodium bicarbonate or N-acetylcysteine is recommended for clinical use to reduce the risk of contrast nephropathy. Sodium bicarbonate begun within 1 h of the procedure has shown a significant benefit in randomized controlled trials.

Patients with chronic kidney disease, diabetes mellitus, heart failure, multiple myeloma, and volume depletion are at the highest risk of contrast-induced nephropathy. Hydration with normal saline is an effective measure to prevent contrast nephropathy. Dopamine and fenoldopam have been proven an ineffective agent to prevent contrast nephropathy. Although several small clinical studies have suggested a clinical benefit to the use of N-acetylcysteine, a meta-analysis has been inconclusive. In addition, N-acetylcysteine should be given well in advance of 4 h as is needed here.

Reference

Merten G, Burgess W, Gray L, Holleman J, Roush T, Kowalchuk G, Bersin R, Van Moore A, Simonton C, Rittase R, Norton H, Kennedy T. Prevention of contrast-induced nephropathy with sodium bicarbonate: a randomized controlled trial. JAMA. 2004;291(19):2328–34.

86. A 72-year-old man is admitted to the hospital because of worsening shortness of breath during the past 2 days due to an exacerbation of chronic obstructive pulmonary disease. He has not had an increased in temperature but reports increased sputum production. He initially responds to breathing treatments, but after arriving on the floor, you are called to see him for shortness of breath.

On physical exam, the patient is in respiratory distress with some accessory muscle usage. Temperature is 37.1 C (98.8 F), pulse rate is 100 per minute, respirations are 20 per minute, and blood pressure is 120/82 mmHg. There is minimal air movement. No crackles are heard. Arterial blood studies on 6 L/min oxygen by nasal cannula are pH of 7.34 PCO_2, of 78 mmHg, and PO2 of 72 mmHg. Repeat chest X-ray is clear. Antibiotics and intravenous corticosteroids have been started.

Which of the following is indicated for managing this patient's respiratory status?
A) Continued monitoring on 6 L/min oxygen by nasal cannula
B) 50 % oxygen via facemask
C) Invasive mechanical ventilation
D) 100 % Nonrebreathing mask
E) Noninvasive mechanical ventilation (NPPV)

Answer: E

This patient is in respiratory distress. Continued current oxygen via nasal cannula or nonrebreathing mask is not appropriate. It is unlikely that increasing delivered oxygen will resolve this patient's ventilation issues. Avoidance of intubation is desired as well.

This patient has several factors that make NPPV the best option. In patients who have severe exacerbations of COPD defined as $PCO_2 > 45$ mmHg, use of NPPV resulted in decreased mortality, decreased need for intubation, and reduction in treatment failure compared to standard therapy. Factors that predict success with NPPV include higher pH, lower $PaCO_2$, and higher FVC.

Poor outcomes were associated with a diagnosis of pneumonia, decreased compliance with the apparatus, and severe accessory muscle use. There is no guarantee that NPPV will resolve the respiratory distress. Close observation is needed after initiation.

References

Berkius J, Fredrikson M, Nilholm L, Sundh J, Walther SM. What determines immediate use of invasive ventilation in patients with COPD? Acta Anaesthesiol Scand. 2013;57(3):312–319.

Delclos GL, Lee W, Tsai C, et al. Comparative effectiveness of noninvasive ventilation vs invasive mechanical ventilation in chronic obstructive pulmonary disease patients with acute respiratory failure. J Hosp Med. 2013;8(4):165–72.

87. A 35-year-old diabetic man presents 2 days after obtaining a puncture wound to his left arm which occurred while gardening 2 days ago. Initially, he reported some mild erythema of the arm which was stable. Over the past 24 h, he has developed increasingly intense pain and swelling in the arm. He also reports an increased temperature and mild shortness of breath.

On physical exam, the arm is noted to be markedly swollen. It is extremely tender to mild touch. His temperature is 38.8 °C (101.8 °F), BP is 110/60.

Initial therapy should includes:

A) Surgical consultation
B) Irrigation of the wound with sterile saline
C) Incision and drainage in the emergency department
D) Urgent CT scan of the arm
E) MRI of the arm

Answer: A

This patient has an abscess or necrotizing fasciitis, possibly caused by *Clostridium* species due to exposure of decomposing biomaterial. Clostridial gangrene is a highly lethal necrotizing soft tissue infection of skeletal muscle caused by toxin- and gas-producing *Clostridium*. Exotoxins as opposed to an immune reaction are the primary cause of tissue swelling. Frank pus is often absent. Swelling, pallor, and tenderness rapidly develop. Crepitus may also be present. Patients with necrotizing fasciitis have pain out of proportion to their physical exam findings. Necrosis can spread as fast as 2 cm/h. This may result in systemic toxicity and shock that can be fatal within 12 h.

Clostridium perfringens is prevalent in soil and is the most common species associated with infection. Treatment is urgent with aggressive surgical debridement as well as intravenous antibiotics. Consultation with a surgeon should not be delayed by imaging. Hyperbaric oxygen has been utilized as an adjuvant therapy in many situations.

Reference

Larson CM, Bubrick MP, Jacobs DM, West MA. Malignancy, mortality, and medicosurgical management of *Clostridium septicum* infection. Surgery. 1995;118(4):592–7; discussion 597–8.

88. A 36-year-old female with type 1 diabetes mellitus is admitted to the hospital with fever, urinary urgency, and nausea.

On physical examination, the temperature is 38.6 °C (101.5 °F), blood pressure is 110/80 mmHg, and respiration rate is 90 bpm. She is noted to have right flank pain. Otherwise, physical exam is within normal limits.

Laboratory studies reveal blood urea nitrogen is 40 mg/dL, creatinine is 1.9 mg/dL, sodium is 135 mEq/L, potassium is 5.0 mEq/L, chloride is 105 mEq/L, bicarbonate is 16 mmol/L, and glucose is 258 mg/dL. Her urine is noted to be positive for ketones.

She is admitted for a urinary tract infection. Prior to admission, she was on an insulin pump, which was discontinued in the emergency room.

Which of the following is the most appropriate step in her management?

A) Restart her insulin pump
B) Sliding scale insulin
C) Insulin drip
D) Scheduled insulin with sliding scale
E) Insulin pump and sliding scale

Answer: C

This patient has developed diabetic ketoacidosis (DKA). This has occurred despite her glucose being only 258 mg/dL. Her insulin pump is not adequate for titration and should be stopped. An insulin drip should be started and monitored, with glucose and electrolyte levels being measured every 1–2 h per DKA protocols. After resolution of her DKA, she should be transitioned to her basal insulin.

In her case, the use of an insulin pump may require consultation with her clinic endocrinologist to determine her discharge home dose.

Reference

Wallace TM, Matthews DR. Recent advances in the monitoring and management of diabetic ketoacidosis. QJM. 2004;97(12):773–80.

89. A 37-year-old male is evaluated for a 2-week history of painful swallowing. He was diagnosed with HIV 4 years ago and started on antiretroviral therapy but has been noncompliant.

On physical examination, the temperature is 97.7 F (36.5), blood pressure is 130/70 mmHg, pulse rate is 90/min, and respiration rate is 12/min. Cardiac and lung examination are unremarkable. Examination of the oral cavity reveals thick cream-colored deposits on the posterior tongue. Pertinent lab findings include CD4 count of 75 cells/microL.

Which of the following is the most appropriate management?

A) Schedule for esophagogastroduodenoscopy.
B) Start topical treatment with clotrimazole or nystatin.
C) Start amphotericin B.
D) Start diflucan.
E) Reassurance.

Answer: D

Oral fluconazole is the initial treatment of choice for this patient due to its efficacy, better side effect profile, and low cost. Treatment with clotrimazole or nystatin can be administered in mild oropharyngeal candidiasis. This patient is immunocompromised and presents with odynophagia, which is a hallmark of esophageal candidiasis. Amphotericin B is effective but it is given intravenously and is associated with increased toxicity. Endoscopy is not necessary for presumed esophageal candidiasis unless symptoms do not improve in 72 h.

References
Braykov NP et al. Assessment of empirical antibiotic therapy optimization in six hospitals: an observational cohort study. The Lancet Infect Dis. 2014;14(12):1220–7.
Porro GB, Parente F, Cernuschi M. The diagnosis of esophageal candidiasis in patients with acquired immune deficiency syndrome: is endoscopy always necessary?. Am J Gastroenterol. 1989;84(2):143–6.

90. A 52-year-old female is transferred from a rural hospital for new onset abdominal pain and right leg weakness. In the initial workup there has been non-diagnostic including a CT scan of abdomen, head, and spine.

    On physical examination, she is awake, alert, and speaking in full sentences. Temperature is 37.2 °C (99.0 °F). The lungs are clear upon auscultation. She is using accessory muscles, and breath sounds are decreased at the lung bases. Diffuse symmetrical weakness is noted throughout her lower extremities. A diagnosis of Guillain–Barré is suspected, and the patient is transferred to the intensive care unit for close monitoring of her respiratory status. Routine measurements of patient's bedside vital capacity are initiated.

    Which of the following is the best management strategy to prevent respiratory failure in this patient?
    A) Continuous positive airway pressure.
    B) Bilateral transcutaneous phrenic nerve pacing.
    C) Plasma exchange.
    D) Methylprednisolone.
    E) Ciprofloxacin.

Answer: C
Plasma exchange and intravenous immunoglobulin (IVIG) are the recommended treatment options for Guillain–Barré. Trials have demonstrated that plasma exchange and IVIG reduce the incidence and duration of mechanical ventilation in patients with Guillain–Barré syndrome as opposed to supportive care. The efficacy of plasmapheresis and IVIGs appears to be about equal in shortening the average duration of disease. Combined treatment has not been shown to produce an additional reduction in disability. Systemic corticosteroids by themselves or in conjunction with immunoglobulin are no longer indicated based upon previous trials that demonstrated no benefit.
This patient is at a high risk for respiratory failure. Approximately one-third of patients require admission to an ICU, primarily because of respiratory failure. Her vital capacity and ability to maintain adequate oxygenation indicate that mechanical ventilation is not currently

needed but should be closely followed. Stool culture for *Salmonella* may be considered as well.

References
Raphaël JC, Chevret S, Hughes RA, Annane D. Plasma exchange for Guillain-Barré syndrome. Cochrane Database Syst Rev. 2012;7:CD001798.
Walgaard C, Lingsma HF, Ruts L, Drenthen J, van Koningsveld R, Garssen MJ, et al. Prediction of respiratory insufficiency in Guillain-Barré syndrome. Ann Neurol. 2010;67(6):781–7.

91. A 47-year-old man with chronic obstructive pulmonary disease (COPD) presents with shortness of breath, purulent sputum, fever, and dyspnea increasing over the past 5 days. He has had multiple COPD exacerbations. His most recent admission was 9 months ago. He reports a 50-pack-year smoking history and still continues to smoke.

    On physical examination, he appears moderately ill. He can speak in full sentences without significant shortness of breath. His pulse rate is 90 per minute, temperature is 37.5 °C(99.4 °F), respirations are 22 per minute, and oxygen saturation is 86 % on room air. He is placed on 3 l nasal cannula, and oxygenation improves to 92 %.

    Chest X-ray reveals no significant infiltrates. Laboratory studies: leukocyte count is 11,000; basic metabolic panel is within normal limits; hemoglobin is 14.0 g/dl. He is admitted and placed on bronchodilators and corticosteroids. Which of the following approach is best in this patient?
    A) Observation without antibiotic therapy
    B) Doxycycline or azithromycin for 5 days
    C) Doxycycline or azithromycin for 14 days
    D) Zosyn (piperacillin and tazobactam) and vancomycin

Answer: B
This patient has a moderate exacerbation of COPD. Three clinical factors may be considered in determining the severity of COPD exacerbation: dyspnea, sputum volume, and sputum purulence. Antibiotic treatment is recommended for moderate or severe exacerbations. This includes greater than two clinical factors. Several studies have shown improved clinical response with the use of the antibiotics in this group. Long-term antibiotics show no additional benefits and increase both expense and risk. Without evidence of sepsis or the need for an intensive care unit admission, broad-spectrum antibiotics is not indicated. Focused antibiotics, perhaps on a rotating basis if there are multiple exacerbations, are the best option.

Reference
Quon BS, Gan WQ, Sin DD. Contemporary management of acute exacerbations of COPD. Chest. 2008;133:756–766.

92. A 72-year-old man is readmitted with acute dyspnea and hemoptysis. Seven days prior to this current admission, the patient underwent emergency surgery for a ruptured diverticula that required an open procedure. He was discharged from the hospital 2 days ago. CT pulmonary angiography shows two pulmonary emboli in the right pulmonary artery branches to the upper and middle lobes.

On physical exam, his weight is 80 kg. Heart rate is 110 beats/min, respirations are 22 per minute, and blood pressure is 105/68 mmHg. Oxygen saturation by pulse oximetry ranges from 90 to 93 % on oxygen at 6 L/min.

Laboratory values are significant for hemoglobin of 10.2 g/dL, a platelet count of 68,000/µL, and serum creatinine of 0.9 mg/dL. A preoperative platelet count was 177,000/µL.

Which of the following treatment choices should be considered now?

A) Enoxaparin, subcutaneously
B) Fondaparinux, subcutaneously
C) Unfractionated heparin, by continuous intravenous infusion
D) Alteplase, intravenously

Answer: B

It is possible that the patient has heparin-induced thrombocytopenia, as his platelet count decreased by more than 50 %, and he has had exposure to subcutaneous heparin, starting 72 h after surgery, thus making fractionated and unfractionated heparin compounds dangerous. HIT antibodies should be drawn. The pentasaccharide fondaparinux can be used in patients with thrombocytopenia, since the drug does not appear to interact with platelets. No routine platelet monitoring is needed. Fondaparinux is contraindicated in patients with creatinine clearance less than 30 mL/min.

References

Blackmer AB, Oertel MD, Valgus JM. Fondaparinux and the management of heparin-induced thrombocytopenia: the journey continues. Ann Pharmacother. 2009;43:1636–46.
Konstantinides S. Clinical practice: acute pulmonary embolism. N Engl J Med. 2008;359:2804–13.

93. A 18-year-old high school football player presents with a chief complaint of erythema to his right thigh which he has had for the past 3 days. He denies any puncture wounds to the area but does report the usual trauma associated with football practice.

On physical examination, the thigh appears moderately swollen. He has a fever of 102.1 °F. His pulse rate is 110 beats per minute. His blood pressure is 95/68.

Some mild lymphangitic spread is noted on the right surface of the thigh extending down to the posterior aspect of his calf. In the emergency room, 1 g of ceftriaxone has been administered, and you are consulted for admission.

Which of the following is the most appropriate for this patient now?

A) Intravenous vancomycin, 1 g every 12 h
B) IV clindamycin
C) Consultation to surgery for urgent incision and drainage, followed by intravenous vancomycin
D) IV ceftriaxone 1 g every 12 h

Answer: C

This patient has cellulitis with evidence of sepsis. In this particular case, community-acquired methicillin-resistant *Staphylococcus aureus* (CA-MRSA) is probable. CA-MRSA is an emerging cause of necrotizing fasciitis. CA-MRSA infections have become more common in athletes.

It is important that urgent surgical consultation be obtained in cases where there is suspicion of an underlying fasciitis, as in this case. The Laboratory Risk Indicator for Necrotizing Fasciitis (LRINEC) score can be utilized to risk stratify people having signs of cellulitis to determine the likelihood of necrotizing fasciitis being present. It uses six serologic measures: C-reactive protein, total white blood cell count, hemoglobin, sodium, creatinine, and glucose. A score greater than or equal to 6 indicates that necrotizing fasciitis should be seriously considered.

Many patients with necrotizing fasciitis who undergone debridement should return to the operating room 24–36 h after the first debridement and then daily thereafter until the surgical team finds no further need for debridement. Antibiotics, such as vancomycin, should be administered.

References

Benjamin HJ, Nikore V, Takagishi J. Practical management: community-associated methicillin-resistant Staphylococcus aureus (CA-MRSA): the latest sports epidemic. Clin J Sport Med. 2007;17(5):393–7.
Stevens DL, Bisno AL, Chambers HF, et al. Practice guidelines for the diagnosis and management of skin and soft tissue infections: 2014 update by the Infectious Diseases Society of America. Clin Infect Dis. 2014;59(2):e10–52.

94. A 72-year-old woman is seen for cellulitis of her left leg. Her history is remarkable for a significant allergy to vancomycin. On presentation, her temperature is 39.6 °C (103.3 °F). Her pulse rate is 100 per minute. Respirations are 18 per minute. Her blood pressure is 110/70 mmHg. Daptomycin is started.

Which of the following tests should be ordered?
A) Complete blood count
B) Serum ALT
C) Serum calcium
D) Serum creatine kinase
E) Serum creatinine

Answer: D

Daptomycin is known to cause rhabdomyolysis. Weekly serum creatine kinase tests are recommended. If the CK level is greater than or equal to five times the upper limit of normal, or if the patient develops symptoms suggestive of rhabdomyolysis, daptomycin should be discontinued.

In addition in July 2010, the FDA issued a warning that daptomycin could cause life-threatening eosinophilic pneumonia.

Reference

Vilhena C, Bettencourt A. Daptomycin: a review of properties, clinical use, drug delivery and resistance. Mini Rev Med Chem. 2012;12:202–9.

95. A 44-year-old female is admitted for severe alcoholic hepatitis and is started on prednisolone. Her last alcoholic drink was 3 days prior to admission. At hospital day 7, she is not responding to corticosteroids based on calculation of her Lille score.

What is the most appropriate next step in management?
A) Stop prednisolone, start pentoxifylline.
B) Palliative care consultation.
C) Continue prednisolone, start octreotide.
D) Continue prednisolone, refer to liver transplantation.
E) Continue prednisolone, start plasmapheresis.

The Lille score is a predictor of response to therapy in acute alcoholic hepatitis. This patient is a nonresponder as determined by Lille score and there is little clinical benefit for continuing prednisolone. Her prognosis is poor given that she is a nonresponder to corticosteroids and it is reasonable to involve palliative care. Switching to pentoxifylline has been evaluated in a prospective randomized trial and has no proven clinical benefit. The overall 30-day mortality rate in patients hospitalized with alcoholic hepatitis is approximately 15 %. In patients with severe chronic liver disease, the rate approaches or exceeds 50 %. Liver transplantation would not be an option in the United States for fulminant alcoholic hepatitis given his recent alcohol use. A consultation with the liver transplant service may be needed to review and communicate these issues.

Reference

Louvet A, Naveau S, Abdelnour M, et al. The Lille model: a new tool for therapeutic strategy in patients with severe alcoholic hepatitis treated with steroids. Hepatology. 2007;45:1348–54.

96. A 35-year-old female veterinarian is admitted for a 2-week history of abdominal pain, increased abdominal girth, and peripheral edema. Her past medical history is significant for multiple sclerosis for which she has received interferon treatments.

On physical examination, temperature is normal, blood pressure is 130/65 mmHg, pulse rate is 60/min, and respiration rate is 22. Cardiopulmonary examination discloses normal heart sounds without murmur and symmetric breath sounds. She has 2+ pitting edema of the lower extremities. Abdominal distension is noted. Laboratory studies show hematocrit of 47 %, leukocyte count 10,000/μL, platelet count 125,000/μL L, and total bilirubin 6.0 mg/dL. A Doppler ultrasound of the abdomen shows occlusion of the hepatic veins.

Which of the following is the most appropriate next step in the evaluation of this patient?
A) Antiphospholipid antibody assay
B) Antithrombin activity assay
C) Flow cytometry for paroxysmal nocturnal hemoglobinuria
D) JAK2 V617F mutational analysis
E) Protein C activity assay

Answer: D

This patient has Budd-Chiari syndrome, which is characterized by thrombosis of the hepatic veins, upper quadrant pain, and hepatomegaly. Rapid development of jaundice and ascites often occur. Sixty percent of patients with this syndrome have or eventually will be diagnosed with a myeloproliferative disorder. Polycythemia vera and essential thrombocytosis are the two most common underlying disorders.

The JAK2 V617F gene mutation is present in 97 % of patients with polycythemia vera and in 50 % of those with essential thrombocythemia. It should be measured in all patients with Budd-Chiari syndrome. Positive findings indicate a myeloproliferative disorder and suggest the need for cytoreductive therapy.

There are several options in the treatment of Budd-Chiari including anticoagulation, thrombolytics, and surgery. Consultation with hepatology for the management, guidance, and possible need for transplantation should be first undertaken. In addition, consultation with interventional radiologists, hematologists, oncologists, gastroenterologists, and general surgeons may be required to coordinate the most effective approach.

Reference

Patel RK, Lea NC, Heneghan MA, et al. Prevalence of the activating JAK2 tyrosine kinase mutation V617F in the Budd-Chiari syndrome. Gastroenterology. 2006;130(7):2031–8.

97. A 38-year-old man was diagnosed with *Pneumocystis jiroveci* pneumonia associated with human immunodeficiency virus (HIV) infection. This is his first opportunistic infection. He was treated with trimethoprim–sulfamethoxazole. Severe dermatitis and fever subsequently developed, and the drugs were stopped.

The patient was then treated with pentamidine, but this medication was also discontinued because of the development of abdominal pain with elevations in serum amylase and lipase levels. Clindamycin–primaquine was then started. On the third day of treatment, he developed jaundice and dark urine.

Which of the following tests would most likely provide the etiology of this patient's syndrome?

A) Serum indirect bilirubin
B) Serum lactate dehydrogenase
C) Blood glucose-6-phosphate dehydrogenase
D) Serum trypsin

Answer: C

Side effects of treatment regimens are often seen in the primary treatment of *Pneumocystis jiroveci* pneumonia. Second-line salvage treatment also has high incidences of side effects. This patient has first developed a rash and fever due to trimethoprim–sulfamethoxazole. He then developed pancreatitis due to pentamidine. Both of these occur with some frequency.

Primaquine can cause hemolytic anemia in patients with G6PD deficiency, and patients should be tested when possible prior to starting treatment. The patient has developed clinical evidence of hemolysis, and although bilirubin, erythropoietin, and LDH assessment would suggest the diagnosis, actual measurement of G6PD level is indicated.

References

Benfield T, Atzori C, Miller RF, Helweg-Larsen J. Second-line salvage treatment of AIDS-associated Pneumocystis jirovecii pneumonia: a case series and systematic review. J Acquir Immune Defic Syndr. 2008;48:63–7.

Kim T, Kim SH, Park KH, et al. Clindamycin-primaquine versus pentamidine for the second-line treatment of Pneumocystis pneumonia. J Infect Chemother. 2009;15(5):343–6.

Smego RA Jr, Nagar S, Maloba B, Popara M. A meta-analysis of salvage therapy for Pneumocystis carinii pneumonia. Arch Intern Med. 2001;161(12):1529–33.

98. A 37-year-old male is admitted for acute alcohol intoxication and the desire to seek help for his alcohol dependency. He denies any history of delirium tremens. However, he states that he has attempted to quit drinking several times in the past, which results in prolonged withdrawal symptoms requiring sedation. He denies any other past medical history, and he is on no medications.

On physical examination, he appears alert and slightly diaphoretic. He is oriented to person, place, and time. His temperature is 37.6 °C (99.6 °F), pulse rate is 100 per minute, and respirations are 12 per minute. Blood pressure is 138/74. Lungs are clear upon auscultation. He has a mild tremor. Laboratory data is within normal range. He is admitted for acute intoxication and consultation with a substance abuse service is ordered.

Which of the following is the most appropriate treatment for the patient's alcohol withdrawal?

A) Schedule diazepam 10 mg every 4 h
B) Oral chlordiazepoxide 50 mg every 6 h
C) Oral chlordiazepoxide 50 mg every 6 h and lorazepam 2 mg every 4 h based on symptoms
D) Oral chlordiazepoxide 50 mg every 6 h and Haldol 2.5 mg every 4 h as needed for symptoms
E) Oral diazepam 10 mg every 4 h based on symptoms

Answer: E

This patient demonstrates no symptoms of delirium tremens and is experiencing moderate withdrawal symptoms from alcohol. Symptom-triggered therapy as opposed to fixed dose is appropriate. The most objective and best-validated tool to assess the severity of alcohol withdrawal is the Clinical Institute Withdrawal Assessment for Alcohol, Revised (CIWA-Ar). This survey consists of ten items and can be administered rapidly by trained personnel at the bedside in about 5 min. Therapy is based upon the score. The CIWA-Ar scale has its limitations and is not universally used. It has not been validated in complex medical patients, postsurgical patients, and critically ill patients.

Fixed dose therapy can be instituted if symptoms are not controlled, erratic, or escalate despite symptom-based therapy. Haloperidol is not recommended in alcohol withdrawal in the absence of hallucinations. It may be used in psychosis or agitation nonresponsive to benzodiazepines.

References

Daeppen JB, Gache P, Landry U, et al. Symptom-triggered vs fixed-schedule doses of benzodiazepine for alcohol withdrawal: a randomized treatment trial. Arch Int Med. 2002;162:1117–21.

Sullivan JT, Sykora K, Schneiderman J, Naranjo CA, Sellers EM. Assessment of alcohol withdrawal: the revised clinical institute withdrawal assessment for alcohol scale (CIWA-Ar). Br J Addict. 1989;84(11):1353–7.

99. A 56-year-old male is admitted for a COPD exacerbation. This is his second admission this month. He complains of shortness of breath, "coughing up yellow stuff," and fatigue. He has a past medical history of COPD,

diabetes mellitus II, hypertension, and dyslipidemia. He smokes ½ pack per day and drinks 1–2 beers nightly.

He is on the following medications at home: Insulin detemir 25 units SQ BID, insulin aspart 3 units SQ with meals, tiotropium 18 mcg 2 puffs once daily, fluticasone/salmeterol 250/50, 1 inhalation BID, albuterol HFA 90 mcg 2 puffs every 4–6 h as needed for SOB, lisinopril 5 mg PO daily, rosuvastatin 20 mg PO daily, hydrochlorothiazide 12.5 mg PO daily, and gabapentin 300 mg PO TID. He is started on moxifloxacin 400 mg PO daily and prednisone 40 mg PO daily during admission. He continued on his home insulin dose. On the day following his admission, his accu-check readings are as follows: 0600: 130, 0900: 220, 1230: 245, 1730: 251, 2100: 139.

What medication adjustments would you make after seeing these readings?
A) Increase meal-time insulin
B) Increase basal insulin
C) Increase both meal-time and basal insulin
D) No change

Answer: A

Glucocorticoid use is associated with the risk of hyperglycemia. Effects are greater in the fed rather than fasting state. Insulin regimens need to take into account that glucocorticoids typically have greater effects on postprandial glucose levels rather than on fasting levels. Thus, the patient's initiation of prednisone is likely the culprit of those increased accu-check readings. B is incorrect because the target blood glucose goal in the non-critical patient in the hospital is typically 100–140 mg/dl and 140–180 mg/dl in critically ill patients. Thus, the fasting level of 130 mg/dl is appropriate and does not require dose adjustment. C is incorrect as referenced above – no basal adjustments are needed. Lastly, D is incorrect because a change is required for the meal-time dosing regimen as the values range from 220 to 251 mg/dl.

References

Hoogwerf B, et al. Drug selection and management of corticosteroid-related Diabetes Mellitus. Rheum Dis Clin North Am. 2000;3:489–505.
AACE Diabetes Care Plan Guidelines. Endocr Pract. 2011;17(Suppl 2):26–7.

100. A 57-year-old male presents with a chief complaint of an acute onset of chest pain that began approximately 20 min prior to presentation. ECG reveals acute elevations in the anterior leads consistent with an evolving anterior myocardial infarction. He has a history of peptic ulcer disease for which he was admitted to the hospital 1 month ago, at which time he underwent an EGD which revealed gastritis with no active bleeding sites.

On physical examination, he is afebrile. Blood pressure is 140/70. Heart rate is 90. Respiration rate is 18. Cardiovascular examination reveals normal S1 and S2 without an S3.

Serum troponin is pending. The hematocrit is 44 %. Which of the following is the most appropriate treatment?
A) Thrombolytic therapy.
B) Await laboratory results.
C) Antiplatelet therapy.
D) Consult cardiology for urgent cardiac catheterization(PCI) and intervention.

Answer: D

Treatment options include percutaneous coronary intervention, thrombolytic therapy, and medical management. If available, the patient should undergo urgent percutaneous coronary intervention. PCI performed within 90 min of a patient's arrival is superior to fibrinolysis with respect to combined endpoints of death, stroke, and reinfarction.

He has an ECG consistent with acute anterior myocardial infarction. Therapy for an acute MI presenting with 12 h of symptoms should be thrombolytic therapy or percutaneous intervention. This patient has a relative contraindication to thrombolytic therapy with his history of recent peptic ulcer disease. Absolute contraindications to thrombolytic therapy include any history of cerebrovascular hemorrhage, known cerebrovascular lesion, an ischemic stroke within 3 months, significant facial trauma or closed head injury within 3 months. Relative contraindications are poorly controlled hypertension. Medical management of the patient including aggressive anticoagulation should be delayed until definitive percutaneous coronary intervention.

Reference

Rokos IC, French WJ, Mattu A, et al. Appropriate cardiac cath lab activation: optimizing electrocardiogram interpretation and clinical decision-making for acute ST-elevation myocardial infarction. Am Heart J. 2010; 160(6):995–1003.

101. You are asked to see a 60-year-old man in the emergency department for shaking chills, cough, and productive sputum. He has a 37-pack-year history of cigarette smoking but has no other significant medical history.

On physical examination, the temperature is 38.6 °C (101.5 °F), the blood pressure is 160/90 mmHg, the heart rate is 115 bpm and regular, and the respiration rate is 27/min. There is increased dullness upon percussion at the right base, crackles in the right mid-lung field, and diffuse anterior wheezes.

Chest radiograph shows a right lower lobe posterior infiltrate and a moderate-sized pleural effusion. Therapy with ceftriaxone, azithromycin, and inhaled bronchodilators is started in the emergency room.

What is the most appropriate treatment?
A) Admit and perform pleural cavity drainage.
B) Admit and repeat chest radiograph in 2 days.
C) Admit for video-assisted thoracoscopic surgery (VATS).
D) Treat as an outpatient.

Answer: A

This patient has pneumonia with a significant parapneumonic effusion. He should be admitted and diagnostic tap performed. Observation of pleural effusion is reasonable when benign etiologies are likely. This can occur with chronic overt congestive heart failure, viral pleurisy, or recent thoracic or abdominal surgery. Effusions may resolve with antibiotic therapy alone, but complications can occur in about 10 % of parapneumonic effusions. For this reason diagnostic and therapeutic thoracentesis is recommended.

This patient with underlying chronic obstructive pulmonary disease had typical symptoms of an acute bacterial pneumonia with development of a parapneumonic effusion. These factors suggest that the patient may have a poor outcome without immediate pleural space drainage. This patient needs close observation in the hospital. He needs follow-up for possible escalation of therapy, repeat radiographs, and possible repeat thoracentesis.

Reference
Diaz-Guzman E, Dweik RA. Diagnosis and management of pleural effusions: a practical approach. Compr Ther. Winter 2007;33(4):237–46.

102. A 26-year-old female is admitted with diarrhea, abdominal pain, and ten-pound weight loss over the past few months. She has just completed her 18-month basic science training at medical school in the Caribbean islands. She is back in the United States for her clinical rotations. She has been trying to participate in her rotations but is unable to function. She is referred by her attending physician for admission to the hospital. She is on no medicines and reports no other medical history.

Her initial workup is unremarkable. Stool studies are all negative. The patient has mild anemia and increased mean corpuscular volume (MCV).

Which of the following is the most likely diagnosis?
A) Inflammatory bowel disease
B) Irritable bowel disease
C) Tropical sprue
D) Laxative abuse

Answer: C
The symptoms of diarrhea, abdominal pain, and weight loss with recent travel suggest tropical sprue. Findings of steatorrhea, malabsorption, and villous atrophy by biopsy are adequate to make a diagnosis. Response to treatment is considered to be the conclusive evidence that confirms the diagnosis.

An individual needs to be in a tropical country for at least one month to consider this as a diagnosis. The exact etiology of tropical sprue is uncertain. It may be caused by endemic *E. coli* or *Klebsiella*. Other infectious etiologies have been suggested as well. Treatment of tropical sprue is usually with prolonged course of tetracycline. In addition vitamins, particularly folic acid, should be given.

The first description of tropical sprue is attributed to William Hillary's 1759 account of his observations of chronic diarrhea while in Barbados. Subsequently, tropical sprue was described in tropical climates throughout the world.

Reference
Brown IS, Bettington A, Bettington M, et al. Tropical sprue: revisiting an underrecognized disease. Am J Surg Pathol. 2014;38(5):666–72.

103. A 38-year-old male is admitted with the acute onset of fever and headaches for the past two days. He denies any recent sick contacts.

On physical exam, the patient has significant neck stiffness. Temperature is normal. He responds to questions appropriately.

Lumbar puncture is performed in the emergency room and cerebrospinal fluid (CSF) studies are obtained. Opening pressure is noted at 285 mm H_2O. CSF analysis reveals 1700 WBCs/μL, a PMN predominance, 10 RBCs, glucose 22 mg/dL, and protein 104 mg/dL. Serum glucose is 80 mg/dL.

Which of the following is the most likely diagnosis?
A) St. Louis encephalitis
B) Herpes simplex encephalitis (HSV)
C) Early bacterial meningitis
D) West Nile virus
E) Bacterial meningitis

Answer: C
This patient has early bacterial meningitis. Several classic factors point toward this including an elevated opening pressure, high CSF neutrophil count, and low CSF glucose. Symptoms in bacterial meningitis are reliable, with 95 % of patients having two out of the four classical symptoms of fever, headache, stiff neck, and altered mental status.

To determine the time frame of bacterial meningitis, a CSF-to-serum glucose ratio can be calculated. If this ratio is less than 0.4, early bacterial meningitis is likely. This patient's CSF-to-serum glucose ratio is 0.275.

Some consideration could be given to HSV encephalitis that may present with a variable CSF pattern including a high CSF neutrophil count. However, other diagnostic clues such as red blood cells in the CSF are absent. Patients with HSV encephalitis often present with global cognition deficits.

References

Seupaul RA. Evidence-based emergency medicine/rational clinical examination abstract. How do I perform a lumbar puncture and analyze the results to diagnose bacterial meningitis?. Ann Emerg Med. 2007;50(1):85–7.

Thomas KE, Hasbun R, Jekel J, Quagliarello VJ. The diagnostic accuracy of Kernig's sign, Brudzinski's sign, and nuchal rigidity in adults with suspected meningitis. Clin Infect Dis. 2002;35(1):46–52.

van de Beek D, de Gans J, Spanjaard L, Weisfelt M, Reitsma JB, Vermeulen M. Clinical features and prognostic factors in adults with bacterial meningitis. N Engl J Med. 2004;351(18):1849–59.

104. A 62-year-old female with a history of prior abdominal surgery presents with the chief complaint of worsening abdominal pain over the past 24 h.

    On physical exam, the patient has moderate abdominal pain. Increased bowel sounds are noted. Vital signs: BP is 137/85, heart rate is 88, and respirations are 20.

    CT scan of the abdomen is consistent with partial small bowel obstruction. Therapy should include the following:
    A) Surgical consultation for open laparotomy
    B) NG tube placement and fluid resuscitation
    C) Gastrografin enema
    D) NG tube placement with clamping

Answer: B

Conservative therapy will lead to resolution of partial small bowel obstruction in 90 % of cases. The leading cause of SBO in industrialized countries is postoperative adhesions. Patients without alarming symptoms can be managed conservatively. Surgery consultation is usually required on admission and is of benefit as surgery may be indicated at some point during the hospitalization. Having surgery following may decrease the lag time when surgery is indicated. Alarming symptoms where surgery is required emergently include complete obstruction, peritonitis, pneumatosis intestinalis, or strangulation.

Surgery is indicated in patients with small bowel obstructions that have not shown signs of resolution in 24–48 h. NG tube decompression is used to clear gastric contents, decompress the small bowel, and prevent aspiration. The tube should be placed on intermittent suction and output recorded. The NG tube is removed when obstruction is resolved. If resolution is uncertain, the NG tube should be clamped for a 4-h period and can be removed as residuals are <100 mL and no nausea and vomiting is noted.

It is reasonable to admit this patient to a medical service with surgery consult. Suspected complete obstruction or those where surgery is anticipated should be admitted to a surgical team.

Reference

Diaz JJ Jr, Bokhari F, Mowery NT, Acosta JA, Block EF, Bromberg WJ, et al. Guidelines for management of small bowel obstruction. J Trauma. 2008;64(6):1651–64

105. A 72-year-old female is admitted with sepsis, pneumonia, and hypotension. In the emergency room, the patient has received 0.9 % saline at a rate of 150 cm³/h. Broad-spectrum antibiotics have been administered. Laboratory studies on admission reveal a hematocrit of 30 %, a serum creatinine of 1.9, and a serum lactate level of 3.7 mm/l. A serum albumin is 2.7 g/dL. Her blood pressure is noted to be 90/50 with decreased urine output.

    Which of the following should be selected for ongoing volume resuscitation?
    A) 0.9 % saline
    B) 6 % hydroxyethyl starch (HES) solution
    C) Packed red blood cells
    D) Normal saline with 5 % albumin infusion
    E) D5 1/2 normal saline

Answer: A

Several studies have looked at fluid resuscitation in sepsis. Among ICU patients, 90-day mortality was observed between patients resuscitated with 0.9 % saline and with 6 % hydroxyethyl starch (HES) solution. In the study, no significant difference was noted.

Other studies have looked at crystalloid and albumin for fluid resuscitation and have found no benefit as compared to 0.9 % saline.

In this particular case, blood products should not be employed for volume expansion unless there is a specific need.

Reference

van Haren F, Zacharowski K. What's new in volume therapy in the intensive care unit? Best Pract Res Clin Anaesthesiol. 2014;28(3):275–83.

106. A 35-year-old female presents with fulminant hepatic failure. She is 8 months pregnant and recently arrived from Honduras. Her past medical history is unknown, but per family she has not had hepatic disease.

Which of the following viral causes of acute hepatitis is most likely to cause fulminant hepatitis in this pregnant woman?
A) Hepatitis A
B) Hepatitis B
C) Hepatitis C
D) Hepatitis D
E) Hepatitis E

Answer: E

Hepatitis E usually has a mild presentation. However, pregnant women are highly susceptible to fulminant hepatic failure in the setting of acute hepatitis E infection. This RNA virus is an enteric virus that is endemic in India, Asia, Africa, the Middle East, and Central America. It is spread via contaminated water supplies.

In pregnant women fulminant hepatic failure is as high as 10–20 %. Hepatic failure is rare with most infectious cause of hepatitis. Hepatitis A and C have fulminant hepatic failure is about 0.1 %. It is slightly higher for hepatitis B at around 0.1–1 %.

Hoofnagle, J. H.; Nelson, K. E.; Purcell, R. H. (2012). "Hepatitis E". New England Journal of Medicine 367 (13): 1237–1244. 306)

107. An 80-year-old female presents to the emergency room with a one-week history of weakness, fatigue, nausea, and anorexia. Past medical history is significant for metastatic squamous cell carcinoma of the lung, which has been treated with chemotherapy.

On physical examination, temperature is 38.2 °C (100.8 °F), blood pressure is 100/70, and pulse rate is 125 per minute. Laboratory studies reveal blood urea nitrogen of 52 mg/dL, calcium level of 14.4 mg/dL, creatinine of 1.9 mg/dL, and phosphorus of 2.2 mg/dL.

Which of the following is the most appropriate therapy?
A) 0.5 % saline infusion with furosemide
B) 0.9 % saline infusion
C) 0.9 % saline infusion with furosemide
D) 0.45 % saline infusion

Answer: B

This patient should receive volume replacement with 0.9 % saline. In the treatment of acute hypercalcemia, aggressive volume expansion with an intravenous normal saline is the first step. Normal saline, as opposed to 0.5 % saline or saline, with furosemide, is the current recommended treatment. Increased excretion of calcium can be achieved by inhibition of proximal tubular and loop sodium reabsorption, which is best achieved by aggressive volume expansion.

Reference

Makras P, Papapoulos SE. Medical treatment of hypercalcaemia. Hormones 2009;8(2):83-95å

108. Proton-pump inhibitors (PPI) have been associated with the following conditions:
A) *Cl*ostridium difficile colitis
B) Hospital-acquired pneumonia
C) Osteoporosis-related fractures
D) Myopathy
E) All of the above

Answer: E

The evidence for PPI adverse events is limited by the absence of randomized controlled trial studies. The best evidence supports *Clostridium difficile* infections and bone fractures. Other studies show a correlation between proton-pump inhibitors and each of the conditions mentioned.

In general PPI should be prescribed for overt indications only and discontinued when no longer indicated. They should be used with caution in the elderly and in patients with other risk factors for bone fractures or *C. difficile* infection.

Reference

Corleto VD et al. Proton pump inhibitor therapy and potential long-term harm. Curr Opin Endocrine Diabetes Obes. 2014;21(1):3–8.

109. A 52-year-old male is admitted with fever, headache, and mild nuchal rigidity. He reports exposure to several children with respiratory tract infections.

On physical exam, he appears in mild distress. He has mild neck stiffness and photophobia. Otherwise, the exam is normal.

A lumbar puncture reveals a white blood cell count of 44, of which 98 % are lymphocytes. Glucose is 64 mg/dl. Protein is 46 mg/dl. He is admitted overnight and started on IV vancomycin and ceftriaxone. The following day, PCR for herpes simplex is negative. He is afebrile overnight and feels markedly better.

Which of the following is the most appropriate management?
A) Continue with antibiotics until cultures are negative.
B) Observe for 48 h.
C) Discontinue current medications and observe.
D) Discharge home.
E) Discharge home with Augmentin.
F) Start acyclovir.

Answer: D

This patient has aseptic meningitis. The term aseptic is frequently a misnomer, implying a lack of infection. Many cases of aseptic meningitis represent infection with viruses, many of which are known causes of generalized viral illnesses. Polymerase chain reaction testing has increased the ability of clinicians to detect viruses such as enterovirus, cytomegalovirus, and herpes virus in the CSF. However, except for the herpes virus, this is not widely done.

When CSF findings are consistent with meningitis, and microbiological testing is unrevealing, clinicians typically assign the diagnosis of aseptic meningitis. In most instances, morbidity is low. There is no indication for waiting until cultures are negative in obvious cases of aseptic meningitis. In this particular case, the patient can be safely discharged home.

References

Logan, SA; MacMahon, E "Viral meningitis.". BMJ 2008;336 (7634): 36–40.

Khetsuriani, N; Quiroz, ES; Holman, RC; Anderson, LJ "Viral meningitis-associated hospitalizations in the United States, 1988–1999.". Neuroepidemiology 2003 22 (6): 345–52.

110. A 26-year-old white female is admitted for left forearm MRSA cellulitis. She is currently receiving vancomycin 1 g IV every 12 h. A vancomycin trough returns as 41 ug/ml. However, per her MAR, she received her 4th dose of vancomycin at 6:30 A.M. and the trough was drawn at 6:45 A.M.

     Which statement is correct?
     A) Trough drawn inappropriately
     B) Trough drawn appropriately, continue current dose
     C) Trough drawn appropriately, increase current dose
     D) Trough drawn appropriately, decrease current dose

Answer: A

Vancomycin serum trough concentrations should be obtained at steady-state conditions, prior to the fourth or fifth dose. Her trough level was drawn immediately following the fourth dose, likely while the drug was still infusing. Thus this was not considered a trough and was drawn inappropriately.

In the past, it was fairly routine to measure both peak and trough concentrations; now, many clinicians monitor only the trough concentration or do not monitor drug concentrations at all. Using vancomycin concentrations to monitor patients' therapeutic response is not typically suggested if the duration of therapy is expected to be less than 72 h.

References

Liu C et al. Clinical Practice Guidelines by the Infectious Disease Society of America for the Treatment of Methicillin-Resistant Staphylococcus aureus in Adults and Children. CID 2011;52:1–38.

Ryback M et al. Therapeutic Monitoring of Vancomycin in Adult Patients. Am J Health-Syst Pharm 2009;66:82–98.

111. A 19-year-old man presents with lethargy, fever, and decreased appetite. In the past three years, he has been admitted for similar symptoms twice with no obvious source found. Prior extensive diagnostic workup has not found evidence of lymphoma, leukemia, or other malignancies. Further extensive infectious workup has been negative for HIV, tuberculosis, histoplasmosis, Q fever, typhoid fever, Epstein–Barr virus, infectious mononucleosis, cytomegalovirus, human herpes virus (HHV)-6, viral hepatitis, and Whipple's disease. He was born in Honduras and moved to the United States 16 year ago.

     On presentation the only abnormal physical finding is hepatosplenomegaly and possibly an audible pericardial friction rub. The estimated sedimentation rate is 45 and there are mild elevations of his liver function studies. He is noted to have fever as high as 39.6 °C (103.3 °F), which occurs twice per day.

     The most likely diagnosis is:
     A) Lymphoma
     B) Juvenile arthritis
     C) Somatoform disorder
     D) Endocarditis

Answer: B

The most difficult causes of fever of unknown origin (FUO) involve those without specific diagnostic tests, many autoimmune diseases such as juvenile rheumatoid arthritis (JRA) adult Still's disease fall into that category. In a young adult with a prolonged or recurrent FUO, an ongoing negative workup suggests autoimmune or somatoform disorder. One of the key goals of an FUO admission is the controlled observation of fever curves. Several factors can be accomplished during the admission: is it factitious, what is the fever's pattern, and does the fever respond to antipyretics. In this case, the double quotidian pattern is suggestive of JRA. Other clues to the diagnosis include hepatosplenomegaly, serositis, and mild hepatitis. Other clues include tenosynovitis, lymphadenopathy, and transient salmon pink macules.

References

Hoffart C and Sherry DD Early identification of juvenile idiopathic arthritis. Journal of Musculoskeletal Medicine. 2010;247 (2).

Ringold S, Burke A, Glass R (2005). "JAMA patient page. Juvenile idiopathic arthritis". JAMA 294 (13): 1722.

112. A 75-year-old male with a history of heart failure, hypertension, and stage 3 chronic kidney disease is admitted to the hospital with shortness of breath.

On physical exam, the temperature is 36.4 C (97.5 F), pulse rate is 108 per minute, respirations are 24 per minute, and blood pressure is 100/60 mmHg. Crackles are heard halfway up both lungs. Edema (2+ to 3+) is noted in the legs. Serum creatinine is 1.8 mg/dL.

Home medications are furosemide 40 mg orally twice daily, lisinopril 20 mg daily, and a beta-adrenergic blocking agent.

Radiograph of the chest reveals diffuse pulmonary edema. Electrocardiogram shows left ventricular hypertrophy but no acute ischemia.

Which of the following furosemide treatment strategies is most likely to result in a shorter hospital stay for this patient?

A) There is no difference among dosages and administration routes.
B) Intravenous furosemide through continuous infusion, 80 mg daily.
C) Intravenous furosemide through continuous infusion, 200 mg daily.
D) Intravenous furosemide, 100 mg every 12 h dosage.
E) Intravenous furosemide, 40 mg every 12 h.

Answer: A

A large randomized trial looked at low dose, based on home furosemide dose versus high (2.5 times the home dose) furosemide treatment strategies and bolus versus continuous infusion. There was no difference in in-hospital or overall mortality or length of hospital stay.

There was a very slight benefit for patients in the high-dose strategy group who had dyspnea.

Reference

Felker GM, Lee KL, Bull DA, et al. Diuretic strategies in patients with acute decompensated heart failure. N Engl J Med. 2011;364(9):797–805.

113. A 58-year-old woman who has COPD was admitted for an acute exacerbation. She is now ready for discharge. You bring up the issue of smoking cessation.

The patient has smoked one pack of cigarettes daily for 30 years. In the hospital she expresses a desire to quit smoking, but she is unwilling to set a definite quit date. The patient is physically active, and she has no other medical problems. Her COPD symptoms have been well controlled with inhaled tiotropium. One year ago, FEV1 was 60 % of predicted, and FVC was 80 % of predicted.

Which of the following should you recommend for smoking cessation?

A) Recommend she try to quit "cold turkey."
B) Recommend that she try nonprescription nicotine replacement and use a telephone quit line.
C) Recommend she return to the office when she is ready to set a quit date.
D) Prescribe varenicline and recommend that the patient try to set a quit date sometime between one and five weeks, scheduling a return visit to the office a week after her quit.

Answer: D

A hospitalization is an excellent opportunity to address a variety of lifestyle interventions. Obviously smoking cessation is the most important. The patient has time and possibly new motivation to undertake this endeavor. It is important to stay up-to-date on new methods.

A stop date should be suggested. An opportunity exists while the patient is in the hospital to clean the house of triggers of smoking as well as bring in family members to support the decision.

Individuals willing to make a quit attempt should be given the best chance possible. In general, this may require pharmacotherapy combined with counseling support. Varenicline has greater efficacy than either nicotine replacement or bupropion. A variable stop date strategy has been studied with varenicline with favorable results.

Reference

Rennard S et al. A randomized placebo-controlled trial of varenicline for smoking cessation allowing flexible quit dates. Nicotine Tob Res 2012;14:343–350.

114. A 20-year-old college student presents to the emergency room with a chief complaint of diarrhea, nausea, vomiting, abdominal pain, fever, and chills. He also reports decreased urine output. He recently returned from Central America where he has been taking an archaeology course.

On physical examination, his temperature is 38.3 °C,(101 °F), blood pressure is 120/80, and pulse rate is 120. Oral mucosa is dry. He has diffuse abdominal pain with mild guarding.

Laboratory studies reveal hemoglobin of 8.5 g/dL, leukocyte count of 16,000 μl, and a platelet count of 38,000 μl. Peripheral blood smear reveals many schistocytes. Urinalysis reveals many erythrocytes and erythrocyte casts. Urine protein-to-creatinine ratio is 0.6.

Which of the following is the most likely cause of the patient's acute kidney injury?

A) Hemolytic uremic syndrome
B) Acute tubular necrosis
C) Post-infectious glomerulonephritis
D) Scleroderma renal crisis
E) Sepsis

Answer: A

This patient has hemolytic uremic syndrome. It was probably caused by *Escherichia coli*, in particular the O157: H7 strain. This strain produces a *Shigella*-like toxin that is effective against small blood vessels, like those found in the digestive tract and kidneys.

In developing countries, infections usually develop after ingesting contaminated food or water. In developed countries sporadic outbreaks have occurred, often associated with food vendors.

This patient has the triad of microangiopathic hemolytic anemia, schistocytes, and thrombocytopenia. Patients with acute tubular necrosis are more likely to present with muddy brown casts. Post-infectious glomerulonephritis commonly occurs after Streptococcal and Staphylococcal infections. Scleroderma renal crisis is characterized by an acute onset of hypertension, kidney failure, and microangiopathic hemolytic anemia. Scleroderma renal crisis is not associated with bloody diarrhea. In addition, the absence of skin findings makes this diagnosis unlikely.

Reference

Safdar N, Said A, Gangnon RE, Maki DG. Risk of hemolytic uremic syndrome after antibiotic treatment of Escherichia coli O157:H7 enteritis: a meta-analysis. JAMA. 2002;288(8):996–1001.

115. A 74-year-old man with a history of cirrhosis and ascites presents with spiking fevers, abdominal pain, and progressive abdominal distention over the last week. He is immediately started on broad-spectrum antibiotics and albumin for possible spontaneous bacterial peritonitis (SBP).

What is the demonstrated benefit of adjuvant albumin treatment in this patient?

A) Improvement in underlying cirrhosis
B) No published data to support benefit
C) Prevention of worsening renal failure and
D) Improvement in 1 and 3-month survival
E) C and D

Answer: E

Current guidelines call for adjuvant albumin therapy in the treatment of SBP. Based on a large prospective randomized trial, albumin infusion (1.5 g/kg on day 1 and 1 g/kg on day 3) along with antibiotics prevented worsening renal failure with 1 and 3-month survival advantage.

Reference

Runyon BA. Management of adult patients with ascites due to cirrhosis: an update. Hepatology 2009;49:2087–107.

116. A 57-year-old oyster fisherman is admitted with severe pain in his right hand and arm. Past medical history is positive for hemochromatosis and cirrhosis of his liver.

On physical exam his vitals reveal a pulse of 110 bpm, a blood pressure of 90/60 mmHg, and a temperature of 38.3 °C(101 ° F). His right hand is very swollen and is red with blackened hemorrhagic bullous lesions. It is extremely tender.

What is the likely cause of the above condition?

A) Group A β-hemolytic streptococcus
B) Staphylococcus aureus
C) Aeromonas hydrophila
D) Clostridium perfringens
E) Vibri*o vulnificus*

Answer: E

V. vulnificus is usually found in warm, shallow, coastal salt water in temperate climates. It can be found estuaries from the Gulf of Mexico, along most of the East Coast of the United States, and along much of the West Coast of the United States. Filter feeders such as oysters pose a particularly high risk. *V. vulnificus* septicemia is the most common cause of death from seafood consumption in the United States.

Necrotizing fasciitis caused by *V. vulnificus* is extremely aggressive. It progresses more rapidly than either methicillin-resistant *Staphylococcus aureus* or methicillin-sensitive *S. aureus* infection. Most patients infected with *V. vulnificus* have bullous skin lesions. Effective antibiotics include tetracycline, third-generation cephalosporins, and imipenem. Often two agents are used. Early surgical consultation is advised.

Reference

Choi HJ, Lee DK, Lee MW, Choi JH, Moon KC, Koh JK. Vibrio vulnificus septicemia presenting as purpura fulminans. J Dermatol. 2005;32(1):48–51.

117. A 77-year-old woman who has been admitted to the hospital for community-acquired pneumonia has developed palpitations that began approximately one-half hour ago. She has a history of hypertension and preserved cardiac function. Ejection fraction is 65 %. Medications are hydrochlorothiazide, aspirin, and ceftriaxone.

On physical examination, she is afebrile. Blood pressure is 110/70 mmHg. Heart rate is 160 bpm.

Respiration rate is 25. Oxygen saturation is 90 %. Cardiac auscultation reveals a regular, tachycardic rhythm. Mild expiratory wheezes are heard throughout her lung fields.

Which of the following is the most appropriate acute treatment?
A) Adenosine
B) Amiodarone
C) Cardioversion
D) Diltiazem
E) Metoprolol

Answer: A

The patient presents with a supraventricular tachycardia that may or may not be atrial fibrillation. She is hemodynamically stable but requires semi-urgent conversion to normal sinus rhythm. Considerations would include beta-blockers, but as she is currently experiencing a moderate degree of reactive airway disease. Beta-blockers may not be the best option. Adenosine may be useful for diagnosing and treating supraventricular tachycardia. It can treat atrioventricular node-dependent tachycardias such as atrioventricular reentrant tachycardia. It is not useful in the treatment of atrial fibrillation.

Urgent electrocardioversion may be considered if needed urgently, but this must be weighed against the risk of a thrombotic event occurring in a patient who is not anticoagulated. Diltiazem could be considered; however, this may lower her blood pressure. Adenosine may control her rate or reveal atrial fibrillation and is an appropriate choice in this situation.

The recommended initial dose is 6.0 mg. In patients who fail to convert to normal sinus rhythm, the dose may be increased to 12.0 mg.

Reference
Link MS. Clinical practice. Evaluation and initial treatment of supraventricular tachycardia. N Engl J Med. 2012; 367(15):1438–48

118. A 40-year-old male presents to the emergency department with 2-day history of hemoptysis. He reports that he has been coughing up 2–5 tablespoons of blood each day. He reports mild chest pain, low-grade fevers, and weight loss. He reports that he has had similar mild symptoms for about one year. This has included frequent epistaxis and purulent discharge. He has been treated with several courses of antibiotics. He is otherwise healthy. His only medications are daily aspirin and lovastatin.

On physical examination, he has normal vital signs, and the upper airway is notable for saddle nose deformity and clear lungs. A CT of the chest shows multiple cavitating nodules, and urinalysis shows red blood cells.

Which of the following tests offers the highest diagnostic yield to make the appropriate diagnosis?
A) Deep skin biopsy
B) Surgical lung biopsy
C) Pulmonary angiogram
D) Percutaneous kidney biopsy
E) Upper airway biopsy

Answer: B

This patient has granulomatosis with polyangiitis, formerly known as Wegner's. The diagnosis is made by demonstration of necrotizing granulomatous vasculitis on biopsy. Pulmonary tissue offers the highest yield. The patient presents with classic symptoms for granulomatosis with polyangiitis. The average age of diagnosis is 40 years and there is a male predominance. Upper respiratory symptoms including sinusitis and epistaxis often predate lung or renal findings. This may present with septal perforation. Biopsy of the upper airway usually shows the granulomatous inflammation. Lung biopsy is often needed to demonstrate vasculitis. Renal biopsy may show the presence of pauci-immune glomerulonephritis.

References
Falk RJ, Gross WL, Guillevin L et al. Granulomatosis with polyangiitis (Wegener's): An alternative name for Wegener's granulomatosis. BMJ. 2011; Ann. Rheum. Dis. 70: 74
Fauci AS, Haynes BS, Katz P, Wolff SM. Wegener's granulomatosis: prospective clinical and therapeutic experience with 85 patients for 21 years. Ann Intern Med. 1983; 98(1):76–85.

119. A 78-year-old male presents with worsening confusion and progressive memory loss over the past four weeks. He has a history of mild dementia but has been living independently. Family members report that his mild memory loss has been stable for the past two years until now. He has been in the hospital for one week and despite extensive workup including computed tomography of the head, EEG, and cerebrospinal fluid analysis, no definitive diagnosis has been found.

By the second week of his hospitalization, his mental status has deteriorated further. Myoclonus not present on admission is now seen in his right arm.

The most likely diagnosis is:
A) Creutzfeldt–Jakob disease (CJD)
B) Multi-infarct dementia
C) Recurrent seizure disorder
D) Catatonic depression
E) Herpes simplex encephalitis

Answer: A

The differential diagnosis of a rapidly progressive dementia is limited. The clues to CJD in this patient are the relatively normal head imaging, the unexplained rapid onset of dementia, and the eventual appearance of myoclonus.

Initially, individuals experience problems with muscular coordination; personality changes, including impaired memory, judgment, and thinking; and impaired vision. EEG, which may initially be normal, but often demonstrates a typical triphasic spike pattern. Criteria have been developed to confirm the diagnoses. A confirmatory protein can be measured in cerebrospinal fluid. CJD remains a diagnostic challenge with an average of seven months passing before initial symptoms and confirmation of a diagnosis.

Imaging studies are emerging as valuable tools in diagnosing CJD, with evidence that diffusion-weighted imaging (DWI) and magnetic resonance imaging (MRI) sequences are more useful than electroencephalography. Paraneoplastic syndromes which can cause a rapid diffuse encephalopathy can present in a similar picture. A focused workup for malignancy would be warranted in this case as well.

There are investigational therapies available, but treatment is primarily supportive. Rapid progression of the disease and death are the usual outcome.

Reference
Takada LT, Geschwind MD. Prion diseases. Semin Neurol. 2013;33(4):348–56.

120. A 38-year-old female with a history of heroin addiction is admitted for withdrawal symptoms consisting of diarrhea, nausea, and vomiting. On admission, her pulse is 120 beats per minute, respirations are 20 per minute, and blood pressure is 120/70. Oxygen saturation is 94 %. She is mildly agitated. Her agitation and mild psychosis is treated with benzodiazepines and haloperidol. Her nausea is treated with Phenergan.

On her second day of hospitalization, you are urgently called to her bedside. On physical examination, the patient has marked increased muscle tone. Her eyes are deviated superiorly, and she states that she has difficulty moving them. She appears distressed but can follow commands.

Which of the following treatments is most appropriate?
A) Lorazepam
B) Benztropine
C) Naloxone
D) Phenytoin load

Answer: B

This patient is likely experiencing an acute dystonic reaction. Acute drug-induced dystonia can be treated with anticholinergic agents such as benztropine or diphenhydramine. It is unlikely that this patient is experiencing a seizure. Acute dystonic reactions can include ocular dystonia with eye deviation. Typically, this is superior.

Dystonic reactions are rarely life threatening but the adverse effects often cause distress for patients and families. Medical treatment is usually rapidly effective. Motor disturbances resolve within minutes, but they can reoccur over subsequent days. IV is the route of choice.

Reference
Christodoulou C, Kalaitzi C. Antipsychotic drug-induced acute laryngeal dystonia: two case reports and a mini review. J Psychopharmacol. May 2005;19:307–11

121. A 38-year-old female is admitted to the hospital with fever, abdominal pain, and jaundice. She drinks approximately one-half liter of vodka per day. Her family reports a possible recent increase in alcohol intake. She is not taking any medications.

On physical examination, she appears ill and disheveled. Heart rate is 126 beats/min, blood pressure 92/56 mmHg, respiratory rate 22 bpm, temperature 38.4 °C (101.1 °F), and oxygen saturation 94 % on room air. She has scleral icterus, and spider angiomata are present on the trunk. There is a fullness in the right upper quadrant. It is smooth and tender upon palpation. The spleen is not palpable.

Laboratory studies demonstrate an AST of 543U/L, ALT of 215 U/L, bilirubin of 8.7 mg/dL, alkaline phosphatase of 217U/L, and lipase of 38U/L. Total protein is 4.9 g/dL, and albumin is 2.7 g/dL. The prothrombin time is 30.2 (control is 11) seconds. What is the best approach to the treatment of this patient?
A) Administer IV fluids, thiamine, and folate, and observe for improvement in liver function studies.
B) Administer IV fluids, thiamine, folate, and broad-spectrum antibiotics.
C) Administer prednisone 40 mg daily for 4 weeks.
D) Perform abdominal ultrasound.
E) Perform an abdominal CT with IV contrast to assess for necrotizing pancreatitis.

Answer: C

This patient has severe acute alcoholic hepatitis. Treatment with prednisone 40 mg daily for four weeks should be initiated. If steroids are contraindicated, pentoxifylline 400 mg three times daily for four weeks can also be used.

A discriminate function (DF) can be calculated as (4.6 × the prolongation of prothrombin time above control) + serum bilirubin. A DF greater than 32 is associated with a poor prognosis and is an indication for treatment with steroids. The Model for End-Stage Liver Disease (MELD) score can also be used in acute alcoholic hepatitis, with a score greater than 21 being an indication for treatment as well.

References

McCullough AJ, O'Connor JF. Alcoholic liver disease: proposed recommendations for the American College of Gastroenterology". Am. J. Gastroenterol.1998 93 (11): 2022–36.
Akriviadis E, Botla R, Briggs W, Han S, Reynolds T, Shakil O Pentoxifylline improves short-term survival in severe acute alcoholic hepatitis: a double-blind, placebo-controlled trial. Gastroenterology.2000; 119 (6): 1637–48.

122. A 47-year-old male is involved in a boating accident. He sustains multiple injuries to the face, chest, and hips. He was unresponsive on presentation and is intubated for airway protection. He is started on antibiotics. The patient is admitted to the intensive care unit (ICU) with multiple orthopedic injuries. He is stabilized medically and undergoes successful open reduction and internal fixation of the right femur and right humerus. He is transferred to the floor.

   He develops an unexplained elevated heart rate. Thyroid function is ordered. After his TSH is 0.2 mU/L, and the total T4 level is normal. T3 is 0.7 µg/dL.

   What is the most appropriate next management step?
   A) Initiation of levothyroxine
   B) Initiation of prednisone
   C) Observation
   D) Radioiodine uptake scan
   E) Thyroid ultrasound
   F) Stress dose steroids

Answer: C

This patient has euthyroid sick syndrome. Euthyroid sick syndrome is defined as abnormal findings on thyroid function tests that occur in the setting of a nonthyroidal illness. This can commonly occur in the setting of any severe illness. The most common hormone pattern is a decrease in total and unbound T3 levels as a peripheral conversion of T4 to T3 is impaired. Replacement therapy in critically ill patients has been studied with variable results. Very sick patients may have a decrease in T4 levels. This patient has abnormal thyroid function tests as a result of his injuries from an accident.

Traditionally no thyroid replacement is recommended. Replacement therapy has not been shown to be of benefit in the vast majority of critically ill patients. However, this is an area of active research . There is no prospective study to date demonstrating benefit or harm of thyroid hormone replacement in euthyroid sick states. The most appropriate management consists of observation. Thyroid function studies will return to normal in weeks to months.

Reference

Docter R, Krenning EP, de Jong M, Hennemann G. The sick euthyroid syndrome: changes in thyroid hormone serum parameters and hormone metabolism. Clin Endocrinol (Oxf). 1993;39(5):499–518.

123. Who of the following represents the best candidate for noninvasive positive-pressure ventilation?
   A) A 23-year-old woman with an asthma exacerbation who has been treated with bronchodilators and has dyspnea and bronchospasm despite 4 h of therapy
   B) A 51-year-old woman who is admitted with multilobar pneumonia and SpO2 of 82 % on FIO2 of 1.0 by nonrebreathing mask
   C) An 82-year-old man with dyspnea and pleuritic chest pain following ankle surgery and SpO2 of 78 % on FIO2 of 0.21.
   D) A 67-year-old man with a COPD exacerbation and arterial blood gas studies showing pH of 7.28, PCO2 of 68 mmHg, and PO2 of 60 mmHg on FIO2 of 0.21

Answer: D

Noninvasive positive-pressure ventilation (NPPV) is recommended for patients who have respiratory distress, but do not require emergent intubation. COPD exacerbation with ventilation abnormalities are often the best circumstances for its use.

The 67-year-old man is the best candidate for NPPV because he has hypercapnic acidosis due to a COPD exacerbation and does not require emergent intubation. Patients with moderate hypercapnia PaCO2 greater than 45 mmHg and less than 92 mmHg and moderate acidemia with a pH less than 7.35 and greater than 7.10 have a higher rate of success with NPPV.

Reference

Liesching T, Kwok H, Hill NS. Acute applications of noninvasive positive pressure ventilation. Chest. 2003;124: 699–713.

124. A 67-year-old male is admitted to the intensive care unit for sepsis due to a urinary tract infection. Gram stain of the blood shows a gram-negative rod. The patient receives aggressive fluid resuscitation consisting of 2 l of normal saline and appropriate antibiotics. Five hours after admission, the blood pressure remains at 79/37, and mean arterial pressure is 54 mmHg.

Which of the following vasopressor drugs should you order next?

A) Epinephrine
B) Norepinephrine
C) Phenylephrine
D) Vasopressin

Answer: B.

Norepinephrine and dopamine are considered first-line agents in the setting of septic shock nonresponsive to fluid. Norepinephrine has emerged from the various trials as the first choice of vasopressors based on randomized controlled trials, meta-analyses, and international consensus guidelines.

The surviving sepsis campaign lists norepinephrine as the first-line vasopressor with an evidence grade of 1BA. According to their guidelines, norepinephrine increases MAP due to its vasoconstrictive effects, with little change in heart rate and less increase in stroke volume compared with dopamine. Norepinephrine is more potent than dopamine and may be more effective at reversing hypotension in patients with septic shock.

Reference

Dellinger RP, Levy MM, Carlet JM, et al. Surviving Sepsis Campaign: international guidelines for management of severe sepsis and septic shock: 2008. Crit Care Med. 2008;36:296–327.

125. A 32-year-old man with amyotrophic lateral sclerosis (ALS) is admitted for feeding tube placement. During a preoperative exam, finger pulse oximetry is 86 % on room air, his lungs are clear. He reports feeling at his baseline and is not short of breath. His condition is intact. Chest radiograph shows low lung volumes but is otherwise normal.

On physical exam he appears mildly cachectic, no accessory respiratory muscles are being used. Lung sounds are diminished but clear.

Which of the following is most likely the source of his low oxygen saturation?

A) Atelectasis
B) Mucous plug
C) Elevated PaCO2
D) Pneumonia
E) Methemoglobinemia

Answer: C

The patient has a progressive neuromuscular disease and is at risk for the development of hypoventilation. Many patients with hypoventilation are relatively asymptomatic. Symptoms have a gradual onset, which is typical of

ALS. Further questioning about sleep quality, morning headache, and orthopnea may give clues to the hypoxia.

Elevations of PaCO2 alone can cause hypoxia. An arterial blood gas measurement in this case would show this with elevations in PaCO2, depressed PaO2, and a normal A-a gradient.

Reference

Miller RG, Jackson CE, Kasarskis EJ et al. Practice Parameter update: The care of the patient with amyotrophic lateral sclerosis: Drug, nutritional, and respiratory therapies (an evidence-based review). Report of the Quality Standards Subcommittee of the American Academy of Neurology. Neurology. 2009;73:1218–1226

126. A 35-year-old woman is admitted for worsening chronic elevated temperature and anxiety. She felt well until three months ago when she developed fevers to 38.3 °C (101.0 °F) associated with sweating and pruritus. The fevers last for hours to days and then are absent for five days before recurring. She has been seen by her primary care physician to have the symptoms twice. She underwent a urine test and blood work with no diagnosis. She traveled to Brazil six months ago.

She has no cough, chest pain, joint aches, or rash. She does note anorexia and occasional loose stools. She has lost 25 lbs. She has never lived or worked in an institutionalized setting.

Which clinical feature is most useful in narrowing the differential diagnosis?

A) Weight loss
B) Loose bowel movements
C) Pattern of fever
D) Eating fresh fruit
E) Anxiety

Answer: C

Fever patterns can assist in the diagnosis in fevers of unknown origin. Of the symptoms listed, it may be the most helpful in narrowing the diagnosis. This patient has fever of unknown origin – a fever that lasts three weeks or longer with temperatures exceeding 100.9 °F with no clear diagnosis despite 1 week of clinical investigation.

Fever lasting 3–10 days followed by afebrile periods of 3–10 days (Pel-Ebstein pattern) is seen in some lymphoma patients. In addition, sixteen percent of patients with Hodgkin's disease present with this cyclic. A shaking chill and fever lasting a few hours, improving with profuse sweating and coming every other day or every three days strongly suggests malaria.

She also has several other symptoms that suggest malignancy or chronic inflammation including weight loss and sweats, but these are nonspecific.

Reference

Hayakawa K, Ramasamy B, Chandrasekar PH. Fever of unknown origin: an evidence-based review. Am. J. Med. Sci.2012;344(4), 307–316)

127. A 31-year-old woman present with fever, dysuria and nausea. Her past medical history is unremarkable except for Vaginal delivery of a healthy baby one year ago, she has no known past medical history.

    On physical exam, her temperature is 39.0 °C(102.2 °F). Her pulse is 120 and BP is 160/90. Otherwise, her physical exam is unremarkable.

    Her urine culture is positive for *Staph. aureus*. Her first set of blood cultures are negative.

    Further initial workup and treatment should include:
    A) Oral bactrim
    B) IV vancomycin
    C) Echocardiography
    D) Repeat urine cultures, no antibiotics
    E) B and C

Answer: E

Despite no predisposing factors for *S. aureus* infection, isolation of the organism in the urine should always prompt an evaluation for alternative site of infection. This should include examinations of bone, joint, or vascular sources of infection. Patients with a known *S. aureus* urinary tract infection should have blood cultures drawn prior to the initiation of antibiotics to detect occult bacteremia.

It is not unusual to see a patient who is suspected of having a *S. aureus* UTI that is later shown to have a deep-seated *S. aureus* infection.

Fowler VG Jr., Sanders LL, Sexton DJ, et al. Outcome of Staphylococcus aureus bacteremia according to compliance with recommendations of infectious diseases specialists: experience with 244 patients. Clinical Infect Dis. 1998;27:478–86

128. A 67-year-old female is admitted to the hospital for progressive weakness over the past two months. She states she has been feeling depressed lately and is having a difficult time adjusting to the cold weather. Her family reports that she rarely leaves the house. She has no bowel movements for the past week. She denies any fluctuations of her weight.

    On physical exam, her blood pressure is 94/60 mmHg. She is thin. Her skin appears smooth and tan. Her mood is depressed, but she denies suicidal thoughts.

    Her sodium is 134 mEq/L, potassium 5.9 mEq/L, chloride 106 mEq/L, bicarbonate 19 mEq/L, BUN 10 mg/dL, creatinine 1.0 mg/dL, glucose 54 mg/dL, TSH 18 µU/mL, and free T4 0.1 ng/dL.

Which of the following is the best next step in management?
A) Refer her to a psychiatrist for her depression.
B) Start dexamethasone, and then oral levothyroxine, and perform a cosyntropin stimulation test.
C) Start hydrocortisone, and then oral levothyroxine, and perform a cosyntropin stimulation test.
D) Check cosyntropin stimulation test and start levothyroxine.

Answer: B

This patient has polyendocrine failure. This is likely Schmidt's syndrome, which is also known as autoimmune polyendocrine syndrome. Her labs are consistent with hypothyroidism and adrenal insufficiency. Hypothyroidism is indicated by labs showing an elevated TSH and decreased free T4. Adrenal insufficiency is presenting with a thin body habitus hyperkalemia, hypoglycemia, metabolic acidosis, and hyperpigmentation.

Adrenal insufficiency should be treated urgently before thyroid replacement. Dexamethasone will not interfere with the cosyntropin stimulation test. After starting dexamethasone, levothyroxine will help correct the patient's hypothyroidism. Then a cosyntropin stimulation test should be done to confirm the patient has adrenal insufficiency. If the test indicates that the patient does have adrenal insufficiency, then it would be appropriate to start replacement therapy with hydrocortisone.

Reference

Betterle C, Zanchetta R Update on autoimmune polyendocrine syndromes (APS). Acta Biomed . 2003;74 (1): 9–33.

129. An 89-year-old woman is admitted to the hospital for the evaluation of atypical chest pain. She describes the pain as pressure within the middle of her chest with radiation to the neck. During the past week, she has had several episodes with exertion and rest. Two episodes occurred in the last 24 h for which she took aspirin. ECG on admission was significant for ischemia, but is now normal. She is currently free of pain.

    She and her family request no further invasive cardiac procedures, including a left heart catheterization. They would like to maximize medical therapy. Her medications are aspirin, a multivitamin, and docusate.

    On physical examination, temperature is normal, blood pressure is 135/80 mmHg, pulse rate is 70/min, and respiration rate is 15 bpm.

In addition to aspirin and low-molecular-weight heparin, which of the following is the most appropriate treatment?

A) Diltiazem
B) Diltiazem, clopidogrel
C) Metoprolol
D) Metoprolol, atorvastatin, and clopidogrel
E) No additional therapy

Answer: D

Current American College of Cardiology/American Heart Association (ACC/AHA) guidelines recommend the use of statin therapy before hospital discharge for all patients with acute coronary syndrome (ACS) regardless of the baseline low-density lipoprotein. Recent findings suggested that the earlier the treatment is started after the diagnosis of ACS, the greater the expected benefit.

Despite the non-aggressive approach in this elderly patient here, beta-blockers, statins, and additional and platelet therapy are probably of benefit in this patient and should be well tolerated.

Reference

Angeli, F., Reboldi, G., Garofoli, M., Ramundo, E. and Verdecchia, P. Very early initiation of statin therapy and mortality in patients with acute coronary syndrome. Acute Card Care. 2012; 14: 34–39.

130. A 32-year-old female with chronic lower back pain on naproxen therapy presents to the emergency department following one episode of bright red hematemesis. In addition, she reports a 3-day history of dark, tarry stools. Following stabilization of the patient, gastroenterology was consulted and performed an EGD. The procedure report is pertinent for an ulcer.

    Which of the following is the lowest-risk stigmata for possible re-bleeding?

    A) A visible but non-bleeding vessel
    B) A clean base ulcer located in the duodenum
    C) An adherent clot
    D) Active oozing from the site of ulceration
    E) Non-bleeding clot

Answer: B

Patients with upper gastrointestinal bleed should undergo endoscopy within 24 h upon admission. This should be done after resuscitative efforts.

Stigmata of recent hemorrhage predict risk of further bleeding, length of stay, and management decisions. In descending risk of further bleeding, the lesion is active spurting, non-bleeding visible vessel, active oozing, adherent clot, flat pigmented spot, and clean base. Second-look endoscopy is recommended in certain situations.

Reference

Laine, Loren MD, Jensen, Dennis MD. Management of Patients with Ulcer Bleeding. Guidelines from the American College of Gastroenterology. Am J Gastroenterol 2012; 107:345–360;

131. A 63-year-old male with end-stage liver disease is admitted with spontaneous bacterial peritonitis and possible sepsis. He is started on broad-spectrum antibiotics. Twelve hours after admission, he is noted to be oozing from venipuncture sites. Platelet count is 35,000/µL, international normalized ratio is 2.9, hemoglobin is 6.1 mg/dL, and D-dimer is elevated to 4.8.

    DIC and his underlying liver disease are considered as possible source of his bleeding.

    What is the best way to distinguish between new-onset DIC and his underlying chronic liver disease?

    A) Blood culture
    B) Elevated fibrinogen degradation products
    C) Prolonged aPTT
    D) Serial laboratory analysis
    E) Reduced platelet count

Answer: D

Liver disease and disseminated intravascular coagulation (DIC) can present with similar coagulation profiles. Both entities may present with elevated fibrinogen degradation products, prolonged activated partial thromboplastin time and prothrombin time, anemia, and thrombocytopenia. Both may cause spontaneous bleeding.

When suspecting DIC, these tests should be repeated over a period of 6 h. Abnormalities may change in patients with severe DIC. In chronic liver disease, coagulation profiles would remain relatively stable.

Reference

Levi, M; Toh, C-H et al. (2009). "Guidelines for the diagnosis and management of disseminated intravascular coagulation". British Journal of Haematology 2009 145 (5): 24–33.

132. A 32-year-old female presents to the emergency room with severe pain in her upper back and knees for the past 12 h. She reports that this is typical for her usual sickle cell attacks. She also reports a mild productive cough and moderate shortness of breath. She states she is usually admitted 3–4 times per year.

    On physical examination, her temperature is 39.1 °C (102.4 °F), pulse rate is 100 beats per minute, and respirations are 26 per minute. Her blood pressure is 150/68. Oxygen saturation is 86 % by pulse oximetry. The lungs have diffuse moderate wheezes. No joint infiltration or edema is noted. Chest radiograph reveals a right middle lobe opacity. Laboratory studies are as follows: hematocrit is 22 %; hemoglobin is 6; leukocyte count is 12,800; and platelet count is 170,000.

In addition to intravenous fluids and pain management, which of the following is the next appropriate treatment?
A) Hydroxyurea
B) Exchange transfusion
C) Packed red blood cells
D) Ceftriaxone and erythromycin
E) Bronchodilators
F) D and E

Answer: D

This patient possibly has acute chest syndrome. This is an urgent and lethal complication of sickle cell disease and should be considered when a sickle cell patient is admitted with marked hypoxia. Treatment of acute chest syndrome consists of oxygen, antibiotics, incentive spirometry, simple transfusion, and bronchodilators.

Patients are immunocompromised due to the lack of a functional spleen. In this particular case, antibiotics against *S. pneumonia* and empiric addition of a macrolide antibiotic, because chlamydial and mycoplasmal infections are common, should be urgently given. Bronchodilators, which may be of some benefit, should be started as well. The role of corticosteroids in nonasthmatic patients with acute chest syndrome remains a topic of clinical research.

Exchange transfusions for the treatment of acute chest syndrome should be considered after antibiotics have been administered. This, however, is not the first line of treatment. Hydroxyurea is often given for chronic treatment of sickle cell disease but has no benefit in the acute setting. Transfusion greater than baseline will have no benefit as well.

References

Madden, JM; Hambleton, IR (Aug 2, 2014). "Inhaled bronchodilators for acute chest syndrome in people with sickle cell disease.". The Cochrane database of systematic reviews 8: CD003733.

Rees DC, Olujohungbe AD, Parker NE, Stephens AD, Telfer P, Wright J. Guidelines for the management of the acute painful crisis in sickle cell disease. Br J Haematol. Mar 2003;120(5):744–52.

133. A 65-year-old male with a history of COPD is admitted with a chief complaint of dyspnea, increased cough, and green sputum. The patient states he is on 2 l of oxygen at home. On the first night of admission, you are called to the patient's room where you find him ill-appearing and short of breath. This is a decline from his admission status twelve hours ago.

On physical exam, he has course wheezes. He is in moderate distress. He is able to answer questions with full sentences. O2 saturation is 85 % on 2 L of oxygen.

The most correct initial action is:
A) Immediate intubation.
B) Decrease the oxygen to 2 l.
C) Increase the oxygen to 6 l.
D) Perform an arterial blood gas (ABG).
E) Continue the O2 at 4 l and order a stat respiratory treatment.

Answer: C

Hypoxemia is the most immediate threat to life in patients with a declining COPD exacerbation. This patient's pulse oximetry of 85 % along with increased respiratory rate indicates severe hypoxemia. Although there is a concern for CO2 retention in patients with COPD, it should not stop the immediate goal of improving oxygenation.

This patient's oxygen should be immediately raised while considering further options. A reasonable goal of titrating oxygen is 90 % with continued direct observation. Several other modalities may be urgently considered after the oxygen has been increased. This includes noninvasive measures such as BiPAP and endotracheal intubation.

Reference

Decramer M, Janssens W, Miravitlles M. Chronic obstructive pulmonary disease". Lancet. 2012; 379 (9823): 1341–51.

134. A 62-year-old man is admitted to the hospital for palpitations and paroxysmal episodes of atrial fibrillation. Five days ago, he was discharged after an acute myocardial infarction. At that time, he received a drug-eluting stent in the left anterior descending coronary artery. Medications are lisinopril, digoxin, furosemide, aspirin, clopidogrel, eplerenone, simvastatin, and unfractionated heparin.

On physical examination, the patient is afebrile, blood pressure is 105/65 mmHg, and pulse rate is 83 min. He is in atrial fibrillation. Mild crackles are heard at the base of his lungs. CXR reveals evidence of mild fluid overload. Transthoracic echocardiogram shows left ventricular ejection fraction of 30 %.

Which of the following is the most appropriate treatment for this patient's atrial fibrillation?
A) Amiodarone
B) Disopyramide
C) Dronedarone
D) Flecainide
E) Sotalol

Answer: A

Amiodarone is the best option for managing symptomatic atrial fibrillation in the setting of congestive heart failure (CHF). Patients with heart failure and myocardial infarction are at an increased risk of developing atrial fibrillation. Amiodarone has β-blocking properties that can help with rate control.

Amiodarone has a class IIa recommendation from the American College of Cardiology for use as a rate-controlling agent for patients who are intolerant to other agents. Patients with CHF may not tolerate diltiazem or metoprolol. Caution should be exercised in those who are not receiving anticoagulation, as amiodarone can promote cardioversion. Flecainide is contraindicated after a myocardial infarction because it increases the risk of polymorphic ventricular tachycardia.

Disopyramide has negative inotropic effects, which would detrimental in the setting of reduced left ventricular function and heart failure. It is contraindicated in this setting.

References

McNamara RL, Tamariz LJ, Segal JB, Bass EB. Management of atrial fibrillation: review of the evidence for the role of pharmacologic therapy, electrical cardioversion, and echocardiography. Ann Intern Med. 2003;139(12):1018–33

Siddoway LA. Amiodarone: guidelines for use and monitoring. American Family Physician.2003; 68 (11): 2189–96

135. A 55-year-old man with a past medical history of gallstones presents to the emergency department with acute onset of fever, jaundice, and abdominal pain.

    On physical exam, the temperature is 38.3 °C(101.0 °F), heart rate of 92 bpm, and BP of 98/50. He has diffuse abdominal pain.

    Lab work is pertinent for elevated WBC of 16,500/μL predominantly with neutrophils, lipase of 600 units/L, AST 150 units/L, ALT 165 units/L, and a bilirubin of 4.0 μmol/L.

    Which is the following is the least appropriate next step?

    A) Aggressive hydration with 250–500 ml per hour of isotonic crystalloid solution.
    B) Stat trans abdominal ultrasound
    C) MRCP
    D) Empiric antibiotics
    E) Nasogastric suction

Answer: C

The diagnosis of acute pancreatitis is established by the presence of two of the three following criteria: abdominal pain consistent with the disease, serum amylase and/or lipase greater than three times the upper limit of normal, and/or characteristic findings from abdominal imaging.

Transabdominal ultrasound is the first test of choice and should be performed in all patients with acute pancreatitis. Contrast-enhanced computed tomography of the pancreas should be reserved for patients in whom the diagnosis is unclear. It is also indicated in patients who fail to improve clinically within the first 48–72 h after hospital admission. Aggressive hydration, at 250–500 ml per hour of isotonic solution, should be provided to all patients, unless cardiovascular or renal comorbidities exist. Early aggressive intravenous hydration is most beneficial in the first 12–24 h. Volume status should be assessed every 6 h. Antibiotics should be given for signs of infection, such as cholangitis. In patients with mild acute pancreatitis, found to have gallstones in the gallbladder, a cholecystectomy should be performed before discharge to prevent a recurrence of acute pancreatitis. Enteral nutrition is always preferred over parenteral if available.

Reference

Scott Tenner MD et al. Management of Acute Pancreatitis. American College of Gastroenterology. Am J Gastroenterol 2013; 108:1400–1415

136. A 66-year-old woman presents with a chief complaint of fever, nausea, and vomiting.

    On physical examination, she appears ill. Her temperature is 39.9 °C, blood pressure is 127/878, and pulse rate is 120 per minute. Laboratory studies reveal a leukocyte count of 23,000 with 87 % neutrophils. Urinalysis demonstrates >68 leukocytes/hpf and has a positive leukocyte esterase. Gram-negative rods are seen upon microscopic examination.

    She is admitted to the hospital with a diagnosis of probable urinary tract infection. On the second day of her hospitalization, her urine and blood cultures are positive for *Escherichia coli*, susceptible to piperacillin/tazobactam, ciprofloxacin, imipenem, ampicillin, and ceftriaxone.

    Which of the following is the most appropriate management?

    A) Continue piperacillin/tazobactam.
    B) Discontinue piperacillin/tazobactam and begin ampicillin.
    C) Discontinue piperacillin/tazobactam and begin ciprofloxacin.
    D) Discontinue piperacillin/tazobactam and begin ceftriaxone.

Answer: B

In this patient, broad-spectrum antibiotics on presentation are indicated. However, once the specific organism is isolated and sensitivities are known, it is beneficial to de-escalate therapy to a limited-spectrum antibiotic. De-escalation strategies involve not only changing antibiotics but can reduce dosage as well.

This may present as a challenge in a situation where a patient has responded well to a broad-spectrum antibiotic. However, failure to do so places the patient at additional risk for antibiotic-induced complications. Ciprofloxacin may be considered, but it provides unnecessarily broad-spectrum coverage.

Studies have shown that appropriate de-escalation improves outcomes in cases of sepsis and ventilator-related pneumonia.

References
Duchene E, Montassier E, Boutoille D, Caillon J, Potel G, Batard E. Why is antimicrobial de-escalation under-prescribed for urinary tract infections? Infection. 2013;41(1):211–214.

Garnacho-Montero J, Gutierrez-Pizarraya A, Escoresca-Ortega A, et al. De-escalation of empirical therapy is associated with lower mortality in patients with severe sepsis and septic shock. Intensive Care Med. 2014;40(1):32–40.

137. According to consensus guidelines, when should catheter-directed thrombolysis be considered in deep vein thrombosis?
    A) Patients who have a low bleeding risk
    B) Patients who have a high risk of postthrombotic syndrome
    C) Inferior vena cava thrombosis
    D) Should never be considered
    E) Both A, B, and C together should be present

Answer: E
Catheter-directed thrombolysis can be risky as compared to conventional treatment. Studies have shown conflicting benefits and risks. It should be used cautiously and limited to selected cases. Experts feel it may be reasonable to restrict catheter-directed thrombolysis to patients who have a low bleeding risk and have a high risk of post-thrombotic syndrome.

Some specific indications for thrombolytic intervention include the relatively rare phlegmasia or symptomatic inferior vena cava thrombosis that responds poorly to anticoagulation alone, or symptomatic iliofemoral or femoral popliteal DVT in patients with a low risk of bleeding.

Reference
Bjarnason H, Kruse JR, Asinger DA, Nazarian GK, Dietz CA Jr, Caldwell MD, et al. Iliofemoral deep venous thrombosis: safety and efficacy outcome during 5 years of catheter-directed thrombolytic therapy. J Vasc Interv Radiol. 1997;;8(3):405–18.

138. A 65-year-old female is evaluated for a 3-week history of increasing abdominal girth. She has alcoholic liver disease with cirrhosis. Her only medication is propranolol. At this time, she is not considered to be a transplant candidate.

On physical examination, the patient is alert and oriented. Temperature is 36.2 °C (97.2 °F), blood pressure is 110/58 mmHg, pulse rate is 64/min, and respiration rate is 18/min. There are no focal neurologic deficits. There is no asterixis. Abdominal examination reveals shifting abdominal dullness. There is 1+ lower extremity edema.

Laboratory studies show albumin 1.8 g/dL, blood urea nitrogen 8 mg/dL, serum creatinine 1.6 mg/dL (141 μmol/L), sodium 119 mEq/L. Her last recorded sodium one month ago was 121 mEq/L.

Which of the following is the most appropriate management for this patient's hyponatremia?
    A) 3 % saline
    B) Conivaptan
    C) Demeclocycline
    D) Fluid restriction

Answer: D
Hyponatremia is common in end-stage liver disease patients. Asymptomatic hyponatremia in patients with cirrhosis is a poor prognostic marker. Several studies have shown that hyponatremia is a strong predictor of early mortality, independent of MELD score.

In the absence of neurologic symptoms, rapid correction of sodium is not indicated. Fluid restriction and following sodium concentration are the correct initial treatment options. Some degree of hyponatremia can be allowed. Several guidelines recommend implementing fluid restriction only when the serum sodium level is less than 120 mEq/L.

Reference
Zenenberg, Robert; Carluccio, Alessia; Merlin, Mark. Hyponatremia: Evaluation and Management. Hospital Practice.2010;38 (1): 89–96,

139. A 37-year-old female is admitted to the hospital for fever, cough, and a 20-lb weight loss. An episode of thrush was reported six months ago in her medical history. She was lost to follow-up care.

On physical exam, her temperature is 38.9 C (102.0 F), pulse rate is 90 per minute, respirations are 21 per minute, and blood pressure is 110/85 mmHg. Thrush is still present. Breath sounds are decreased in the left upper lung. HIV antibodies are positive, CD4 lymphocyte count is 65/μL . Two of three acid-fast bacilli (AFB) smears are positive. Chest radiograph reveals an opacity and early cavitation in right upper lung.

The patient is treated with fluconazole for thrush. Four-drug antituberculous therapy is started after the sputum results are reviewed. Arrangements are being made for appropriate follow-up and surveillance of her tuberculosis medicines.

When should antiretroviral therapy be started?

A) Immediately
B) Four weeks after completing antituberculous therapy
C) Eight weeks after initiating antituberculous therapy
D) Three to six months after completing antituberculous therapy

Answer: A

There is often some confusion as to when to start antiretroviral therapy in patients presenting with infections and a new HIV diagnosis. It may be dependent on the type of infection. Often the recommendation is to start therapy after the cause of infection is resolved.

Two studies comparing early and delayed antiretroviral therapy suggest that starting within two to four weeks of initiating therapy for tuberculosis improves survival. This is important for hospitalists who may be tempted to wait to start antiviral therapy until the patient sees an infectious disease specialist several weeks later.

References

Abdool Karim SS, Naidoo K, Grobler A, et al. Integration of antiretroviral therapy with tuberculosis treatment. N Engl J Med. 2011;365(16):1492–1501.189)
Blanc FX, Sok T, Laureillard D, et al. Earlier versus later start of antiretroviral therapy in HIV-infected adults with tuberculosis. N Engl J Med. 2011;365(16):1471–1481.

140. A 68-year-old male is admitted with melena and coffee-ground emesis for the past two days. He has a history of rheumatoid arthritis, for which he takes ibuprofen 400 mg 2–3 times daily. He reports that he has increased his intake of this medicine over the past week due to an increase in his joint pains.

On physical examination, his heart rate is 90 beats per minute, the temperature is 36.0 ° C (98.6 °F), and respirations are 17 per minute. His blood pressure is 115/73 mmHg. He is originally started on intravenous pantoprazole 8 mg/h. The next morning he undergoes endoscopy that shows an active ulcer that has some slight oozing.

Which of the following is the most appropriate therapy for this patient?

A) Oral ranitidine 150 mg twice daily
B) Octreotide infusion for 48 h
C) Oral pantoprazole 40 mg by mouth every 12 h
D) Continue with an 8 mg/h pantoprazole infusion

Answer: C

Although IV pantoprazole is often initiated, oral pantoprazole has nearly 100 % bioavailability and may be utilized when the patient is able to take pills, and there is a low risk of rebleeding, as in this case. Investigators compared 30-day rebleeding rates in patients randomized to receive intravenous (IV) versus oral high-dose PPI treatment after successful endoscopic therapy for bleeding peptic ulcers. Rebleeding rates were similar in the IV-PPI and oral-PPI groups at 72 h 7 days and 30 days.

Octreotide is beneficial in acute variceal bleeding and may have a role in severe peptic ulcer disease when endoscopy is deferred or not available. H2-receptor antagonists are inferior to proton-pump inhibitors in the management of acute gastrointestinal bleeds.

Reference

JY Sung, Bing-Yee Suen, Justin CY Wu, James YW Lau, Jessica YL Ching, Vivian WY Lee, Philip WY Chiu, Kelvin KF Tsoi and Francis KL Chan. Effects of Intravenous and Oral Esomeprazole in the Prevention of Recurrent Bleeding from Peptic Ulcers after Endoscopic Therapy. The American Journal of Gastroenterology. 2014; 109, 1005–1010

141. A 37-year-old woman is admitted for dysphagia. She has not seen a physician in many years. She says her swallowing difficulty started two weeks ago. She has lost 20 lb in the past 6 months. She also complains of diarrhea and blurry vision. She has had occasional fevers for the past 4 or 5 months.

On physical exam, there is no thrush. The patient's chest and abdominal examinations are unremarkable; her cardiovascular examination shows tachycardia and her stools are heme positive. HIV rapid screen is positive.

What is the most likely diagnosis?

A) Epstein–Barr
B) Herpes simplex
C) Candida
D) Cytomegalovirus (CMV)
E) Kaposi's sarcoma

Answer: D

This patient has CMV esophagitis and probable CMV retinitis. The gastrointestinal tract is a major site of disease in HIV infection. Almost half of HIV-infected patients have GI symptoms as their first complication. In addition most HIV patients develop GI complications at some point. Endoscopy is the diagnostic test of choice for upper gastrointestinal HIV-associated esophageal disease.

Diseases commonly found include candidiasis, cytomegalovirus and herpes simplex virus infection (HSV), and Kaposi's sarcoma.

CMV typically presents with distal esophageal ulceration. HSV infection presents with multiple vesiculation and ulcerations. The lesions are round, multiple, well circumscribed, uniform, and smaller than those in CMV disease.

CMV is the most common cause of intraocular infection in patients with AIDS and should be considered with any visual complaint. This disease represents a reactivation of latent CMV infection. Before the advent of highly active antiretroviral therapy (HAART), CMV was the most common opportunistic infection in AIDS patients with a CD4+ cell count below 50/mL.

Reference
Springer KL, Weinberg A. Cytomegalovirus infection in the era of HAART: fewer reactivations and more immunity. J Antimicrob Chemother. 2004;54(3):582–6.

142. A 28-year-old female presents to the emergency room with a chief complaint of new-onset bruises to her thighs and some mild bleeding of her gums. She reports that she is otherwise feeling well and has no past medical history. Her menstrual periods are reported to be normal. She reports taking no medications.

On physical exam, she appears well except for the reported bruises on her lower legs and arms. Some petechial is noted in her gums. Laboratory studies revealed a hemoglobin of 13, a leukocyte count of 6,500/μL, and a platelet count of 14,000/μL. A peripheral blood smear is normal. Rapid HIV screening is normal.

Which of the following is the most appropriate management?
A) Platelet transfusions
B) Prednisone 1 mg/kg daily
C) Plasmapheresis
D) Rituximab
E) Immunoglobulin

Answer: B
This patient has idiopathic thrombocytopenic purpura (ITP). ITP often occurs in an otherwise healthy person. On complete blood cell count, isolated thrombocytopenia is the hallmark of ITP. Anemia or neutropenia may indicate other diseases. ITP has no cure, and relapses may occur years after successful initial medical or surgical management. The most frequent cause of death in association with ITP is spontaneous or accidental trauma-induced intracranial bleeding. Most adult cases are diagnosed in women aged 30–40 years, although it may be seen in a wide age distribution in adults. Onset in a patient older than 60 years is uncommon, and a search for other causes of thrombocytopenia is warranted. The primary treatment for this is oral prednisone and it is usually responsive. Platelet transfusion is reserved for incidences of life-threatening bleeding. Plasmapheresis is not first-line therapy for ITP nor is rituximab, which may be considered as second-line therapy. Splenectomy is reserved for resistant cases and should not be considered at this time. HIV screening is appropriate as ITP commonly occurs in this group and may be the first sign of HIV infection.

Reference
Stasi R, Evangelista ML, Stipa E, et al. Idiopathic thrombocytopenic purpura: current concepts in pathophysiology and management. Thromb Haemost. 2008;99(1):4–13.

143. A 56-year-old woman is admitted with worsening confusion. She has a history of hepatitis C virus infection. She currently takes phenytoin 100 mg TID for seizure disorder. She has been on the same dose for many years. Lactulose 30 g TID and spironolactone 25 mg daily are taken for her liver disease.

On physical examination, her blood pressure is 110/65 mmHg, heart rate is 87 beats/min, respiratory rate is 22 breaths/min, and oxygen saturation is 97 % on room air. She is afebrile. She is minimally responsive to voice and follows no commands. Her abdomen is distended with a positive fluid wave but without tenderness. She does not appear to have asterixis. She has a horizontal nystagmus on examination. The white blood cell count is 12,000/μL with a normal differential. Her liver function tests are unchanged from baseline with the exception of an albumin that is now 2.1 g/dL compared with three months ago when her level was 2.9 g/dL. The ammonia level is 15 μmol/L, and her phenytoin level is 17 mg/L. A paracentesis shows a white blood cell count of 90/μL.

What test would be most likely to demonstrate the cause of the patient's change in mental status?
A) CT scan of the head
B) Free phenytoin level
C) Electroencephalogram (EEG))
D) Gram stain of ascites fluid
E) Gram stain of cerebrospinal fluid (CSF)

Answer: B
This patient has phenytoin toxicity due to her chronic liver disease. Signs and symptoms of phenytoin toxicity include slurred speech, horizontal nystagmus, and altered mental status that can progress to obtundation and coma. Worsening hypoalbuminemia can lead to increased free levels of drugs that are more highly protein bound. This can lead to drug toxicity at total drug levels that are not typically considered toxic.

Medications that are bound to plasma proteins include phenytoin, warfarin, valproic acid, and amiodarone. Although phenytoin is not contraindicated in those with mild liver disease, it should be discontinued in individuals with evidence of cirrhosis.

Reference
De Schoenmakere G, De Waele J, Terryn W, Deweweire M, Verstraete A, Hoste E, et al. Phenytoin intoxication in critically ill patients. Am J Kidney Dis. 2005;45(1):189–92.

144. A 55-year-old female not on any medication presents with a 3-month history of worsening rash, fever to 38.2 °C (100.8 °F), weight loss, and worsening loss of sensation in her feet.

On physical examination, you note tender palpable purpura of the bilateral lower leg. In addition, tract marks on the arms are present. Her laboratories indicate a Hg of 9.5 g/L and a creatinine of 2.5 mg/dL. Gross proteinuria is noted on urinalysis. Baseline creatinine is 1.2 mg/dL from 6 months ago.

Which lab abnormality would you expect?
A) Positive hepatitis B surface antigen
B) Positive anti-SSA and SSB
C) Positive antihistone antibody
D) Elevated TSH and low ferritin
E) Positive P-ANCA

Answer: A

The patient's clinical scenario is consistent with a systemic vasculitis. Symptoms are consistent with nephrotic syndrome and polyarteritis nodosa (PAN); both of which occur in hepatitis B-induced vasculitis. HBV-associated vasculitis almost always takes the form of PAN.

Dermatologic symptoms are very common in PAN. Skin involvement, which can be painful, occurs most frequently on the legs.

While lupus may be a possibility, antihistone antibody is most commonly associated with drug-induced lupus and this patient is no medications. In addition, drug-induced lupus is less likely to cause renal disease.

The presence of injection marks or history of intravenous drugs makes the acquisition of hepatitis B more likely.

Reference
Trepo C, Guillevin L. Polyarteritis nodosa and extrahepatic manifestations of HBV infection: the case against autoimmune intervention in pathogenesis. J Autoimmun. 2001;16(3):269–74

145. A 55-year-old white man with a history of hypertension and diabetes mellitus is admitted for diverticulitis. He presents with left lower quadrant abdominal pain. He undergoes an ultrasound in the emergency room which reveals an incidental finding of three gallstones measuring 1×1 cm were seen. The gallbladder and biliary tract is otherwise normal.

In the hospital, he has a good response to antibiotics and is ready for discharge. This was his first episode of diverticulitis. He reports no other episodes of abdominal pain to suggest biliary disease.

What is the correct advice concerning management of his gallstones?
A) Recommend not having surgery and continue to monitor clinically
B) Recommend in patient cholecystectomy
C) Recommend surgery in four weeks
D) HIDA scan

Answer: A

Prophylactic cholecystectomy is not indicated for this patient. Observation is the appropriate management. The consensus is that with a few exceptions asymptomatic gallstones should be followed. Most patients with asymptomatic gallstones will never develop symptoms.

There are instances where prophylactic cholecystectomy should be considered. These are when a patient is immunocompromised, awaiting organ transplantation, sickle cell disease, calculi greater than 3 cm in diameter, or when gallbladder cancer is likely. Cholecystectomy can be considered when other biliary tract abnormalities are present.

In the past patients with diabetes mellitus were thought to be at higher risk, and prophylactic cholecystectomy was often recommended. Studies have shown that prophylactic cholecystectomy is of no clear benefit and should not be routinely recommended for diabetics.

Patients with no other risk factors but who are going to be living or traveling for a long period of time in a location that is far from basic medical care such as missionary work, scientific expeditions, or space travel may be advised to have cholecystectomy prophylactically.

Reference
Gupta SK, Shukla VK. Silent gallstones: a therapeutic dilemma. Trop Gastroenterol. 2004;25(2):65–8.

146. A 34-year-old man presents to the physician complaining of yellow eyes. For the past week, he has felt ill with decreased oral intake, low-grade fevers, fatigue, nausea, and occasional vomiting. With the onset of jaundice, he has noticed pain in his right upper quadrant. He has a prior history of injection drug use with cocaine.

On physical examination, he appears ill and has obvious jaundice with scleral icterus. His liver is 14 cm upon percussion and is palpable 6 cm below the right costal margin. The edge is smooth and tender upon palpation. The spleen is not enlarged. There are no stigmata of chronic liver disease. His AST is 1475 U/L, ALT is 1678 U/L, alkaline phosphatase is 547 U/L, total bilirubin is 13.8 mg/dL, and direct bilirubin is 13.2 mg/dL. His INR is 2.4, and aPTT is 49 s. Serologic tests for hepatitis B surface antigen (HBsAg) and hepatitis B core antibody (anti-HBc) immunoglobulin M (IgM) are positive.

Which of the following is the correct treatment?

A) Administration of anti-hepatitis A virus IgG.
B) Administration of lamivudine.
C) Administration of pegylated interferon α plus ribavirin.
D) Administration of prednisone
E) Do nothing and observe

Answer: E

No treatment is recommended for acute hepatitis B in most individuals. Close observation is warranted with possible hepatology consultation. Full recovery is the expected outcome. 99 % of infected individuals recover without intervention.

However, patients with hepatitis B disease and fulminant hepatic failure should be hospitalized in the intensive care unit and be considered as liver transplant candidates in the event that they do not recover.

Reference

Sorrell MF, Belongia EA, Costa J, Gareen IF, Grem JL, Inadomi JM, et al. National Institutes of Health Consensus Development Conference Statement: Management of hepatitis B. Ann Intern Med. 2009;150(2):104–10.

147. A 63-year-old woman with primary biliary cirrhosis which is being considered for liver transplantation is admitted for worsening ascites and shortness of breath. She has been followed closely by the hepatology service.

In the past six weeks, she has had three paracenteses performed. Today, the shortness of breath has returned, but she has no fever, cough, or chills. She reports meticulous attention to her sodium-restricted diet.

On physical examination, she is afebrile. Pulse rate is 90 per minute, respirations are 24 per minute, and blood pressure is 108/57 mmHg. Breath sounds are absent in the lower half of the right lung field; other pulmonary findings are normal. The abdomen is distended, with a prominent fluid wave. She exhibits no confusion or asterixis.

Ultrasonography of the liver reveals a nodular liver with patent hepatic vasculature; no focal mass was detected. Labs reveal an of INR 1.5, a serum creatinine of 1.4 mg/dL, and a sodium of 140. Her MELD score is 18.

Which of the following should you recommend?

A) Serial paracenteses
B) Serial thoracenteses
C) Chest tube placement on the right side
D) Transjugular intrahepatic portosystemic shunt (TIPS)

Answer: D

Refractory ascites may be treated with a TIPS procedure. Previous meta-analysis shows possible benefit, especially in those listed for transplant. Indications for TIPS include uncontrolled variceal hemorrhage from esophageal, gastric, and intestinal varices that do not respond to endoscopic and medical management, refractory ascites, and hepatic pleural effusion (hydrothorax). Repeat paracentesis is unlikely to be of benefit in this patient. Chest tube placement is not recommended in patients with end-stage liver disease.

All patients undergoing transjugular intrahepatic portosystemic shunt placement should receive prophylactic antibiotics. Resuscitation with fluid and blood products is indicated prior to the procedure. Portal vein patency should be confirmed prior to attempts at TIPS placement.

References

Fidelman N, Kwan SW, LaBerge JM, et al. The transjugular intrahepatic portosystemic shunt: an update. AJR Am J Roentgenol. 2012;199(4):746–755.

Krok KL, Cardenas A. Hepatic hydrothorax. Semin Respir Crit Care Med. 2012;33(1):3–10. Epub 2012 Mar 23.

148. A 71-year-old woman is admitted from a nursing home with confusion, fever, and flank pain. She has a presumed urinary tract infection.

On physical exam, temperature is 38.8 °C (101.8 °F), blood pressure is 86/52 mmHg, pulse rate is 130/min, and respiration rate is 23/min. Mucous membranes are dry and tender, and poor skin turgor is noted. She is oriented to name and place.

Hemoglobin concentration is 9.5 g/dL and leukocyte count is 15,600/μL; urinalysis reveals 100 to 150 leukocytes/hpf and many bacteria/hpf. The patient has an increase anion gap metabolic acidosis. The patient is admitted to the intensive care unit and antibiotic therapy is started.

Which of the following is the first goal of therapy?

A) Aggressive fluid resuscitation
B) Hemodynamic monitoring with a pulmonary artery catheter
C) Maintaining hemoglobin concentration above 12 g/dL (120 g/L)
D) Maintaining PCO2 below 50 mmHg
E) Initiation of vasopressor drugs

Answer: A

The patient has severe sepsis from pyelonephritis. Initial treatment includes respiratory and circulatory support. The first 6 h of resuscitation of a critically ill patient with sepsis or septic shock are the most critical. Resuscitation of the circulation should target a central venous oxygen saturation or mixed venous oxygen saturation of at least 70 %.

This often requires of 5 to 6 L of fluid. The time required to achieve resuscitative goals matters to survival. Early goal-directed therapy that within the first 6 h maintains a SCVO2 of greater than 70 % and resolves lactic acidosis results in higher survival rates than more delayed resuscitation attempts.

Blood transfusion may be part of resuscitation for anemic patients in shock. In stable patients who are not in shock, a transfusion threshold of 7 g/dL is acceptable. There are no data to support that maintaining a lower PCO2 is of any benefit. Placement of a pulmonary artery catheter would not help to increase survival in this patient.

Reference

Rivers, E; Nguyen, B; Havstad, S; Ressler, J et al.. Early goal-directed therapy in the treatment of severe sepsis and septic shock. The New England Journal of Medicine 345 (19): 1368–77

149. A 63-year-old female smoker presents to the emergency department with an onset of worsening dyspnea, wheezing, and coughing x 3 days. She denies any fever or chills. She has not been treated for COPD in the past. The results of her spirometry test three week ago are FEV1 < 60 % of predicted and DLCO was decreased.

    She is on short-acting inhaled beta agonists at home. She is admitted for COPD exacerbation and improves to her baseline respiratory status with steroids and nebulized albuterol treatments. Her oxygen saturation on discharge is 89 % on room air with a PaO2 of 54 mmHg.

    Which of the following are appropriate treatment modalities to initiate for this patient upon discharge?
    A) Initiate long-acting inhaled B-agonist in conjunction with break through inhaled short-acting anticholinergic agent.
    B) Prescribe continuous supplemental oxygen therapy.
    C) Recommend wearing oxygen supplementation only during exertion.
    D) Begin inhaled corticosteroids as monotherapy.
    E) All of the above.
    F) A and B.
    G) B and D.

Answer: F

Guidelines suggest that clinicians may administer a combination of long-acting inhaled anticholinergics, long-acting inhaled β-agonists, or inhaled corticosteroids for symptomatic patients with stable COPD and FEV1 < 60 % predicted.

The American College of Chest Physicians recommends that clinicians should prescribe continuous oxygen therapy in patients with COPD who have severe resting hypoxemia defined as Pao2 ≤ 55 mmHg or Spo2 ≤ 88 %.

Spirometry is used to diagnose obstructive airway disease in a patient with respiratory symptoms. Spirometry is best assessed outside of periods of exacerbation. A diagnosis of obstructive airway disease is defined as a FEV1 < 80 % or an FEV1/FVC ratio < 70 % of predicted.

Reference

Amir Qaseem, MD, PhD, MHA; Timothy J. Wilt, MD, MPH et al. Diagnosis and Management of Stable Chronic Obstructive Pulmonary Disease: A Clinical Practice Guideline Update from the American College of Physicians, American College of Chest Physicians, American Thoracic Society, and European Respiratory Society. Ann Intern Med. 2011;155(3):179–191.

150. An 81-year-old man is admitted to the hospital for altered mental status. He was found at home, confused and lethargic, by his son. His medical history is significant for metastatic prostate cancer.

    On physical examination, he is afebrile. Blood pressure is 110/50 mmHg, and the pulse rate is 115 bpm. He is lethargic and minimally responsive to sternal rub. He has bitemporal wasting, mucous membranes are dry and poor skin turgor is noted. He is obtunded. The patient has an intact gag reflex and withdraws to pain in all four extremities. The rectal tone is normal. Laboratory values are significant for a creatinine of 4.2 mg/dL, a calcium level of 14.6 meq/L, and an albumin of 2.6 g/dL.

    All of the following are appropriate initial management steps EXCEPT:
    A) Normal saline
    B) Dexamethasone
    C) Pamidronate
    D) Furosemide when the patient is euvolemic
    E) Calcitonin

Answer: B

In vitamin D toxicity or extrarenal synthesis of 1,25(OH) D3 such as sarcoid or lymphoid malignancies steroids may help reduce plasma calcium levels by reducing intestinal calcium absorption. However, in this patient with prostate cancer, dexamethasone will have little effect on the calcium level.

Several methods can lower calcium in the acute setting. Volume depletion results from uncontrolled symptoms leading to decreased intake and enhanced renal sodium loss. Hypercalcemia resolves with hydration alone, and when possible this should be begun immediately. Euvolumeia should be obtained first. When euvolemia is achieved, furosemide may be given to increasing calciuresis. This can usually decrease serum calcium by 1–3 mg/dL within 24 h.

Bisphosphonates, which can be given IV or oral, stabilize osteoclast resorption of calcium from the bone and are quite effective. However, their effects may take 1 to 2 days to occur.

Calcitonin can be given intramuscularly or subcutaneously, but it becomes less effective after several days of use.

When other measures fail, hemodialysis against calcium-free or lower calcium concentration dialysate solution is highly effective in lowering plasma calcium levels.

Reference

Ariyan CE, Sosa JA. Assessment and management of patients with abnormal calcium. Crit Care Med. 2004;32(4 Suppl):S146-54.

151. A 58-year-old female with no past medical history presents to the emergency room with complaints of fever 39 °C (102.2 °F), headache, confusion, and lethargy. Symptoms began with an abrupt onset of unusual behavior reported by her husband. This was followed by fever and progressive lethargy.

    Empiric antibiotics and steroids are started for possible community-acquired meningitis. CT scan is performed which is negative. The patient undergoes a lumbar puncture that reveals a white blood cell count of 325/mm3, of which 97 % are lymphocytes. Protein is 110 mg/dL.

    The correct initial therapy should include:
    A) Ampicillin, vancomycin, and ceftriaxone
    B) Acyclovir
    C) Dexamethasone
    D) Amphotericin
    E) Observation alone

Answer: B

This patient's presentation is consistent with a viral encephalitis. Herpes simplex encephalitis (HSE) is the most common cause of severe encephalitis in the United States. The most common symptoms are fever, headache, and psychiatric symptoms. HSE has a predication for the temporal lobe, which accounts for the typical symptoms seen. Other specific symptoms include focal deficits and seizures.

Empiric acyclovir therapy should be started promptly in patients with suspected HSE. Acyclovir, the drug of choice, is relatively nontoxic and the prognosis for untreated HSE is poor. Initiation within 48 h of symptom onset improves outcomes. Despite early recognition, long-term neurologic damage of varying degrees occurs in over half of survivors. Relapses after HSE have been reported to occur in 5–26 % of patients. Most relapses occur within the first three months after completion of treatment.

PCR examination for HSV 1 and HSV 2 of the cerebrospinal fluid is the diagnostic test for the confirmation of HSE. Arboviruses, such as the West Nile virus, also continue to be prevalent in the United States and currently have no proven antiviral medicinal therapy.

References

Whitley RJ. Herpes simplex encephalitis: adolescents and adults. Antiviral Res. Sep 2006;71(2–3):141–8.

Whitley RJ, Gnann JW Viral encephalitis: familiar infections and emerging pathogens". Lancet. 2002 359 (9305): 507–13.

152. A 72-year-old man is admitted to the hospital with generalized fatigue and easy bruising. After a rapid workup, he is diagnosed with acute myelomonocytic leukemia. The hematology service is planning induction chemotherapy to start in the morning.

    His physical examination is notable for normal vital signs and no focal findings other than some bruising. On the night prior to transfer, you are called. He is confused and somnolent. He has been drinking water constantly. Over the last hour, despite frequently urinating, he has not been able to drink water due to somnolence.

    Laboratory studies are notable for a serum sodium of 159 mg//dl.

    Which of the following therapies should be administered immediately?
    A) All-trans retinoic acid (ATRA)
    B) Hydrochlorothiazide
    C) Hydrocortisone
    D) Desmopressin
    E) Lithium

Answer: D

This patient has acute central diabetes insipidus (DI). Diabetes insipidus (DI) is defined as the passage of large volumes (>3 L/24 h) of dilute urine (<300 m Osm/kg).

In patients with central DI, desmopressin is the drug of choice. It can be given nasally or intravenously with rapid onset. IVF should be administered as well. It is recommended that fluid replacement should be provided at a rate no greater than 500–750 mL/h. Serum sodium should be reduced no greater than by 0.5 mmol/L (0.5 mEq/L) every hour. This is to avoid hyperglycemia, volume overload, and overly rapid correction of hypernatremia,

Altered mental status is likely due to the hypernatremia, which typically develops in central DI as water intake cannot keep up with urine output. This can exceed 5 L/d. Immediate replacement of ADH in the form of desmopressin will be both diagnostic and therapeutic. Hydrochlorothiazide may be used in nephrogenic DI to increase proximal sodium and water reabsorption. Lithium is a well-known cause of nephrogenic DI.

Reference

Vande Walle J, Stockner M, Raes A, Nørgaard JP. Desmopressin 30 years in clinical use: a safety review. Curr Drug Saf. Sep 2007;2(3):232–8339)

153. A 62-year-old woman has been admitted for pneumonia 48 h ago. She is responding well to antibiotics. Her breathing has improved, and her white blood cell count is declining. She has no other past medical history other than occasional palpitations. Other than antibiotics she is on no medicines. You are called to see her for sudden onset of palpitations.

On physical exam, her heart rate is 178 beats/min on telemetry, and blood pressure is 100/65 mmHg with normal oxygen saturation. She is alert. She has marked venous pulsations in her neck. ECG shows a narrow complex tachycardia without identifiable P waves.

Which of the following is the most appropriate first step to managing her tachycardia?

A) 5 mg metoprolol IV
B) 6 mg adenosine IV
C) 10 mg verapamil IV
D) Carotid sinus massage
E) DC cardioversion using 100 J

Answer: D

The patient has probable AV nodal reentrant tachycardia. She has prominent venous pulsations in the neck due to cannon A waves, as seen in AV dissociation. This occurs with simultaneous atrial and ventricular contraction. First-line therapy for these reentrant narrow complex tachyarrhythmias is carotid sinus massage to increase vagal tone. Often this simple maneuver is all that is required to return the patient to sinus rhythm.

Carotid sinus massage is a bedside vagal maneuver technique involving digital pressure on the richly innervated carotid sinus. It takes advantage of the accessible position of this baroreceptor for diagnostic and therapeutic purposes. Its main therapeutic application is for termination of SVTs owing to paroxysmal atrial tachycardia (PAT).

Carotid massage is contraindicated in patients with known or suspected carotid artery disease. It also should be done with caution in the elderly.

The carotid sinus should be massaged firmly. In training, it has been described as the amount of pressure needed to indent a tennis ball. The duration should last five seconds. Carotid sinus massage should be discontinued immediately if the ECG shows asystole for more than three seconds. If that is not successful, IV adenosine 6 mg may be attempted. This can be repeated. If adenosine fails, intravenous beta-blockers or calcium channel blockers may be used. In hemodynamically compromised patients or those who have failed to respond to previous measures, DC cardioversion with 100–200 J is indicated.

References

Lim SH, Anantharaman V, Teo WS, Goh PP, Tan AT. Comparison of treatment of supraventricular tachycardia by Valsalva maneuver and carotid sinus massage. Ann Emerg Med. 1998 Jan;31(1):30–5.

O'Shea D, Parry SW. The Newcastle protocol for carotid sinus massage [Letter]. J Am Geriatr Soc. February 2001;49:236–7.

154. An 82-year-old female is admitted with a diagnosis of urosepsis. She was noted to be hypotensive with an admitting blood pressure of 80/60 mmHg. During the first 24 h of her admission, her blood pressure has improved to 110/60 mmHg, but she is noted to have decreased urine output.

Which of the following tests would be the most accurate for predicting the development of ongoing acute kidney injury?

A) Serum creatinine
B) Urinalysis
C) Neutrophil gelatinase-associated lipocalin (NGAL)
D) Ultrasound
E) Urinary tubular enzyme assay

Answer: C

NGAL may aid in the diagnosis of early acute tubular necrosis (ATN) and differentiate it from prerenal disease. NGAL is a novel urinary biomarker for ischemic injury.

This patient has decreased urine output secondary to either prerenal azotemia or acute tubular necrosis (ATN). Acute tubular necrosis generally results in muddy brown, granular, and epithelial casts. The formation of these may not be prominent in the early stages and may take several hours or days to develop.

NGAL has been validated in multiple studies of patients at risk for AKI. NGAL levels were demonstrated to improve risk classification prior to fulminant

AKI. NGAL in patients who later developed AKI occurred before any change in serum creatinine level. NGAL has also shown some potential to aid in the diagnosis of early acute tubular necrosis and differentiate it from prerenal disease. It is still to be determined if NGAL is cost effective for routine use in the hospital.

Reference

Koyner JL, Garg AX, Coca SG, Sint K, Thiessen-Philbrook H, Patel UD, et al. Biomarkers predict progression of acute kidney injury after cardiac surgery. J Am Soc Nephrol. 2012;23(5):905–14.

155. A 33-year-old man and his 29-year-old wife present with acute respiratory failure. Over the past four days, they both have had a fever, myalgias, and gastrointestinal symptoms that included abdominal pain, back pain, nausea, and vomiting. Two days ago, they were seen in the emergency room and diagnosed with gastroenteritis.

    Two weeks prior to the onset of symptoms, they returned from a camping trip where they had rented a cabin in the midwest United Sates for two weeks.

    On physical exam, both patients have similar symptoms consisting of coarse crackles, abdominal tenderness, and marked tachycardia.

    The most likely diagnosis is:
    A) Hantavirus
    B) Coccidiomycosis
    C) Leptospirosis
    D) Tularemia

These patients have *Hantavirus* cardiopulmonary syndrome (HCPS). Because symptoms initially referable to the respiratory tract are minimal or absent, the physician may conclude that the patient has viral gastroenteritis. The rapidly progressive cardiopulmonary phase is initiated by dyspnea, nonproductive cough, and circulatory collapse.

Mortality from HCPS is about 50 %. Most deaths are caused by intractable hypotension and associated dysrhythmia. The causative agent is a hantavirus. The principal animal reservoir is the deer mouse. Human infections occur by inhalation of aerosols of infectious excreta. Most HCPS cases have occurred in healthy young to middle-aged adults who have no underlying disease. The mean age of patients with HCPS is 37 years. Less than 7 % of cases occur in persons younger than 17 years, and disease is very rare in those younger than ten years.

The largest numbers of cases have occurred in New Mexico, Arizona, and California. The incubation period of *Hantavirus* pulmonary syndrome ranges from 1 to 4 weeks. A history of exposure to a rural setting, rodents or their dwellings, or agricultural work may suggest the diagnosis.

Ribavirin has been used to treat *Hantavirus* infections, but its efficacy in HCPS remains unproven.. Corticosteroids are also of uncertain value. There is currently no clinically available vaccine to prevent *Hantavirus* infections.

Other species of hantavirus, such as the Bayou virus identified in Louisiana and found in the Marsh rat, have been reported to cause a similar HCPS.

References

Duchin JS, Koster FT, Peters CJ, et al. Hantavirus pulmonary syndrome: a clinical description of 17 patients with a newly recognized disease. The Hantavirus Study Group. N Engl J Med. 1994;330(14):949–55.

Morzunov, S. P.; Feldmann, H.; Spiropoulou, C. F.; Semenova, V. A.; Rollin, P. E.; Ksiazek, T. G.; Peters, C. J.; Nichol, S. T.). A newly recognized virus associated with a fatal case of hantavirus pulmonary syndrome in Louisiana. Journal of virology. 1995 69 (3): 1980–1983.

156. A 38-year-old man is admitted for evaluation of epigastric pain, diarrhea, and reflux. He reports frequent similar episodes and has undergone multiple endoscopies at several different hospitals. He has persistent five bowel movements per day for the past few years. In each encounter, he was told that he had an ulcer. His current medications are high-dose omeprazole, oxycodone, and acetaminophen.

    Old records were obtained that reveal that he has had six endoscopies in the past four years, each with evidence of PUD and each was *H. pylori* negative. No specific cause was found for the diarrhea.

    Which of the following is the most appropriate next step in his diagnostic evaluation?
    A) CT scan of the abdomen.
    B) Discontinue omeprazole for 1 week and measure plasma gastrin level.
    C) Gastric pH measurement.
    D) Screen for parathyroid hyperplasia.
    E) Emperic *H. pylori* treatment.

Answer: C

The patient has Zollinger-Ellison syndrome. Zollinger-Ellison syndrome (ZES) is caused by a non-beta islet cell, gastrin-secreting tumor of the pancreas that stimulates maximum acid secretion. This leads to mucosal ulceration.

This patient presents with recurrent peptic ulcers without evidence of *H. pylori* infection. Additional features that suggest nonclassic ulcer disease include the presence of diarrhea, which is present in 73 % in Zollinger-Ellison syndrome. Fasting serum gastrin is the best single screening test. Because PPI use suppresses gastric acid production, it should be discontinued for at least 1 week prior to the measurement of gastrin in plasma.

Once hypergastrinemia is confirmed, the presence of low gastric pH must be confirmed. The most common cause of elevated gastrin is achlorhydria due to pernicious anemia. Imaging of the abdomen is indicated after demonstration of hypergastrinemia. Zollinger-Ellison syndrome may be associated with multiple endocrine neoplasia type 1. Elevated serum calcium levels with Zollinger-Ellison should prompt a search for MEN 1 syndrome.

References

Cadiot G, Jais P, Mignon M. Diagnosis of Zollinger-Ellison syndrome. From symptoms to biological evidence. Ital J Gastroenterol Hepatol. Oct 1999;31 Suppl 2:S147-52.

Campana D, Piscitelli L, Mazzotta E. Zollinger-Ellison syndrome. Diagnosis and therapy. Minerva Med. Jun 2005;96(3):187–206.

157. You are called to see a 76-year-old male in consultation for acute kidney injury. The patient is four days post-op abdominal aneurysm repair. For the past 3 days, urine output has decreased. On your review fluid has been matched appropriately with output. He is now oliguric. A bladder scan shows minimal urine. An indwelling catheter is in place. It flushes without complications. The patient has received two doses of vancomycin postoperatively.

   On physical examination, temperature is 37.8 °C (100.1 °F), blood pressure is 117/68, pulse rate is 114, and respirations are 17 per minute. Abdominal examination reveals a tense and distended abdomen. Bowel sounds are decreased.

   Laboratory data reveals a blood urea nitrogen of 57 mg/dL and a serum creatinine of 3.8 mg/dL. A baseline of 1.0 mg/dL is noted in the record. Fraction excretion of sodium is 1.7 %. A kidney ultrasound is ordered which reveals normal-sized kidneys and no hydronephrosis.

   Which of the following is the most likely cause of this patient's condition?
   A) Aminoglycoside toxicity
   B) Abdominal compartment syndrome
   C) Prerenal acute injury
   D) Urinary obstruction
   E) Ischemic bowel

Answer: B

This patient has an abdominal compartment syndrome. Abdominal compartment syndrome is increasingly recognized as the cause of morbidity such as metabolic acidosis, decreased urine output, and decreased cardiac output.

The syndrome occurs when there is an abnormal increase in abdominal pressure resulting in new organ dysfunction. This occurs when abdominal pressure is greater than 12 mmHg. Patients often have an abdomen clearly out of proportion to their body habitus. The exact pathophysiol-

ogy of acute compartment syndrome is uncertain. Other risk factors for the acute compartment syndrome include aggressive fluid resuscitation, which can occur with surgery. Measurement of intravesicular pressure through a bladder catheter is a common method for assessing intra-abdominal pressure. However, this may not correlate directly with measured intra-abdominal pressure.

Surgical depression through various methods of the abdomen is the definitive treatment. Temporizing measures include removing any constricting garments and not placing anything on the patient's abdomen. Aggressive fluid resuscitation should be avoided.

Reference

Malbrain ML, Chiumello D, Pelosi P, Bihari D, Innes R, Ranieri VM. Incidence and prognosis of intraabdominal hypertension in a mixed population of critically ill patients: a multiple-center epidemiological study. Crit Care Med. 2005;33(2):315–22.

158. A 75-year-old woman with a history of mechanical aortic valve repair is admitted with several days of intermittent melena with intermixed brown stool. She is currently on warfarin. She is hemodynamically stable and asymptomatic. Her Hb is 9.3 g/dL and her INR is 3.4. She does not have any further melena. The gastroenterologist would like to perform a colonoscopy.

   What is the best pre-endoscopic management of this patient?
   A) Hold warfarin and administer IV vitamin K.
   B) Proceed with no changes.
   C) Hold warfarin and start heparin once INR is less than 2.5 and continue through the procedure.
   D) Hold warfarin and start heparin once INR is less than 2.5 and hold 4–6 h before the procedure.
   E) Hold warfarin and administer two units of fresh frozen plasma.

Answer: D

This patient is considered a high-risk for bleeding, as she may require endoscopic hemostasis. A mechanical aortic valve requires that she be on anticoagulation to prevent thrombus formation. A mechanical valve that is in the aortic position makes this lower risk for thromboembolism than a mechanical mitral valve, but still requires bridging.

The best option given the non-emergent nature of her bleeding is to hold warfarin and start heparin with plans to hold 4–6 h pre-procedure.

Reference

Jaffer AK, Brotman DJ, Chukwumerije N. When patients on warfarin need surgery. Cleve Clin J Med. Nov 2003;70(11):973–84.

159. A 77-year-old woman presents to the emergency department with a 6-week history of a progressive worsening headache. She states the headache occurs daily and is diffuse. She denies any localization of symptoms. She also reports fatigue and malaise during the same period. She has taken acetaminophen for the headaches with mild relief.

On physical examination, the temperature is normal. Blood pressure is 140/70 mmHg. Pulse is 70 beats per minute. Respirations are 16 per minute. Scalp tenderness is noted bilaterally over the temporal parietal area. No papilledema is noted. CT scan is performed which reveals no abnormalities.

Significant laboratory data reveals a sedimentation rate of 80 mm/h, and leukocyte count is within normal limits.

Which of the following is the most appropriate next step?

A) Cerebral angiography
B) MRI of the head
C) Referral for temporal artery biopsy
D) Prednisone therapy

Answer: D

This patient has giant cell arteritis (GCA). The onset of GCA may be either abrupt or insidious. GCA may begin with constitutional manifestations such as anorexia, fever, myalgia, night sweats, and weight loss. These symptoms may occur for a few days or weeks.

Patients suspected of GCA should undergo immediate treatment with prednisone therapy, followed by temporal artery biopsy. Patients who present with visual symptoms have a 22-fold increased chance of visual improvement if therapy is started within the first day.

Further diagnostic workup should not delay the initiation of steroid therapy. In this patient who is >50 years of age who develops new-onset headaches with elevated sedimentation rate, temporal arteritis is the probable diagnosis. Available data suggests that when the biopsy is performed within four weeks of initiating corticosteroid therapy, the results will be unaffected.

Few studies exist regarding the efficacy of different dosing protocols for corticosteroids in GCA. Several dosing regimens are recommended depending on the severity of symptoms.

References
Bhatti MT, Tabandeh H. Giant cell arteritis: diagnosis and management. Curr Opin Ophthalmol. 2001;12(6):393–9
Borchers AT, Gershwin ME. Giant cell arteritis: a review of classification, pathophysiology, geoepidemiology and treatment. Autoimmun Rev. 2012;11(6–7):A544-54.

160. A 55-year-old man is in the hospital for the evaluation of ongoing fevers and weight loss. He first developed symptoms 3 months previously. He reports daily fevers to as high as 39.2 °C (102.6 °F) with night sweats and fatigue. He has lost 37 lb compared with his weight at his last annual examination.

Diagnostic tests have been negative so far with exception of an elevated calcium at 11.6 g/dL. The serum protein electrophoresis demonstrated polyclonal gammopathy. HIV, Epstein–Barr virus (EBV), and cytomegalovirus (CMV) testing are negative. Blood cultures for bacteria have been negative on three separate occasions. Chest radiograph and purified protein derivative (PPD) testing results are negative. A CT scan of the chest, abdomen, and pelvis has borderline enlargement of lymph nodes in the abdomen and retroperitoneum to 1.4 cm.

What would be the next best step in determining the etiology of fever in this patient?

A) Empiric treatment with corticosteroids
B) Exploratory laparotomy
C) Needle biopsy of enlarged lymph nodes
D) PET-CT imaging
E) Serum angiotensin-converting enzyme levels
F) Flow cytometry of leukocytes

Answer: C

The next step in the workup of this patient would be to obtain a sample from an enlarged lymph node for cultures and pathology. His elevated calcium with prominent lymph nodes suggest granulomatous diseases, including disseminated tuberculosis, fungal infections, or sarcoidosis.

Before treatment can begin, every effort should be made to confirm a diagnosis. Sarcoid is a possibility. However, serum angiotensin-converting enzyme levels are neither appropriately sensitive nor specific for diagnosis of sarcoidosis and should not be used to determine if therapy is needed.

Reference
Bleeker-Rovers CP, Vos FJ, de Kleijn EM, Mudde AH, Dofferhoff TS, Richter C, et al. A prospective multicenter study on fever of unknown origin: the yield of a structured diagnostic protocol. Medicine (Baltimore). 2007;86(1):26–38.

161. A 62-year-old white male admitted to the hospital medicine service for right wrist cellulitis. The appearance is purulent, and a specimen is sent for culture. Empirically, he is started on piperacillin/tazobactam IV 4.5 g every 8 h and vancomycin IV 15 mg/kg every 12 h (weight=96 kg). The vancomycin trough returns as 22 ug/ml.

Cultures are positive for MRSA. What would you do next?

A) De-escalate to vancomycin only but keep the current dose.
B) Continue both piperacillin/tazobactam and vancomycin at current doses.

C) De-escalate to vancomycin only, check if trough drawn appropriately, and decrease dose.

D) De-escalate to vancomycin only, check if trough drawn appropriately, and change interval to every 24 h.

Answer: D

For hospitalized patients with complicated skin and soft tissue infections (SSTI's), including purulent cellulitis, the following antibiotics can be considered for empirical therapy covering presumed MRSA: IV vancomycin, oral or IV linezolid, daptomycin, telavancin, and clindamycin. Piperacillin/tazobactam does not cover MRSA.

Vancomycin 15 mg/kg every 8–12 h for complicated infections, including MRSA, a trough of 15–20 mcg/ml is recommended (10–15 mcg/ml for uncomplicated skin infections). Thus, a trough of 22 mcg/ml is considered elevated for this type of infection. Vancomycin is a time-dependent drug; hence, it is preferred to adjust the interval rather than decrease the dose in order to maintain therapeutic levels.

References

Liu C et al. Clinical Practice Guidelines by the Infectious Disease Society of America for the Treatment of Methicillin-Resistant Staphylococcus aureus in Adults and Children. CID 2011;52:1–38.

Ryback M et al. Therapeutic Monitoring of Vancomycin in Adult Patients. Am J Health-Syst Pharm 2009;66:82–98.

162. A 26-year-old female is admitted for severe abdominal pain. She reports that over the last five years, she has had several bouts of severe abdominal pain that has resulted in admission. No cause was identified, and the symptoms spontaneously resolved after about a day. Two of these episodes were accompanied by delirium. After each attack, she reports bilateral leg weakness.

On physical exam, the pain is diffuse with distention and not accompanied by vomiting or diarrhea. She is otherwise healthy and active. She reports no past medical history and only medicines are birth control pills which she has been on for five years.

Which of the following is the next most appropriate step in his evaluation?

A) Endoscopy and colonoscopy
B) Measurement of P-ANCA
C) Prescription of hyoscyamine
D) Referral to psychiatry
E) Measurement of urine porphobilinogen during attack

Answer: E

The patient has acute intermittent porphyria. It is most commonly associated with attacks of abdominal pain and neurologic symptoms that develop after puberty. Often a precipitating cause of symptomatic episodes can be iden-

tified such as steroid hormone use, oral contraceptives, systemic illness, reduced caloric intake, and many other medications.

Although not common, the diagnosis is often considered in any individual with unexplained abdominal pain especially when accompanied by neuropsychiatric complaints. The abdominal symptoms are often more prominent. The abdominal pain often is epigastric and colicky in nature. Additional findings may include peripheral neuropathy, sensory changes, and delirium. Patients can have a wide variety of psychiatric symptoms. Diagnosis is made by measurement of urine porphobilinogens measured during an attack. Therapy for an acute attack is with carbohydrate loading, narcotic pain control, and possibly IV hemin.

Reference

Kuo HC, Huang CC, Chu CC, Lee MJ, Chuang WL, Wu CL, et al. Neurological complications of acute intermittent porphyria. Eur Neurol. 2011;66(5):247–52.

163. An 82-year-old woman is admitted with a stroke. She awoke at home five hours ago with mild left hemiparesis. A CT scan of the head confirmed a right hemispheric infarction.

On physical examination, blood pressure is 154/75 mmHg, pulse rate is 80/min, and respiration rate is 18/min. Neurologic assessment reveals left facial droop and left hemiparesis. No dysarthria is noted.

Which of the following is the most appropriate first step in assessing the patients swallowing after transfer is completed?

A) Bedside screening for dysphagia immediately
B) Nasogastric tube placement
C) No further studies
D) Modified Barium Swallow immediately
E) Cautious liquids

Answer: A

Aspiration is one of the foremost complications of stroke patients, and its evaluation should be undertaken as a primary step in stroke management. Despite the lack of dysarthria in this patient, all stroke patients are at significant risk of aspiration. Some degree of dysphagia occurs in 45 % of all hospitalized patients with stroke. This patient should be NPO until a dysphagia screen is undertaken.

The American Heart Association/American Stroke Association recommends a water swallow test performed at the bedside. A trained observer should perform this. A prospective study of the bedside water swallow test demonstrated a significantly decreased risk of aspiration pneumonia.

Reference

Jauch EC, Saver JL, Adams HP Jr, Bruno A, Connors JJ, Demaerschalk BM. Guidelines for the early management of patients with acute ischemic stroke: a guideline for healthcare professionals from the American Heart Association/American Stroke Association. Stroke. 2013;44(3):870–947.

164. A 47-year-old man has been admitted for an asthmatic exacerbation. Over the past 2 days, he has developed fever and erythema at the site of a peripherally inserted central catheter. He had a catheter placed upon admission. Medical history is also significant for the vancomycin hypersensitivity reaction characterized by urticaria, bronchospasm, and hypotension.

On physical examination, the temperature is 39.0 °C (102.2 °F), blood pressure is 110/80 mmHg, pulse rate is 107/min, and respiration rate is 21/min. Erythema and tenderness are noted at the catheter insertion site in the left antecubital fossa.

Laboratory studies show hemoglobin 8.0 g/dL, leukocyte count 3500/μL, with 70 % neutrophils and platelet count 20,000. Blood cultures reveal growth of methicillin-resistant *Staphylococcus aureus*. The vancomycin MIC is >1 μg/mL. A chest radiograph and electrocardiogram are unremarkable. A transthoracic echocardiogram reveals vegetation on the tricuspid valve.

Which of the following is the most appropriate treatment?

A) Cefazolin
B) Clindamycin
C) Daptomycin
D) Nafcillin
E) Vancomycin

Answer: C

This patient has nosocomially acquired methicillin-resistant *Staphylococcus aureus* (MRSA) bacteremia, and endocarditis. In addition to catheter removal, this patient requires a 6-week course of intravenous antibiotics. Daptomycin is currently approved for treatment for bacteremia and right-sided endocarditis.

Daptomycin has been shown to be non-inferior to standard therapies in the treatment of bacteremia and right-sided endocarditis caused by *S. aureus*. Daptomycin resistance is still uncommon.

Clindamycin is not included in the consensus guidelines for treatment of MRSA-associated infective endocarditis. Clindamycin has a primarily bacteriostatic effect. It has been associated with treatment failure and relapse when used to treat methicillin-susceptible *S. aureus* bacteremia and infective endocarditis.

Results from studies support the practice of switching from vancomycin to daptomycin for the treatment of MRSA bacteremia when the vancomycin MIC is >1 μg/mL. Treatment with daptomycin results in significantly improved outcomes with the patients.

Reference

Fowler VG, Boucher HW, Corey GR. Daptomycin versus standard therapy for bacteremia and endocarditis caused by Staphylococcus aureus". N Engl J Med.2006; 355 (7): 653–65.

165. A 27-year-old man is evaluated for the third time in the past two months for recurrent nausea, vomiting, and cramping epigastric pain. Since his symptoms began six months ago, the patient has lost 10 kg (22 lbs). He vomits several times weekly, usually in the morning. He reports that his nausea persists until he takes a hot bath, which he does every day for greater than one hour.

Symptoms are not exacerbated by any particular food and are not alleviated by eating, bowel movements, or nonprescription proton-pump inhibitors. The patient does not smoke cigarettes or drink alcoholic beverages. Comprehensive metabolic panel and serum amylase and lipase levels were normal two months ago.

On physical exam temperature is 36.7 C (98.0 F), pulse rate is 70 per minute, respirations are 16 per minute, and blood pressure is 127/4 mmHg. Minimal epigastric tenderness without rebound is noted. The comprehensive metabolic panel, complete blood count, and serum amylase, and lipase levels are normal.

Which of the following should be ordered to confirm the diagnosis?

A) Urine test for cannabis
B) Serum alpha-fetoprotein and human chorionic gonadotropin levels
C) Mesenteric artery Doppler ultrasonography
D) Magnetic resonance cholangiopancreatography
E) Upper endoscopy

Answer: A

This is a classic case of cannabis-induced hyperemesis. In this otherwise healthy male, excessive cannabis use may be suspected as a potential cause of unexplained symptoms of nausea. This occurs most commonly in men younger than age 50 and is associated with cyclic vomiting and occurs in the morning. Compulsive bathing is the most common home remedy. Most patients are nonsmokers, do not use other illicit drugs, and do not drink alcoholic beverages. The most prominent developers of this syndrome are the recreational cannabis users who began using cannabis from a very early age and also those who use it chronically or daily. Criteria have been suggested to confirm the diagnosis.

Reference
Simonetto DA, Oxentenko AS, Herman ML, Szostek JH. Cannabinoid hyperemesis: a case series of 98 patients. Mayo Clin Proc. 2012;87(2):114–119.

166. A 54-year-old woman is admitted with episodes of diaphoresis, asthenia, near syncope, and confusion. She reports these symptoms for several months. These episodes most commonly occur several hours after she eats. She has no other significant medical history and takes no medications. She has checked her glucose with her husband's glucometer and at times it has been below 50 mg/dl.

She is admitted for the confirmation of hypoglycemia. A prolonged fast is begun. During this period the patient becomes symptomatic. Her serum glucose concentration at the time is 41 mg/dl. The insulin level is elevated, and no insulin antibodies are present. The C-peptide level is high. Tests for the use of sulfonylureas and meglitinides are negative.

What is the diagnosis and most effective therapy for this patient's condition?
A) Factitious insulin use, psychiatric consultation.
B) Observe the patient and schedule a follow-up fast 2 to 3 months from now.
C) Begin diazoxide 400 mg TID and verapamil 180 mg QD.
D) Refer the patient to surgery for imaging and resection.
E) Begin phenytoin and octreotide.

Answer: D

This patient has an insulinoma. C-peptide levels are high in patients with insulinomas as well as with sulfonylurea ingestion. Insulinoma is characterized by hypoglycemia caused by elevated levels of endogenous insulin. Insulinomas are rare and alternative diagnosis should be actively pursued in cases of hypoglycemia.

Once a clinical and biochemical diagnosis of insulinoma is made, the next step is localization. There are several effective modalities. They include abdominal ultrasound, triple-phase spiral computed tomography, magnetic resonance imaging, and octreotide scan. This should be guided by a surgical consultation.

The treatment of choice for insulinomas is surgical removal. Approximately 90–95 % of insulinomas are benign, and long-term cure with total resolution of preoperative symptoms is expected after complete resection on the lesion.

Medical therapy is less effective than tumor resection but can be used in patients who are not candidates for surgery. Diazoxide is the drug of choice because it inhibits insulin release from the tumor. Adverse effects must be treated with hydrochlorothiazide. In patients not responsive to or intolerant of diazoxide, somatostatin may be indicated to prevent hypoglycemia.

References
Phan GQ, Yeo CJ, Hruban RH, et al. Surgical experience with pancreatic and peripancreatic neuroendocrine tumors: review of 125 patients. J Gastrointest Surg. 1998;2(5):472–82.
Mathur A, Gorden P, Libutti SK. Insulinoma. Surg Clin North Am. 2009;89(5):1105–21

167. A 31-year-old woman is admitted with episodes of dizziness, lightheadedness, palpitations, sweats, anxiety, and confusion. On the morning of admission, she reports that she almost passed out. Her husband checked her blood sugar level and noted it to be low. Her symptoms resolved after drinking some orange juice.

Physical exam is unremarkable and she is admitted for glucose monitoring. A prolonged fast is started. After 18 h, she becomes symptomatic, and her blood is drawn. The serum glucose concentration is 48 mg/dl, the serum insulin level is high, and test results are negative for insulin antibodies. The C-peptide level is low, and tests for sulfonylurea and meglitinides are negative.

Which of the following is the most likely diagnosis for this patient?
A) Insulinoma
B) Factitious hypoglycemia
C) Noninsulinoma pancreatogenous hypoglycemia syndrome (NIPHS)
D) Insulin autoimmune hypoglycemia

Answer: B

A review of the medical literature indicates a considerable increase in the frequency of recognized factitious disorders. This has a significant impact on the practice of hospital medicine. Factitious hypoglycemia should be considered in any patient who requires a fasting glucose test. Factitious hypoglycemia, one of the best-characterized factitious diseases, is a deliberate attempt to induce hypoglycemia by means of insulin or oral hypoglycemic drugs. Diagnosis of sulfonylurea-induced hypoglycemia requires the measurement of the drug in the serum or urine. When a diagnosis of factitious hypoglycemia is suspected, the patient's medical records should be reviewed for similar hospital admissions.

Factitious hypoglycemia is more common in women. It occurs most often in the third or fourth decade of life. Many of these patients work in health-related occupations.

Reference
Grunberger G, Weiner JL, Silverman R, et al. Factitious hypoglycemia due to surreptitious administration of insulin. Diagnosis, treatment, and long-term follow-up. Ann Intern Med. 1988;108:252–257

168. A 37-year-old female with a history of intravenous drug use presents with fever and decreased urine output. She is noted to have a new cardiac murmur, and a transthoracic echocardiogram reveals vegetation on the tricuspid valve. She is started on antibiotics. Acute renal failure does not resolve. On initial workup complement, levels are checked and are low. Hepatitis C serology is positive. A renal biopsy is pursued.

What is the most likely finding on kidney histology?

A) Normal biopsy
B) "Tram-track" double-layered basement membrane
C) "Spike and dome" granular deposits at the basement membrane
D) Subendothelial immune complex deposition
E) Apple-green birefringence under polarized light

Answer: B

Membranoproliferative glomerulonephritis (MPGN) is the most likely diagnosis. Several factors suggest this including hepatitis C infection and endocarditis, along with low complement levels. A biopsy will likely show classic "tram-tracking" of the basement membrane. Normal biopsies may be seen with minimal change disease. Granular spike and dome deposits are more characteristic of membranous nephropathy. Subendothelial immune complexes are seen in lupus nephritis. Apple-green birefringence is characteristic of amyloidosis.

Reference

Sethi S, Fervenza FC. Membranoproliferative glomerulonephritis–a new look at an old entity. N Engl J Med. 2012;366(12):1119–31.

169. A 20-year-old female presents with diarrhea, nausea, and fever. She reports greater than ten stools in the past 24 h. In addition, she has a temperature of 38.9 C (102.0 °F). She is started on ciprofloxacin. Stool cultures are sent. Clostridium difficile is negative. On the second day of her hospitalization, the patient has a grand mal seizure.

Which of the following is the most likely cause?

A) Salmonella
B) Shigella
C) Yersinia
D) Campylobacter
E) Vibrio

Answer: B

This patient has gastroenteritis consistent with an enteroinvasive bacterial infection. Shigella is the most common bacterial cause of acute gastroenteritis in the United States and has been associated with seizures. Shigella infection presents with the sudden onset of severe abdominal cramping, high-grade fever, emesis, anorexia, and large-volume watery diarrhea. Seizures may be an early manifestation. Campylobacter and Yersinia may cause a febrile illness that mimics appendicitis. Vibrio species usually cause a nonspecific gastroenteritis.

Reference

Khan WA, Dhar U, Salam MA, et al. Central nervous system manifestations of childhood shigellosis: prevalence, risk factors, and outcome. Pediatrics. 1999;103(2):E18.

170. A 37-year-old man form a nursing home is evaluated for the acute onset of headache, nausea, and lethargy. He has a history of obstructive hydrocephalus for which he underwent ventriculoperitoneal shunt placement approximately 3 months ago. Per family, he has baseline mental retardation but currently has had subtle changes in his behavior. This has occurred with prior urinary tract infections.

On physical examination, the temperature is 38.0 ° C (100.4 ° F), blood pressure is 115/70 mmHg, pulse rate is 95 bpm, and respiration rate is 14/min. Examination of the scalp reveals the presence of the shunt catheter without tenderness or erythema along the site. He is oriented only to person and place as is his baseline. The remainder of the physical examination is normal.

Laboratory studies indicate a leukocyte count of 15,000/μL (11×109/L) with a normal differential. Urinalysis is within normal limits. Blood cultures are pending. Neurosurgery is consulted for tapping of the shunt.

Pending culture results, which of the following antimicrobial regimens should be initiated in this patient?

A) Trimethoprim–sulfamethoxazole
B) Trimethoprim–sulfamethoxazole plus rifampin
C) Vancomycin
D) Vancomycin, ampicillin, plus ceftriaxone
E) Vancomycin plus cefepime

Answer: E

This patient may have a cerebrospinal fluid (CSF) shunt infection. Ventriculoperitoneal shunt infections can be difficult to diagnose owing to the mild and variable clinical presentation. Symptoms may reflect increased intracranial pressure and may be subtle, such as lethargy, nausea, and headache. Classic meningeal symptoms may be absent, and fever may or may not be present. Patterns may be consistent with previous infections.

The recent placement of a shunt warrants antibiotic coverage for a possible infection. The most likely causative microorganisms of a shunt infection are coagulase-negative staphylococci *S. aureus*, diphtheroids including *Propionibacterium acnes*, and gram-negative bacilli such as *Pseudomonas aeruginosa*.

Empiric therapy with vancomycin to cover staphylococci and diphtheroids and ceftazidime, cefepime, or meropenem to treat the gram-negative bacilli is appropriate pending CSF tap results.

A shunt tap should only be considered after imaging of the brain and a shunt series is performed. Other infections should also be excluded, since shunt infections are less likely less than 3 months after placement.

References

Noetzel MJ, Baker RP. Shunt fluid examination: risks and benefits in the evaluation of shunt malfunction and infection. J Neurosurg. 1984;61(2):328–32.

Wong, GK; Wong, SM; Poon, WS Ventriculoperitoneal shunt infection: intravenous antibiotics, shunt removal and more aggressive treatment?.2011; ANZ J Surg 81 (4): 307170.

171. A 27-year-old female presents to the emergency room with complaints of cough and left-sided chest pain.

    On physical exam temperature is 38.8 °C(100.8°), heart rate is102 bpm, blood pressure is 108/80 mmHg, and oxygen saturation of 92 % on room air at rest. Decreased breath sounds and dullness upon percussion are noted at the left lung base.

    Chest radiograph reveals a significant pleural effusion. A thoracentesis is performed at the bedside.

    Which of the following results from the fluid analysis match the accompanying diagnosis?
    A) Pleural protein LDH of 260, a serum LDH of 100, WBC count differential 80 % neutrophils; parapneumonic effusion
    B) Pleural protein of 1.5 with a serum protein of 4; tuberculosis
    C) Pleural amylase of 250; pancreatitis
    D) A and C
    E) A and B

Answer: D

In the evaluation of pleural fluid, the initial diagnostic consideration is distinguishing transudates from exudates. Although a number of chemical tests have been proposed to differentiate pleural fluid transudates from exudates, the tests first proposed by Light have become the standard.

Common causes of exudative pleural effusions include parapneumonic effusions from typical bacterial infections, tuberculosis, connective tissue diseases, malignancy, and

pancreatitis. A high pleural amylase level (>200) may indicate pancreatitis or esophageal rupture.

The criteria from Light identify nearly all exudates correctly, but they misclassify approximately 20–25 % of transudates as exudates. This usually occurs in patients on long-term diuretic therapy for congestive heart failure. This tends to concentrate the protein and LDH levels within the pleural space.

Reference

Jose C. Yataco MD, Raed Dweik MD. Pleural effusions: Evaluation and management. Cleveland Clinic Journal of Medicine. 2005;72: 854–872.

172. A 57-year-old male with a known 35-year history of alcohol abuse presents with jaundice, ascites, and a left shoulder fracture following a bar room brawl last night. On admission his liver functions are elevated but not markedly different from baseline. Due to intoxication and possible management of alcohol withdrawal, he is admitted to the hospital medicine service. He has been followed by hepatology for possible liver transplant but has not been abstinent from alcohol. He is in moderate to severe pain.

    In reference to pain control, which of the following should be avoided in this patient?
    A) Acetaminophen 325 mg every 6 h
    B) Hydrocodone 5 mg every 6 h
    C) Hydromorphone 0.5 mg iv every 6 h
    D) NSAIDS

Answer: D

Analgesia in cirrhotic patients can be challenging. Few prospective studies have offered an evidence-based approach. End-stage liver disease patients have important issues that make analgesia potentially risky. These include hepatic impairments in drug metabolism, chronic mental status changes, and renal dysfunction.

Most agents can be used with caution. Acetaminophen is the most common cause of fulminant hepatic failure in the United States. Despite this, it can be used with caution. NSAIDS may be contraindicated in cirrhotic patients because of decreased renal blood flow and ensuing hepatorenal syndrome. If possible they should be avoided.

The approach to analgesia in the cirrhotic population should be cautious but practical. Frequent monitoring is needed, including mental status, hepatic function, and renal function.

Reference

Chandok N, Watt KDS. Pain Management in the Cirrhotic Patient: The Clinical Challenge. Mayo Clinic Proceedings 2010;85(5):451–458.

173. You are called to see a 67-year-old man to evaluate a change in his mental status. He was admitted 36 h ago for treatment of community-acquired pneumonia. On a brief review of his past medical and social history, you note that he has been on no prior medications and reports alcohol intake of no greater than one beer daily. On admission his mental status was normal.

On physical exam his blood pressure is 160/85 mmHg, heart rate of 92 beats/min, respiratory rate of 20 breaths/min, temperature of 37.4 °C (99.3 °F), and SaO2 of 92 % on oxygen 2 L/min. He is agitated and restless in bed. He has removed his IV and oxygen tubing from his nose. He is noted to be somewhat tremulous and diaphoretic.

Which of the following is most likely to be beneficial in establishing the diagnosis?

A) Arterial blood gas testing
B) MRI or head CT
C) Fingerstick glucose testing
D) Review of the patient's alcohol intake with his wife
E) Review of the recent medications received by the patient

Answer: D

This patient has features of acute delirium, which can be precipitated by many causes in hospitalized patients. The clinical picture is most consistent with alcohol withdrawal. Alcohol withdrawal is common and despite minimal reported use in this patient, it is the most likely diagnosis. Further discussion with a second source may reveal his actual alcohol use.

Although commonly ordered, brain imaging is often not helpful in the evaluation of delirium.

Patients vastly underestimate and report the actual amount of alcohol consumed. Overall underestimation may be on average as high as 75 %. It has been suggested that asking if alcohol has been ingested in the past 24 h is a better, nonthreatening screening question to identify heavy drinkers.

References
Del Boca FK, Darkes J. The validity of self-reports of alcohol consumption: state of the science and challenges for research. Addiction 2003;98(S2):1–12.
Gleason OC . Delirium. Am Fam Physician. 2003; 67 (5): 1027–34. 313)

174. A 67-year-old female presents with confusion and slurred speech. The mother who brought the patient to the emergency room says that they went out to eat the previous night and developed symptoms this morning.

Other than a jejunoileal bypass many years ago, the patient has enjoyed good health. There is no history of alcohol or substance abuse. She is on no medicines.

On examination, the patient has appearance of being intoxicated. Temperature is 37.4 C (99.3 F), pulse rate is 96 per minute, respirations are 24 per minute, and blood pressure is 130/80 mmHg. The lungs are clear. The abdomen is soft and nontender, and a healed midline scar is noted. No edema, cyanosis, or clubbing of the extremities is noted. The patient is oriented to person only.

Plasma glucose is 152 mg/dL, blood urea nitrogen is 17 mg/dL, serum ammonia is 18 ug/dL, and bicarbonate is mEq/L 13 mEq/L. Arterial blood gas studies reveals a pH 7.26 a PCO2 0f 227 mmHg. Venous blood lactate is 1.3 mmol/L. Blood ethanol is negative. Urine drug screen is negative. CT imaging of her head is normal.

A) Serotonin syndrome
B) Salicylate poisoning
C) D-lactic acidosis
D) Vitamin B1 deficiency
E) Vitamin B6

Answer: C

D-lactic acidosis can occur in patients with jejunoileal bypass or short bowel syndrome. Symptoms typically present after the ingestion of high-carbohydrate feedings. In abnormal bowel, the overgrowth of gram-positive anaerobes such as lactobacilli is able to produce excessive lactate from carbohydrates. These patients develop the appearance of intoxication including confusion, ataxia, and slurred speech.

Jejunoileal bypass was a surgical weight loss procedure performed for the relief of morbid obesity. Many patients developed complications secondary to malabsorption. As a consequence of all these complications, jejunoileal bypass is no longer a recommended bariatric surgical procedure. Many patients have required reversal of the procedure.

References
PW, Wright EC, Baumgartner TG, Bersin RM, Buchalter S, Curry SH, et al. Natural history and course of acquired lactic acidosis in adults. DCA-Lactic Acidosis Study Group. Am J Med. 1994;97(1):47–54
Colquitt JL, Pickett K, Loveman E, Frampton GK. Surgery for weight loss in adults. Cochrane Database Syst Rev. 2014

175. A 72-year-old man presents to the emergency department with severe abdominal distention and pain. He is found to have a palpable bladder, and after Foley catheter placement, 2.0 L of urine passes. His BUN is 85 mg/dL and creatinine is 7.2 mg/dL on admission.

Over the next 3 days of hospitalization, his BUN and Cr fall. On the second day, his urine output is found to be rising. He is not receiving intravenous fluids. He passes 6.5 L of urine on the third and fourth hospital days.

The patient is at risk for which of the following complications?

A) Erythrocytosis
B) Hyperchloremic metabolic acidosis
C) Hyperkalemia
D) Prerenal azotemia
E) Systemic hypertension

Answer: D

Postobstructive diuresis is defined as high urine output exceeding 0.5 L per hour occurring after an obstruction is relieved. This happens particularly in patients with chronic obstruction. Severity ranges from a self-limiting physiologic process lasting 48 h to a pathologic sodium-wasting form. Postobstructive diuresis is usually self-limited. It usually lasts for several days to a week.

Urea diuresis is the most common and resolves by itself within 24–48 h. The next in frequency is sodium diuresis, which may last longer, over 72 h.

Management involves avoiding severe volume depletion, hypokalemia, hyponatremia, hypernatremia, and hypomagnesemia. In the first 24 h, urine output should be checked and approximately matched hourly. If the urine output is over 200 mL/h, then 80 % of the hourly output should be replaced intravenously with either 0.9 % saline or 2/3–1/3 solution. Overhydration can prolong the polyuria phase.

After 24 h of persistent diuresis, total fluids infused should be about 1 L less than the previous day's output. Once the urine output is less than 3 L per day, oral fluids should suffice.

Reference
Loo MH, Vaughan ED. Obstructive nephropathy and postobstructive diuresis. AUA Update Series. 1985;4:9.

176. An 86-year-old woman is admitted to the intensive care unit with depressed level of consciousness, hypothermia, sinus bradycardia, hypotension, and hypoglycemia. She was previously healthy with the exception of a history of hypothyroidism and systemic hypertension. She recently ran out of her medicines. Her serum chemistries reveal hyponatremia and a glucose of 52. TSH is above 100 mU/L.

All of the following statements regarding this condition are true, EXCEPT:

A) External warming is a critical feature of therapy in all patients.
B) Hypotonic intravenous solutions should be avoided.
C) IV levothyroxine should be administered with IV glucocorticoids.

D) Sedation and narcotics should be avoided if possible.
E) This condition occurs almost commonly in the elderly and often is precipitated by infection.

Answer: A

The patient has myxedema coma. Management includes rapid repletion of thyroid hormone through IV levothyroxine and glucocorticoids. There may be a lack of adrenal reserve in severe hypothyroidism.

Warming is not indicated in all circumstances and must be done with caution. It is only recommended for a temperature of less than 30 °C. Care must be taken with rewarming as it may precipitate a cardiovascular collapse.

Profound hypothyroidism most commonly occurs in the elderly. It can be precipitated by an underlying condition such as myocardial infarction or infection. Clinical manifestations include an altered level of consciousness, bradycardia, and hypothermia. Hypertonic saline and glucose may be used if hyponatremia or hypoglycemia is severe. Hypotonic solutions should be avoided as they may worsen fluid retention.

References
Klubo-Gwiezdzinska J, Wartofsky L. Fam Physician..2000;62(11):2485–90 Thyroid emergencies.
Med Clin North Am. Mar 2012;96(2):385–403

177. A 42-year-old woman is admitted with a temperature of 38.9 °C (102 °F), sweats, shaking chills, headache, and slight constipation for the past two days. She has just returned from rural Thailand where she was on a teaching assignment for the past year. She had not taken malaria prophylaxis during her stay in that country.

On the physical exam, her temperature is 39.4 °C (103 °F), and she has tenderness in the right upper quadrant of the abdomen.

Her white blood cell count is 28,000 per mm3 (28 × 109 per L) with a left shift. Serum electrolyte and transaminase levels are unremarkable. A chest radiograph showed minimal blunting of the right costophrenic angle.

Computed tomographic (CT) scanning of the abdomen revealed four large abscesses in the right lobe of the patient's liver. The two largest abscesses were each 4 cm in diameter.

CT-guided catheter drainage was undertaken. Thick, nonmalodorous, brown fluid was withdrawn. Cultures of fluid are negative.

What is the most likely diagnosis?

A) Malaria
B) *Entamoeba histolytica*
C) *Echinococcus*
D) Leishmaniasis

Answer: B

Amebic liver abscess is the most common extraintestinal manifestation of infection with *Entamoeba histolytica*. Untreated, it is associated with significant morbidity and mortality. It has a worldwide distribution, but amebiasis is more prevalent in tropical areas. *E. histolytica* is transmitted via the fecal-oral route. It is generally acquired by the ingestion of contaminated food and water containing the infective cysts. The incubation period for *E. histolytica* infection is commonly 2–4 weeks but may range from a few days to years. Most patients with amebic liver abscess present within 2–4 weeks of infection and almost all within 5 months. Some cases may present years after travel to endemic areas.

The mainstay of therapy is metronidazole, which is usually effective in eliminating the intestinal and extraintestinal amoeba. Amebic liver abscess of up to 10 cm can be cured with metronidazole without drainage. Indications for percutaneous drainage include large liver abscess, abscesses in the left hepatic lobe at risk for rupturing into the pericardium, and treatment failure. This is defined as fever and pain persist for 3 to 5 days after the initiation of therapy.

Reference

Stanley SL Jr. Amoebiasis. Lancet 2003;361:1025–1034.

178. An 80-year-old woman presents with a two-day history of persistent vomiting. She is lethargic and weak and has myalgia. Her mucous membranes are dry. She is diagnosed as having gastroenteritis and dehydration and is admitted.

Measurement of arterial blood gas shows pH 7.51, PaO2 86 mmHg, PaCO2 46 mmHg, and HCO3 38 mmol/L.

What acid–base disorder is shown?
A) Metabolic alkalosis/respiratory acidosis
B) Metabolic alkalosis
C) Respiratory alkalosis
D) Metabolic alkalosis/respiratory alkalosis
E) None of the above

Answer: B

The primary disorder is metabolic alkalosis. Contraction alkalosis is by far the most common cause in the hospitalized patient. CO2 is the strongest driver of respiration. It generally will not allow hypoventilation as a full compensation for metabolic alkalosis. An elevated serum bicarbonate concentration may also be observed as a compensatory response to primary respiratory acidosis. If continuous removal of gastric contents occurs, gastric acid secretion can be reduced with H2-blockers or more efficiently with proton-pump inhibitors.

This patient should be treated with normal saline and electrolyte replacement. This should be delivered slowly, to expand the extracellular fluid volume. In this elderly patient, evidence of volume overload should be followed closely. As the body rehydrates, the kidneys will excrete the excess HCO3 and correct the alkalosis.

Reference

HJ, Madias NE. Secondary responses to altered acid–base status: the rules of engagement. J Am Soc Nephrol 2010;21:920-3ty.

179. A 72-year-old woman has been admitted during the day for a bronchitis. You are called to see her urgently for chest pain that night. On physical exam, she has developed acute pulmonary edema. Blood pressure is 110/60 mmHg. Evidence of myocardial ischemia is seen on telemetry. An ECG shows ST segment elevation of 3 mm in the precordial leads.

She has no known prior contraindications to thrombolytic therapy.

Which of the following statements regarding thrombolytic therapy is true?
A) Thrombolytic therapy or direct revascularization is indicated.
B) Thrombolytic therapy is contraindicated because of her age.
C) Thrombolytic therapy is contraindicated because of the presence of cardiogenic shock.
D) Thrombolytic therapy will establish antegrade coronary artery perfusion in 75 % of cases.
E) Thrombolytic therapy is contraindicated because of her low blood pressure.

Answer: A

This patient's age or underlying medical condition is not a contraindication to thrombolytic therapy nor is the presence of cardiogenic shock. Direct revascularization is preferable if it can be obtained quickly.

Patients who develop cardiogenic shock because of a myocardial infarction have high mortality rates. Mortality can be lowered from 85 % to less than 60 % if flow can be reestablished in the infarct-related artery. Thrombolytic therapy is able to achieve this in only 50 % of cases. Percutaneous angioplasty has a higher success rate. If angioplasty is not available or delayed, thrombolytic therapy is indicated.

O'Gara PT, Kushner FG, Ascheim DD, et al. 2013 ACCF/AHA Guideline for the Management of ST-Elevation Myocardial Infarction: A Report of the American College of Cardiology Foundation/American Heart Association Task Force on Practice Guidelines. Circulation. 2013;127:e362-e452.

180. A 25-year-old woman is admitted with cellulitis. She states that she was working in the garden outside of her house the evening before and felt a sharp pain on the back of her left hand.

On physical examination, you note an area of pallor with surrounding erythema over the dorsum of the patient's left hand. You suspect that she was bitten by a brown recluse spider.

Which of the following therapies may benefit the victim of a brown recluse spider bite?

A) Administration of dapsone in patients who do not have glucose-6- phosphate dehydrogenase deficiency

C) Use of antibiotics if there are signs of infection at the bite site

D) Administration of steroids within 24 h of the bite

E) All of the above

Answer: E

Brown recluse spiders are found under rocks, woodpiles, and in gardens. Characteristic violin-shaped markings on their backs have led brown recluse spiders to also be known as fiddleback spiders. They are most active at night in moderate temperature.

Bites can cause pain within the first few hours. Physical findings are a ring of pallor surrounded by erythema. Typically, at 24–72 h, a single clear or hemorrhagic vesicle develops at the site, which later forms a dark eschar. Treatment with systemic steroids within 24 h of bite is beneficial. Dapsone has been shown to be helpful in treating the local damage caused by the venom. However, dapsone can cause a serious hemolytic reaction in those with glucose-6-phosphate dehydrogenase deficiency. Antibiotics are useful if there is evidence of infection.

Reference

King LE Jr, Rees RS. Dapsone treatment of a brown recluse bite. JAMA. 1983;250(5):648

181. A 67-year-old man presents to the emergency department complaining of intense abdominal pain, nausea, and vomiting for the past 48 h. He reports occasional alcohol use, but no prior episodes of similar abdominal pain.

On physical examination, the patient is uncomfortable, a temperature of 38.4 °C (101.1 °F) is noted. On abdominal exam, he has diffuse moderate tenderness. T. bili is 2.8 mg/dl and amylase is 567 units/L.

What is the most appropriate test to determine the cause of the patient's pancreatitis?

A) Plain film

B) Ultrasonography

C) CT scan

D) Endoscopic retrograde cholangiopancreatography

E) ETOH level

Answer: B

This patient has gallstone-induced pancreatitis. Ultrasonography of the abdomen is the most useful initial test in determining the etiology of pancreatitis. It is more sensitive than CT for the diagnosis of gallstone disease.

CT is better at demonstrating morphologic changes in the pancreas caused by inflammation. It is generally indicated in those with severe pancreatitis. Findings on plain film are of little benefit. ERCP can be useful in the management of pancreatitis but has no role in diagnoses.

His age and elevated total bilirubin make alcohol a less likely cause. The median age at onset depends on the etiology. For alcohol, it is 39 and for biliary tract disease it is 69.

References

Telem DA, Bowman K, Hwang J, Chin EH, Nguyen SQ, Divino CM. Selective management of patients with acute biliary pancreatitis. J Gastrointest Surg. 2009;13(12):2183–8.

Tenner S, Baillie J, Dewitt J, et al. American College of Gastroenterology Guidelines: Management of Acute Pancreatitis. Am J Gastroenterol. Jul 30 2013

182. A 75-year-old male presents with bright red blood per rectum. He states he has had bleeding for the past eight years for which he has been admitted several times to various hospitals outside of the current state. He occasionally is transfused during these admissions. He has had several colonoscopies but reports they are always normal. He reports no weight loss and, otherwise, is enjoying good health.

The most likely diagnosis is:

A) Diverticula

B) Arterial venous malformations

C) Malignancy

D) Hemorrhoids

Answer: B

Arterial venous malformations (AVM) are a common cause of lower intestinal bleeding. Over half are located in the right colon, and approximately 50 % of patients experience painless hematochezia. Colonic lesions most often bleed chronically and slow. However, as many as 15 % of patients present with acute massive hemorrhage. AVMs can be acute, chronic, and intermittent in nature. Angiography is considered the gold standard in diagnosing arterial venous malformations.

Management of AVMs is often difficult. Electrocautery has been used to obliterate angiodysplasias. However, bleeding recurs in approximately 50 % of subjects. A reduction in the posttherapy transfusion requirements in patients' cauterized was not reported to be statistically superior to no therapy.

Currently, no medical therapy has been proven to effectively prevent bleeding from AVM. No preventive methods for angiodysplasia have been definitely identified at this time. Avoidance of nonsteroidal anti-inflammatory drugs (NSAIDs) is recommended.

Reference

Regula J, Wronska E, Pachlewski J. Vascular lesions of the gastrointestinal tract. Best Pract Res Clin Gastroenterol. 2008;22(2):313–28.

183. A 78-year-old male presents with worsening confusion and a significant change in personality over the past four weeks. He has a history of mild dementia, as reported by his family but has been living independently. Two months ago he was still working as a fisherman. He has been in the hospital for ten days, and despite extensive workup including computed tomography of the head, EEG, and cerebrospinal fluid analysis, no definitive diagnosis is found.

During the past week, his confusion has become worse. He is now mainly nonresponsive. He has developed a progressive myoclonus starting in his right arm. Repeat computed tomography of his head is still normal. Repeat EEG is pending. The most likely diagnosis is:
A) Creutzfeldt–Jakob disease (CJD)
B) Multi-infarct dementia
C) Recurrent seizure disorder
D) Catatonic depression
E) Herpes simplex encephalitis

Answer: A

This patient has Creutzfeldt–Jakob disease (CJD). The differential diagnosis of rapidly progressive dementia is limited. The clues to CJD in this patient are the appearance of relatively normal imaging, the unexplained rapidly progressive dementia, and the subsequent appearance of myoclonus. Initially, individuals experience problems with muscular coordination and personality changes, including impaired memory suggestive of typical dementia. Most patients die within six months after initial symptoms appear.

The current accepted theory is that CJD is caused by prions. Prions are misfolded proteins that replicate by converting their properly folded counterparts to the same misfolded structure they possess. The disease leads to neurodegeneration, causing the brain tissue to take a more sponge-like texture. Although most patient have a rapidly declining course, there is some variation. 15 % of patients survive for two or more years. Some patients have been known to live 4–5 years.

Clinical testing for CJD has been problematic. Electroencepgraphy may be normal on presentation as was here. Triphasic spikes often occur later on and may be the first clue to diagnosis. Confirmation is often made by a combination of tests, symptoms, and marker proteins found in the CSF.

References

Belay ED, Schonberger LB Variant Creutzfeldt–Jakob disease and bovine spongiform encephalopathy". Clin. Lab. Med.2002; 22 (4): 849–62, v–vi
Ironside, JW; Sutherland, K; Bell, JE; McCardle, L; :Barrie, C; Estebeiro, K; Zeidler, M; Will, RG A new variant of Creutzfeldt–Jakob disease: neuropathological and clinical features.". Cold Spring Harbor symposia on quantitative biology. 1996; 61: 523–30.

184. A 33-year-old woman is admitted because of headache that began suddenly while playing tennis. The headache is diffuse and reached its greatest intensity over three hours. She denies any head trauma, loss of consciousness, or other symptoms. She has had four similar headaches in the past year.

On physical exam, the patient appears uncomfortable. Blood pressure is 160/92 mmHg. She is alert and oriented. No focal deficits are noted. Cranial nerves are normal. Neck flexion is normal.

The only medicine she reports is birth control pills.

Which of the following aspects suggests subarachnoid hemorrhage (SAH)?
A) Onset during exertion
B) Age of 29
C) Peak intensity of headache at three hours
D) Three or more headaches during the past six to 12 months
E) Use of estrogens

Answer: A

Diagnosis of SAH usually depends on a high index of clinical suspicion combined with radiologic confirmation. Noncontrast CT is recommended, followed by lumbar puncture or CT angiography of the brain.

Physical or emotional strain, defecation, coitus, and head trauma contribute to varying degrees in 60–70 % of cases. The central feature of classic SAH is sudden onset of severe headache, often described as the "worst headache of my life." Other factors strongly associated with SAH diagnosis are aged 40 years or older, syncope, complaint of neck pain or stiffness, arrival by ambulance, vomiting, and diastolic blood pressure ≥100 mmHg or systolic blood pressure ≥160 mmHg.

Reference

Perry JJ, Stiell IG, Sivilotti ML, Bullard MJ, Lee JS, Eisenhauer M. High risk clinical characteristics for subarachnoid haemorrhage in patients with acute headache: prospective cohort study. BMJ. 2010;341:c5204.

185. A 72-year-old man who has chronic systolic heart failure presents with increasing shortness of breath. He has gained 5 kg (10 lb) since his last outpatient appointment one month ago. He has not been following sodium and fluid restrictions as prescribed by his cardiologist.

Temperature is 37.7 C (100.0 F), pulse rate is 90 per minute, respirations are 24 per minute, and blood pressure is 150/77 mmHg. Oxygen saturation by pulse oximetry is 88 %. Physical examination is remarkable for jugular venous distention. An S3 gallop is noted. He has bilateral crackles to the mid-lung fields, and 2+ edema in the legs.

Which of the following interventions has not been proven to be beneficial in the treatment of this patient in the inpatient setting?
A) Supplemental oxygen
B) Continuation of the ACE inhibitor
C) Intravenous furosemide
D) Daily weights
E) Strict sodium and fluid restriction

Answer: E

Despite what is recommended for outpatient management of CHF, a randomized controlled trial of patients who have acute decompensated heart failure demonstrated that aggressive sodium and fluid restriction demonstrated no additional weight loss or benefits to heart failure symptoms compared with a liberal standard hospital diet with no restrictions on sodium or fluid intake.

Reference

Aliti GB, Rabelo ER, Clausell N, Rohde LE, Biolo A, Beckda-Silva L. Aggressive fluid and sodium restriction in acute decompensated heart failure: a randomized clinical trial. JAMA Intern Med. 2013;173:1058–1064.

186. An 82-year-old female is admitted to the hospital because of community-acquired pneumonia. She has been living with her husband.

On physical exam, vital signs are normal, and oxygen saturation by pulse oximetry is 90 %. She is oriented to month but not day or date. Leukocyte count is 13,000/μL [4000–11,000]. Radiograph of the chest shows opacity in the base of the left lung.

Treatment with supplemental oxygen, ceftriaxone, and intravenous azithromycin is started. She improves and is weaned off supplemental oxygen during the next two days. Repeat mental status testing shows that she is oriented but is still not to her baseline mental status. There has been some mild agitation in the hospital but she is sleeping through the night. The family inquires if anything can be done to improve cognitive function and control of her mild agitation.

Which of the following is the best option?
A) Magnetic resonance imaging
B) Prescribe donepezil
C) Prescribe lorazepam
D) Prescribe haloperidol
E) Arrange outpatient follow-up to address cognitive function

Answer: E

Delirium is the most common cause of cognitive changes in the inpatient setting. This patient likely has baseline cognitive impairment, which puts her at higher risk for delirium. The most common differential diagnostic issue when evaluating confusion in older adults involves differentiating symptoms of delirium and dementia. It is not possible to accurately diagnose the extent of her dementia in the current setting. Despite the lack of evidence of benefit in the acute setting, nearly 10 % of all new cholinesterase inhibitors are started in the hospital.

Once she has fully recovered from her community-acquired pneumonia, an accurate assessment can be made and treatment considered. Further medications are likely to increase confusion and should be avoided.

Reference

Fong TG, Tulebaev SR, Inouye SK. Delirium in elderly adults: diagnosis, prevention and treatment. Nat Rev Neurol. 2009; 5:210–220.

187. A 52-year-old man is brought to the emergency department by nursing home staff because of polyuria and polydipsia. Over the past week, they have noted increased urination and almost constant thirst. His past medical history is uncertain, he was recently admitted by family members two months ago. His only medication is lithium,

On physical examination, temperature is normal, blood pressure is 120/80 mmHg, pulse rate is 67/min, and respiration rate is 16/min. The remainder of the examination is normal.

Results of laboratory studies show a serum sodium level of 157 mEq/L, random plasma glucose level of 109 mg/dL, and urine osmolality of 110 mOsm/kg. A trial of vasopressin results in no significant increase in urine osmolality within 1 to 2 h.

Which of the following is the most likely cause of this patient's hypernatremia?
A) Central diabetes insipidus
B) Nephrogenic diabetes insipidus
C) Osmotic diuresis
D) Primary polydipsia

Answer: B

The most likely cause of this patient's hypernatremia is diabetes insipidus (DI). Nonresponse to vasopressin indicates a nephrogenic source. Generally, lithium nephrotoxicity will occur within a month of the onset of use of the drug. The first symptoms are usually polyuria and polydipsia. This may also occur in the presence of accelerating dose regimens.

Correcting electrolyte abnormalities is the first step in management. Treatment should be initiated with normal saline at 200–250 cm³/hour to replete hypovolemia This should be followed by administration of hypotonic fluid.

For patients with greater degrees of lithium toxicity, dialysis is indicated. Diuretics and NSAIDs are used in the long-term treatment of stable lithium-induced nephrogenic diabetes insipidus.

Reference

Garofeanu CG, Weir M, Rosas-Arellano MP, et al. Causes of reversible nephrogenic diabetes insipidus: a systematic review. Am J Kidney Dis. 2005;45(4):626–37.

188. A 28-year-old woman is evaluated in the emergency department because of dizziness for the last week. She has not experienced chest pain, dyspnea, or orthopnea. She was ill six weeks ago with fever, fatigue, and myalgias. Her husband reports an erythematous rash on her abdomen that resolved over two weeks. She has no significant medical history and is on no medicines. Her travel history is significant for a camping trip seven weeks ago.

On physical examination, temperature is normal, blood pressure is 126/65 mmHg, and pulse rate is 42/min. The cardiac examination reveals bradycardia. The remainder of the physical examination is normal.

An electrocardiogram shows variable heart block and a junctional escape rate of 50/min. She is admitted to the telemetry unit.

Which of the following would be the initial appropriate treatment?

A) Electrophysiology study
B) Intravenous ceftriaxone
C) Permanent pacemaker placement
D) Temporary pacemaker placement
E) No treatment until further serological testing

Answer: B

This patient should be treated with intravenous ceftriaxone. Patients with atrioventricular (AV) heart block with early Lyme disease may be treated with either oral or parenteral antibiotic therapy for 14 days. Continuous monitoring is advisable for patients with second- or third-degree heart block.

The prognosis is good, usually with the resolution of atrioventricular block within days to weeks. Ceftriaxone is the drug of choice followed by a 21-day course of oral therapy.

Temporary pacing would be required if the patient were hemodynamically unstable with bradycardia. However, this rarely occurs.

Patients with probable erythema migrans and a recent tick exposure should be started with treatment without blood tests. For serologic testing, the CDC recommends a two-tier testing procedure. An ELISA test can be done initially followed by confirmation with Western blot testing.

Reference

Cameron DJ, Johnson LB, Maloney EL. Evidence assessments and guideline recommendations in Lyme disease: the clinical management of known tick bites, erythema migrans rashes and persistent disease. Expert Rev Anti Infect Ther. 2014;12(9):1103–35.

189. A 72-year-old man with a history of COPD and hypertension is admitted for severe lower back pain that began suddenly two days ago. He also reports an unexplained syncopal episode. Since that time, he has had vague lower abdominal and back discomfort.

On physical examination, temperature is 37.4 °C (99.3 °F), blood pressure is 110/65 mmHg, pulse rate is 96/min and regular, and respiration rate is 18/min. Abdominal examination shows moderate tenderness upon palpation in the infraumbilical and suprapubic regions. Some mild local distension is noted in that area. Findings on rectal examination are unremarkable, with guaiac-negative stool.

Laboratory results include hematocrit of 34 %. Results of liver chemistry studies and urinalysis are normal. Plain abdominal radiograph shows no free air or air-fluid levels. Computed tomography of the abdomen is pending.

Which of the following is the most likely diagnosis?

A) Acute myocardial infarction
B) Diverticulitis
C) Nephrolithiasis or renal colic
D) Ruptured abdominal aortic aneurysm
E) Incarcerated hernia

Answer: D

This patient has a classical presentation of a locally contained ruptured aortic abdominal aneurysm. Severe abdominal or back pain with syncope, followed by vague discomfort, is typical. Patients at greatest risk for abdominal aortic aneurysms are those who are older than 65 years and have peripheral atherosclerotic vascular disease. The temporary loss of consciousness is also a potential symptom of rupture. The most typical manifestation of rupture is the acute onset of abdominal or back pain with a pulsatile abdominal mass. The symptoms of a ruptured aneurysm may be confused with renal calculus, diverticulitis, incarcerated hernia, or lumbar spine disease. The prognosis is poor with as many as 65 % of patients dying before arriving at a hospital.

References

Blanchard JF, Armenian HK, Friesen PP. Risk factors for abdominal aortic aneurysm: results of a case–control study. Am J Epidemiol. 15 2000;151(6):575–83.
Von Allmen RS, Powell JT. The management of ruptured abdominal aortic aneurysms: screening for abdominal aortic aneurysm and incidence of rupture. J Cardiovasc Surg (Torino). 2012;53(1):69–76.

190. A 65-year-old woman is admitted for the acute onset of dyspnea, wheezing, and progressive respiratory distress. She has a history of severe chronic asthma. She has been intubated once previously.

    On physical examination, she is in marked distress and is anxious. Temperature is 37.7 °C (100.0 °F), blood pressure is 160/100 mmHg, pulse rate is 127/min, and respiration rate is 28/min; BMI is 33. She has a rapid and regular rhythm with no murmurs. Pulmonary examination reveals very faint wheezing with poor air movement.

    Arterial blood gas studies breathing ambient air show a PCO2 of 84 mmHg, a PO2 of 51 mmHg, and a pH of 7.00. Chest X-ray shows hyperinflation.

    She is intubated and is started on mechanical ventilation.

    Which of the following strategies in establishing ventilator settings is most appropriate for this patient?
    A) Decreased inspiratory flow
    B) Increased minute ventilation
    C) Prolonged expiratory time
    D) Prolonged inspiratory time

Answer: C

Patient with acute asthma exacerbations have primary expiratory flow problem. This limitation results from both anatomic and dynamic obstruction of the airways. As a consequence, these patients require prolonged expiratory times to reach static lung volumes.

Minimizing hyperinflation and avoiding excessive airway pressures are key goals in ventilating the patient with asthma. These goals are best accomplished by selective hypoventilation. This is accomplished by selecting a low respiratory rate and tidal volume in an effort to give the patient sufficient time for exhalation. Suggested initial ventilator settings for intubated patients with asthma are:
- Assist control mode
- Tidal volume: 7–8 mL/kg (using ideal body weight)
- Respiratory rate: 10–12 breaths/min
- FiO2: 100 %
- PEEP: 0 cm H2O

Reference

Archambault PM, St-Onge M. Invasive and noninvasive ventilation in the emergency department. Emerg Med Clin North Am. 2012;30(2):421–49,

191. You are called to see a 24-year-old patient on the floor which has become markedly obtunded. He was recently admitted two hours ago for possible suicide attempt by ingestion of an unknown substance. His respiratory status was good on admission but he is having difficulty handling secretions and a decision is made to intubate him urgently. Chest radiograph on admission was normal.

    Initial tidal volumes (TV) on the ventilator should be set to what setting?
    A) 4 ml/kg
    B) 6 ml/kg
    C) 10 ml/kg
    D) 12 ml/kg

Answer: B

Synchronous intermittent mandatory ventilation (SIMV) and assist-control ventilation (A/C) are versatile modes that can be used for initial settings. Lower tidal volumes (TV) are recommended than in the past years, when tidal volumes of 10–15 mL/kg were routinely used. This is thought to reduce barotrauma.

An initial TV of 5–8 mL/kg of ideal body weight is generally recommended. The lower range is recommended in the presence of obstructive airway disease and ARDS. The goal is to adjust the TV so that plateau pressures are less than 35 cm H2O.

Reference

Hess DR, Thompson BT. Ventilatory strategies in patients with sepsis and respiratory failure. Curr Infect Dis Rep. Sep 2005;7(5):342–8.

192. Clindamycin as compared to trimethoprim–sulfamethoxazole in the treatment of uncomplicated soft tissue infections resulted in what outcomes?
    A) Improved outcome
    B) More side effects
    C) Worse outcomes
    D) Less side effects
    E) None of the above

Answer: E

Outpatients with uncomplicated skin infections who took clindamycin or a trimethoprim–sulfamethoxazole combination (TMP-SMX) experienced similar benefits and risks. This is according to a randomized trial published in the 2015 New England Journal of Medicine. The authors found no significant differences between the efficacy of clindamycin and that of TMP-SMX for the treatment of uncomplicated skin infections in children and adults with few or no major coexisting conditions.

Reference

Miller, Loren et al. Engl J Med. 2015;372:1093–1103, 1164–1165.

193. A 55-year-old hypertensive white male has been admitted with pneumonia. He has responded well to treatment. You are called to see him urgently. He develops the acute onset of palpitations. He then complains of chest pain and shortness of breath. Blood pressure is 90/60 mmHg and heart rate of 165 BPM. The ECG showed atrial fibrillation with rapid ventricular response.

What is your next step in management?
A) IV Amiodarone
B) IV digoxin
C) IV Cardizem
D) Synchronized cardioversion
E) Asynchronized cardioversion

Answer: D

Synchronized electric cardioversion is the treatment of choice in atrial fibrillation patients with rapid ventricular response who are not stable. Anticoagulation is not indicated since the atrial fibrillation started less than 48 h ago. Asynchronized cardioversion may precipitate ventricular fibrillation. Medical management using amiodarone, Cardizem, or digoxin is not appropriate in with hypotension, ischemia, or other signs of instability.

Reference

Wann LS, Curtis AB, January CT, et al. 2011 ACCF/AHA/h focused update on the management of patients with atrial fibrillation (updating the 2006 guideline): a report of the American College of Cardiology Foundation/American Heart Association Task Force on Practice Guidelines. Circulation.2011;123(1):104–23.

194. A 28-year-old male has been admitted for head trauma resulting in a small subdural hematoma. Little is known about his past medical history. He appears intoxicated on admission and his blood is positive for alcohol. 24 h after his admission for observation, he becomes acutely agitated. He pulls his IV out and threatens a nurse with a broken glass. Security is called, and he is physically restrained in bed, which requires four security officers. At this time he continues to hallucinate, is verbally aggressive, and threatens to kill the staff.

What is the correct initial treatment for sedation ?
A) Lorazepam 5 mg by mouth
B) Haloperidol 10 mg intramuscular and lorazepam 2 mg intramuscular
C) Haloperidol 5 mg PO
D) Lorazepam 2 mg intramuscular
E) Place IV first

Answer: B

This is a medical emergency that requires rapid action, for patient, staff, and fellow patient safety. The acutely agitated patient often does not have IV access, and gaining access is often difficult. Both benzodiazepines and atypical antipsychotics have shown similar effectiveness in reducing aggression and time to sedation when use as single agents.

Oral medications have been shown to have similar onset of action compared to intramuscular (IM) administration, are less invasive, and are more widely accepted by patients. However in this situation the risk of harm to patient and the staff is too high that attempting an oral route may not be successful.

A few randomized trials have indicated that the combination of a benzodiazepine with a traditional or classic antipsychotic results in a more rapid onset of sedation with a similar adverse effect profile. In this situation, a combination approach may be the most effective. This approach is commonly used by physicians in correctional facilities. A dose of 10 mg of haloperidol and 2 mg of Ativan intramuscularly is often suggested.

References

MH, Currier GW, Hughes DH, Docherty JP, Carpenter D, Ross R. Treatment of behavioral emergencies: a summary of the expert consensus guidelines. J Psychiatr Pract. Jan 2003;9(1):16–38.

Kansagra SM, Rao SR, Sullivan AF, Gordon JA, Magid DJ, Kaushal R. A Survey of Workplace Violence Across 65 U.S. Emergency Departments. Acad Emerg Med. 25 2008

195. A 46-year-old woman is admitted for nausea, vomiting, headache, and blurry vision which developed 6 h ago. The patient was previously well and takes no medications.

On physical examination, she appears restless and confused with dysarthric speech. Temperature is 38.1 °C (100.5 °F), blood pressure is 150/92 mmHg, pulse rate is 110/min, and respiration rate is 22/min. Oxygen saturation is 95 %. There is mild nuchal rigidity, but no photophobia. Abdominal examination reveals moderate diffuse tenderness without guarding upon palpation. Bowel sounds are present.

Laboratory studies include a hemoglobin of 9.7 g/dL, leukocyte count of 6600/μL, platlet count of 28,000 and lactate dehydrogenase of 546 U/L. P. Prothrombin time and activated partial thromboplastin time are within normal limits. A peripheral blood smear reveals schistocytes.

What is the most likely diagnosis?

A) Aplastic anemia
B) Disseminated intravascular coagulation
C) Thrombotic thrombocytopenic purpura (TTP)
D) Warm autoimmune hemolytic anemia with immune thrombocytopenic purpura
E) Hemolytic uremic syndrome (HUS)

Answer: C

Patients with thrombotic thrombocytopenic purpura (TTP) typically report an acute or subacute onset of neurologic dysfunction, anemia, and thrombocytopenia. Neurologic manifestations are extensive. They include alteration in mental status, seizures, hemiplegia, paresthesias, visual disturbance, and aphasia. Severe bleeding from thrombocytopenia is unusual, although petechiae are common. Other clinical features may include nausea, vomiting, and abdominal pain with or without elevations of serum amylase and lipase levels. Differentiation of hemolytic uremic syndrome (HUS) and TTP can be problematic, although treatment protocols may be the same. Plasma exchange may be considered for both. It is often based on the presence of central nervous system involvement in TTP and the more severe renal involvement in HUS.

A peripheral blood smear is essential to determine whether the anemia is caused by a microangiopathic hemolytic process, as indicated by the presence of schistocytes. This patient has fever in association with neurologic symptoms, anemia, and thrombocytopenia with normal coagulation parameters (prothrombin time and activated partial thromboplastin time) and a peripheral blood smear showing fragmented erythrocytes (schistocytes), the hallmark of a microangiopathic process. Plasma exchange should be instituted emergently at diagnosis because 10 % of patients die of this disease despite therapy.

Reference

Lau DH, Wun T. Early manifestation of thrombotic thrombocytopenic purpura. Am J Med. 1993;95(5):544–5

196. A 68-year-old woman is admitted for a 3-day history of headache, fever, diarrhea, and nausea. Once admitted to the floor, she rapidly becomes confused. Medical history is significant for diabetes mellitus.

On physical examination on the floor, the patient is disoriented. Temperature is 38.7 °C (101.9 °F), blood pressure is 100/65 mmHg, pulse rate is 110/min, and respiration rate is 19/min. Oxygen saturation is 94 % on room air. There are no focal neurologic abnormalities, but neck stiffness is noted.

Empiric treatment is initiated with ampicillin, ceftriaxone, and vancomycin.

Complete blood count reveals a leukocyte count of 21,000/μL. Noncontrast computed tomographic scan of the head is normal. Blood cultures are obtained.

A lumbar puncture is performed, and the cerebrospinal fluid (CSF) examination reveals that leukocyte count is 950/μL with 85 % neutrophils and 20 % lymphocytes; the protein level is 95 mg/dL; and the glucose level is 15 mg/dL. Gram stain of the CSF reveals gram-positive bacillus. She improves in the first 12 h of treatment.

This patient's antibiotic regimen should be narrowed to intravenous administration of which of the following?

A) Ampicillin
B) Ceftriaxone
C) Vancomycin
D) No change of antibiotic regimen

Ampicillin is included in empiric therapy for bacterial meningitis in patients who are at risk for developing invasive infections with this Gram-positive bacillus. *L. monocytogenes* meningitis develops most frequently in neonates, older adults (>50 years of age), and those who are immunocompromised. Cases have been reported in patients with no underlying disorders.

Although *Listeria* may cause a limited gastrointestinal syndrome, there are few clinical features distinguishing the presentation *Listeria* meningitis from other acute bacterial meningitides. Foods that have sometimes caused outbreaks of *Listeria* include hot dogs, deli meats, pasteurized or unpasteurized milk, cheeses, raw and cooked poultry, raw meats, ice cream, raw fruits, and smoked fish.

Gram stain is positive approximately 50 % of the time and culture is positive nearly 100 % of the time. Meningitis is often complicated by encephalitis, a pathology that is unusual for bacterial infections. Patients should be treated for three weeks.

Reference

Cherubin CE, Appleman MD, Heseltine PN, Khayr W, Stratton CW. Epidemiological spectrum and current treatment of listeriosis. Rev Infect Dis. 1991;13(6):1108–14

197. A 72-year-old woman is admitted with worsening behavior that her husband is having a difficult time managing.

She has had progressive behavioral change over the course of two years. Recently, she has begun eating more and had gained 20 lb in 5 months. She has begun to tell lies and makes inappropriate comments. She has developed poor personal hygiene and refused to take a bath. Five years ago she appeared to be completely functional.

On physical examination, vital signs are normal. The patient's appearance is disheveled and unkempt. There is a loss of verbal fluency. Mental status examination shows minimal memory loss and difficulty drawing a complex figure.

Which of the following is the most likely diagnosis?

A) Alzheimer disease
B) Creutzfeldt–Jakob disease
C) Dementia with Lewy bodies
D) Frontotemporal dementia (FTD)
E) Multi-infarct dementia

Answer: E

This patient has the clinical features of frontotemporal dementia (FTD). This includes an emphasis on prominent personality and behavioral changes with less prominent memory loss early in the course.

The approach to treatment may be different with FTD as compared to Alzheimer disease. Generally, cholinesterase inhibitors are not recommended for patients diagnosed with FTD. People with FTD usually tolerate SSRIs well, and they are generally considered the best available medications for controlling problematic behaviors. Antipsychotics should be used with caution. Their potential benefit must be weighed against potential risks including weight gain, slowing of movement and thinking, accelerating heart disease, and, in rare instances, death. Typical antipsychotics should be avoided, since patients with FTD are likely to show muscle stiffness and trembling which may be made worse with typical antipsychotic use.

The main clinical features of CJD are dementia that progresses rapidly over months and startle myoclonus, although the latter may not be present early in the illness. Other prominent features include visual or cerebellar disturbance, pyramidal/extrapyramidal dysfunction, and akinetic mutism.

Dementia with Lewy bodies is accompanied by parkinsonism, visual hallucinations, and fluctuating symptoms. The characteristic cognitive profile of dementia in patients with dementia with Lewy bodies includes impaired learning and attention, psychomotor slowing, and constructional apraxia, but less memory impairment than in similarly staged patients with Alzheimer disease.

Reference

Manning C. Beyond memory: neuropsychologic features in differential diagnosis of dementia. Clin Geriatr Med 2004;20:45–58.

198. A 58-year-old male is transferred from an outside hospital because of ascites and worsening renal function. He has hepatitis C cirrhosis, portal hypertension, and near end-stage liver disease. Contrast-enhanced computed tomography of the abdomen was performed at the outside hospital 3 days before transfer because of abdominal pain. His oral fluid intake has been restricted. Urine output in the past 24 h is 300 mL.

On physical examination today, he is afebrile. Pulse rate is 75 per minute, and blood pressure is 100/70 mmHg. Decreased breath sounds are noted in the bases of both lungs. He has tense ascites, no worse than his baseline and pitting edema (3+) in his legs.

His MELD score is 25. Creatine is 5.1 μg/dl with a baseline of 1.5 two weeks ago.

Paracentesis reveals a peritoneal fluid leukocyte count of 1672/μL.

Which of the following is the most important next step in this patient's management?

A) Trial of octreotide and midodrine
B) Nephrology consultation
C) Listing for emergency liver transplantation
D) Fluid challenge test
E) Hemodialysis

Answer: D

Requirements for the diagnosis of hepatorenal syndrome (HRS) include a doubling of the serum creatinine level and at least a 1.5 L fluid challenge. This should be considered despite the presence of ascites. Urgent transplantation or hemodialysis may be considered after HRS has been established. Octreotide and midodrine may be of some limited benefit once the diagnosis of HRS has been made.

Reference

Hasper D, Jorres A. New insights into the management of hepato-renal syndrome. Liver Int. 2011;31(Suppl 3):27–30

199. A 39-year-old woman is admitted for diarrhea. The purpose of the admission is to quantify and document her diarrhea before and after a fast has begun. She has been seen in clinic for diarrhea many times in the past two months.

She reports that the diarrhea has been present since she developed a presumed food-borne illness three months ago. At that time, she had severe nausea, vomiting, and watery diarrhea for two days. Although her symptoms improved, she has continued to have episodic diarrhea with four to five watery stools each day, often following meals. She also has had excessive flatus and abdominal distension over the past two months. She denies nocturnal stools, weight loss, fever, or blood in her stool. She denies any recent antibiotics. Medical history is notable for diabetes, hypertension, and a cholecystectomy performed two years ago.

On physical examination, vital signs are normal. Abdominal examination reveals normal bowel sounds and a nontender abdomen. Rectal examination is normal.

A complete blood count, stool cultures, stool examination for ova and parasites, and tests for *Clostridium difficile* are negative. Before a fast is begun, the nurses report six bowel movements in one shift. Stool osmotic gap is measured at 170 mOsm/kg.
A) Bile-salt-induced diarrhea
B) Diabetic gastropathy
C) Irritable bowel syndrome
D) Lactose malabsorption
E) Microscopic colitis

Answer: D

This patient has lactose malabsorption that developed as a result of her recent food-borne illness or gastroenteritis. This is a relatively common occurrence, may occur after a nonspecific gastrointestinal event, and is usually self-limited. Estimating the stool osmotic gap using stool electrolytes evaluates for the presence of an osmotic diarrhea. A gap greater than 100 mOsm/kg (100 mmol/kg) indicates an osmotic cause of diarrhea.

Lactose malabsorption is the most common cause of a stool osmotic gap. Reducing this patient's lactose intake will often result in symptom improvement. Lactose intake can slowly be increased as more time elapses and her lactose intolerance improves.

Even though some patients may have an increase in stool frequency after cholecystectomy, this patient's surgery was remote enough that it would not cause her current symptoms. Bile-salt-induced diarrhea tends to cause a secretory diarrhea. A stool osmotic gap is not consistent with the diagnosis of IBS. Microscopic colitis causes a secretory diarrhea.

Reference

Mattar R, de Campos Mazo DF, Carrilho FJ. Lactose intolerance: diagnosis, genetic, and clinical factors. Clin Exp Gastroenterol. 2012;5:113–21.

200. A 68-year-old man is admitted to the ICU for of a 10-day history of fever, headache, diarrhea, and cough productive of yellow sputum. He also has a 2-day history of progressive dyspnea. He has been on oral antibiotics for the past two days.

On physical examination, the temperature is 38.9 °C (101.9 °F), blood pressure is 100/60 mmHg, pulse rate is 120 bpm, and respiration rate is 30/min. Oxygen saturation is 83 % while breathing 100 % oxygen by nonrebreathing mask. Course breath sounds are heard over the left and right lower lung fields.

Laboratory studies show a leukocyte count of 9000/μL, platelet count of 86,000/μL, and serum sodium level of 129 meq/L.

Chest radiograph shows findings consistent with consolidation in the right middle and lower lobes.

The patient is intubated, and mechanical ventilation is initiated. Blood cultures are obtained, empiric antibiotic therapy is begun, and fluid resuscitation is started.

In addition to an endotracheal aspirate for Gram stain and culture, which of the following is the most appropriate next step in the evaluation?
A) Bronchoscopy with quantitative cultures
B) *Legionella* and *Streptococcus pneumonia* urine antigen assays
C) *Legionella* serologic testing
D) No further testing

Answer: B

This patient may benefit from *Legionella* and *Streptococcus pneumonia* urine antigen assays. The clinical value of diagnostic testing to determine the microbial cause of community-acquired pneumonia (CAP) is controversial. This hospitalized patient has severe CAP, defined as CAP in a patient who requires admission to an intensive care unit or transfer to an intensive care unit within 24 h of admission. The 2007 Infectious Diseases Society of America/American Thoracic Society guidelines recommend *Streptococcus pneumonia* and *Legionella* urine antigen assays for hospitalized patients with severe CAP.

The urinary antigen is useful to confirm the presence of *Legionella* or *S. pneumonia*. However, in HCAP the urinary antigen does not seem to be useful.

Legionella should be suspected in this patient, who is older than 50 years of age and presents with severe pneumonia hyponatremia and extrapulmonary symptoms.

Bronchoscopy with quantitative culture can be used as a diagnostic tool in the evaluation of patients with ventilator-associated pneumonia. However, bronchoscopy with quantitative culture has not been prospectively studied for the management of patients with severe CAP.

Serologic testing for atypical pathogens such as *Legionella* species is not recommended because convalescent titers would need to be obtained 6 to 8 weeks after initial testing to establish a diagnosis.

References

Ishida T, Hashimoto T, Arita M, et al. A 3-year prospective study of a urinary antigen-detection test for Streptococcus pneumonia in community-acquired pneumonia: Utility and clinical impact on the reported etiology. J Infect Chemother. 2004;10:359–63.
Mandell LA, Wunderink RG, Anzueto A, et al. Infectious Diseases Society of America/American Thoracic Society consensus guidelines on the management of community-acquired pneumonia. Clin Infect Dis. 2007;44:S27-72..

201. A 76-year-old man is evaluated in the emergency department because of fever, shortness of breath, and productive cough. A month ago, he was hospitalized in the intensive care unit because of respiratory failure and was treated with broad-spectrum antibiotics. He was discharged in fair condition with antibiotics and steroid taper. He has a history of chronic obstructive pulmonary disease. He has a 40-pack-year history of smoking.

On physical examination, temperature is 38.6 °C (101.5 °F), blood pressure is 115/72 mmHg, pulse rate is 116/min, respiration rate is 27/min, and oxygen saturation is 89 % on ambient air. Pulmonary examination shows crackles at the right base.

The leukocyte count is 22,000/μL with 75 % segmented neutrophils and 10 % band forms. Chest radiograph shows a right lower lobe consolidation. Blood cultures are obtained, and treatment with intravenous fluids is initiated.

Which of the following is the most appropriate empiric antibiotic treatment?

A) Vancomycin and ciprofloxacin
B) Ceftriaxone and azithromycin
C) Ceftriaxone and ciprofloxacin
D) Vancomycin, piperacillin/tazobactam, and amikacin

Answer: D

This patient is at high risk for *Pseudomonas* pneumonia. The most appropriate empiric antibiotic therapy for this patient is vancomycin, piperacillin/tazobactam, and amikacin. *Pseudomonas* pneumonia is observed in patients with immunosuppression and chronic lung disease. It can be acquired nosocomially in the intensive care unit (ICU) setting and is associated with positive-pressure ventilation and endotracheal tubes. Other risk factors for *Pseudomonas* pneumonia include broad-spectrum antibiotic use in the previous month, recent hospitalization, malnutrition, neutropenia, and glucocorticoid use.

Most guidelines recommend starting with two anti pseudomonal antibiotics and then de-escalating to monotherapy in five days. It remains controversial whether combination therapy is more efficacious than monotherapy. Combination therapy has been recommended to broaden the empiric coverage and prevent the emergence of antibiotic resistance during therapy.

References

Chamot E, Boffi El Amari E, Rohner P, Van Delden C. Effectiveness of combination antimicrobial therapy for Pseudomonas aeruginosa bacteremia. Antimicrob Agents Chemother. 2003;47(9):2756–64.

Cunha BA. Pseudomonas aeruginosa: resistance and therapy. Semin Respir Infect. 2002;17:231–239.

202. A 75-year-old man is admitted for a 2-day history of fever, vomiting, and dysuria. He has a history of prostatic hypertrophy.

On physical examination, temperature is 39.0 °C (102.2 °F), blood pressure is 100/60 mmHg, and pulse rate is 122/min. Suprapubic tenderness is present. Careful rectal examination shows an enlarged and extremely tender prostate.

Laboratory studies show a leukocyte count of 19,000/μL with 70 % segmented neutrophils. Urinalysis shows more than 50 leukocytes/high-power field and many bacteria. The serum creatinine level is normal.

Treatment with intravenous fluids and parenteral ciprofloxacin is started. Urine culture grows *Escherichia coli* sensitive to fluoroquinolones. Three days after admission, the patient continues to have fever. He develops abdominal and perineal pain. A repeat leukocyte count shows a result of 19,000/μL.

What should be done next?
A) Discontinue ciprofloxacin and start gentamicin.
B) Insert a catheter for bladder drainage.
C) Renal ultrasound.
D) Obtain a transrectal ultrasound.
E) Perform prostate massage.

Answer: D

The patient presents with a clinical picture that is consistent with acute prostatitis. If there is no clinical improvement after 36 to 72 h of treatment, the most likely cause is a complication, such as a prostatic abscess. Appropriate management for this patient is a transrectal ultrasound to evaluate for a prostatic abscess. If a prostatic abscess is identified, ultrasound-guided or surgical drainage may be indicated.

Causative organisms of acute prostatitis in older men are usually Gram-negative bacteria, with *Escherichia coli* being the most common. Transurethral catheterization should be avoided in acute prostatitis. If bladder drainage is necessary, suprapubic drainage may be considered to reduce the risk of prostatic abscess and septicemia. Furthermore, there is no indication for placement of a bladder catheter, such as outflow obstruction.

At one time prostate massage was believed to be therapeutically useful as a treatment for acute prostatitis. Vigorous massage of the prostate should be avoided in acute prostatitis. It is not helpful diagnostically or therapeutically.

Reference

Ludwig M, Schroeder-Printzen I, Schiefer HG, Weidner W. Diagnosis and therapeutic management of 18 patients with prostatic abscess. Urology.1999;53:340–345.

203. An 88-year-old woman has been admitted for a lower gastrointestinal bleed. She is found by imaging and colonoscopy to have a localized adenocarcinoma. Surgery is offered to the patient who is receiving guidance from her family. The patient manages some of her activities of daily living but has help from her daughter. Current medications are metoprolol 25 mg twice daily and acetaminophen 325 mg twice daily as needed. The patient's weight is 50 kg (110 lb) and height is 160 cm (5 ft 3 in).

On physical examination, the patient is alert. Heart rate is 80 beats per minute, and blood pressure is 140/70 mmHg. The abdomen is soft and nontender. On neurologic examination, the patient is oriented to person and place but seems confused concerning the issues of surgery. There is mild weakness of the hip flexors, and normal sensation and reflexes. Before making the decision to have surgery, the family would like to know the risks of postsurgical complications.

Which of the following would best help you determine this patient's risk of complications after surgery?
A) Urinalysis
B) Radiograph of the chest
C) 12-lead electrocardiogram
D) Physical therapy consult
E) Mini mental status exam testing (MMSE)

Answer: E

The most important predictor of functional decline following surgery in the older population is the patient's preexisting mental status. The mini mental status is the best-validated tool to assess that. MMSE scores of 28 or less are associated with more than a twofold increased risk of developing postoperative delirium. The exact correlation with long-term functional and cognitive decline is uncertain. Sharing these factors with families may assist in decision-making and acceptance of postoperative cognitive decline.

References

Chow WB, Rosenthal RA, Merkow RP, et al. American College of Surgeons National Surgical Quality Improvement Program; American Geriatrics Society. Optimal preoperative assessment of the geriatric surgical patient: a best practices guideline from the American College of Surgeons National Surgical Quality Improvement Program and the American Geriatrics Society. J Am Coll Surg. 2012;215:453–466.
Oresanya LB, Lyons WL, Finlayson E. Preoperative assessment of the older patient: a narrative review. JAMA. 2014;311:2110–2120.

204. A 68-year-old female has been mechanically ventilated in the intensive care unit for sepsis. She has received piperacillin/tazobactam and corticosteroids for her past medical history of chronic obstructive pulmonary disease. Vasopressors were needed but now have been stopped. She has been transferred to the floor. The patient now has fluctuating level of consciousness. She has no prior history of dementia. She does not consistently follow commands and, at times, appears confused. She has no focal neurologic findings. Her lungs are cleared upon auscultation. The last time that she received a narcotic and sedatives was in the ICU 2 days ago.

Which of the following should you do now?
A) Obtain an electroencephalogram.
B) Obtain a computed tomography scan of the head.
C) Start an antipsychotic medication.
D) Start a benzodiazepine.
E) Rapidly taper the corticosteroids.

Answer: E

Corticosteroids are associated with delirium and when possible should be either rapidly tapered or stopped. They are often overused in the hospital setting. In this patient, no clear indication exists for continued steroid use and rapid taper may resolve the delirium.

Steroid psychosis may be dose dependent. In one study patients receiving more than 80 mg/day of prednisone or its equivalent had an 18.4 % incidence of steroid psychosis.

Reference

Barr J, Fraser GL, Puntillo K, et al. Clinical practice guidelines for the management of pain, agitation, and delirium in adult patients in the intensive care unit. Crit Care Med. 2013;41:263–306

205. A 58-year-old female presents with right upper quadrant pain, leukocytosis, and fever. CT scan reveals a gangrenous gallbladder and emergency surgery is recommended. She is on warfarin for atrial fibrillation but has not had levels checked in over two months. Her INR is 6. Some bleeding from her gums is noticed. Despite extensive conversations, she refuses any blood product that has any chance of transmitting a virus.

The best agent to administer is:
A) Fresh frozen plasma (FFP)
B) Prothrombin complex concentrate (PCC)
C) Recombinant factor VII
D) Vitamin K

Answer: B

Prothrombin complex concentrates (PCC) may be used as therapy for the patient who has bleeding related to vitamin K antagonists. In 2013, the FDA approved PCC therapy in adult patients needing an urgent surgery or other invasive procedure.

Although not as commonly used and expensive, PCC may have several advantages. PCCs can be administered more rapidly, do not require a crossmatch, and are virally inactivated. In addition, they require less volume. There are no antidotes for many of the novel oral anticoagulants, although PCC and recombinant activated factor VII have been used with some reported success.

Treatment with fresh frozen plasma (FFP) does carry an extremely small risk of virus transmission.

Reference

Ageno W, Gallius AS, Wittkowsky A, et al. Oral anticoagulant therapy: Antithrombotic Therapy and Prevention of Thrombosis, 9th ed: American College of Chest Physicians Evidence-Based Clinical Practice Guidelines. Chest. 2012;141(2 Suppl):e44S–e88S.

206. A 56-year-old man is admitted with pyelonephritis and dehydration. Vascular access has been difficult. Heart rate is 125 beats per minute, and blood pressure is 90/60 mmHg. Several IV attempts have been made without success. An ultrasound-guided vascular access of the right external jugular is planned. By ultrasound, a clot is appreciated in the right internal jugular.

    Which of the following should you do now?
    A) Proceed with the insertion of a line in the right external jugular vein.
    B) Insert a peripherally inserted central catheter (PICC) line on the same side.
    C) Obtain blood cultures.
    D) Consider other options.

Answer: D

Ultrasound has become a valuable tool in line placement, but additional caution must be undertaken with its use. The external jugular connects with the internal jugular. Inserting a line here would not be a good option due to the possibility of dislodging a clot. In addition, the clot may extend to the subclavian, which would make placing a PICC line on the same side risky.

Reference

Troianos CA, Hartman GS, Glas KE, et al.; Councils on Intraoperative Echocardiography and Vascular Ultrasound of the American Society of Echocardiography. Guidelines for performing ultrasound guided vascular cannulation: recommendations of the American Society of Echocardiography and the Society of Cardiovascular Anesthesiologists. J Am Soc Echocardiogr. 2011;24:1291–1318

207. A 35-year-old woman presents with diarrhea, urgency, frequency, and occasional bright red blood per rectum after multiple bowel movements. She reports no weight loss. The patient reports similar symptom on two prior occasions this year. The patient appears well. The abdomen is tender in the left lower quadrant, without rebound.

    Stool cultures are negative. Despite extensive counseling, the patient refuses colonoscopy or sigmoidoscopy.

    Which of the following noninvasive tests is the best way to screen for inflammatory bowel disease in a patient such as this?
    A) ASCA and ANCA
    B) ASCA and anti-CBIR1
    C) ASCA and anti-OmpC
    D) NOD-2 SNP testing
    E) Fecal calprotectin

Answer: A

Currently, no laboratory test is specific enough to adequately and definitively establish the diagnosis of IBD.

Anti-*Saccharomyces cerevisiae* antibodies(ASCA) is the most sensitive serologic marker of Crohn's disease. Antineutrophil cytoplasmic antibodies (pANCA) are a serologic marker of patients with ulcerative colitis. The combination of positive pANCA and negative ASCA has high specificity for ulcerative colitis, whereas a positive ASCA and negative pANCA are more specific for Crohn's disease. There primary use has been in differentiating Crohn's from ulcerative colitis and occasionally as a screening test in select patients.

Reference

Peeters M, Joossens S, Vermeire S, Vlietinck R, Bossuyt X, Rutgeerts P. Diagnostic value of anti-Saccharomyces cerevisiae and antineutrophil cytoplasmic autoantibodies in inflammatory bowel disease. Am J Gastroenterol. 2001;96(3):730–4.

208. A 52-year-old female is admitted for persistent diffuse joint pain. Her symptoms began two and one-half months ago while she was vacationing on a Caribbean cruise. Initially, she had the abrupt onset of high fever, chills, severe malaise, myalgias, headache, and diffuse joint pain. She was diagnosed as having influenza by the ship's doctor but not tested. The symptoms have resolved, but she continues to have moderate joint pain, which is worse on some days. She also notes stiffness and fatigue.

    On physical examination, temperature is 36.8 C (98.2 F), pulse rate is 82 per minute, respirations are 18 per minute, and blood pressure is 132/75 mmHg. Findings of the examination are otherwise normal except for the presence of small effusions in the ankles and knees.

Which of the following is the most likely infecting agent?

A) Dengue virus
B) Malaria
C) Post influenza neuropathy
D) Chikungunya virus
E) B19 infection

Answer: D

Chikungunya fever is a self-remitting febrile viral illness that has been associated with frequent outbreaks in tropical countries and returning travelers. The illness has recently become a concern in Western countries and temperate zones around the world. International travel is one of the major risk factors for the rapid global spread of the disease.

Patients present with abrupt onset of influenza type symptoms. Fever can reach up to 40.5 °C (105°), with shaking chills that last 2–3 days. The fever may return after an afebrile period of 4–10 days.

Chikungunya infection is confirmed via serological tests, which take about 5–7 after the onset of symptoms.

Severe arthralgia is best managed with nonsteroidal anti-inflammatory drugs (NSAIDS) and early physical therapy.

Ribavirin and steroids have been used but no studies have proven their benefit. As of September 2014, there have been seven confirmed cases of chikungunya in the United States in people who had acquired the disease locally.

Reference

McCarthy M. First case of locally acquired chikungunya is reported in US. BMJ. 2014. 349:g4706.

209. A 46-year-old man presents with cough, fever, and sputum production. Six months ago, the patient traveled to Kuwait on business. The patient was well until five days ago, when his symptoms gradually developed. He denies no chills, chest pain, or hemoptysis. He works in the petroleum industry. He has no pets and takes no medications.

On physical exam, his temperature is 38.7 C (101.5 F), pulse rate is 90 per minute, respirations are 14 per minute, and blood pressure is 135/70 mmHg. The skin is warm and dry. Crackles are heard at the left lung base posteriorly.

The leukocyte count is 15,000/μL, with increased bands.

Which of the following is the best next step?
A) Test induced sputum for MERS by RT-PCR
B) Test blood for MERS by RT-PCR
C) Test blood for MERS by serology
D) Treat for community-acquired pneumonia
E) AFB stain of sputum

Answer: A

Middle Eastern respiratory syndrome (MERS) is an emerging concern among recent travelers to the Middle East. The incubation time is 5.2 days. The interval is 7.6 days. It is only a possibility in a patient who has had traveled within 14 days to the Middle East.

MERS presents with a nonspecific triad of cough, fever, and shortness of breath. Most individuals with confirmed MERS have developed significant acute respiratory illness. There has been a reluctance among some countries to provide accurate statistics concerning MERS. Among the probably underreported 536 cases reported through May 12, 2014, the mortality rate has been 30 %.

Diagnosis for MERS is best done using polymerase chain reaction (PCR) testing of induced sputum or blood. Serology, which is not widely available, can identify previous exposure.

References

Arabi YM et al. Clinical course and outcomes of critically ill patients with Middle East respiratory syndrome coronavirus infection. Ann Intern Med 2014;160(6):389–397.

de Groot RJ, Baker SC, Baric RS, Brown CS, Drosten C, Enjuanes L, et al. Middle East respiratory syndrome coronavirus (MERS-CoV): announcement of the Coronavirus Study Group. J Virol. 2013;87(14):7790–2.

210. A 48-year-old man is admitted for increasing shortness of breath. This admission is thought to be multifactorial including volume overload, reactive airway disease, and pulmonary hypertension. He has a history of sleep apnea and he is obese. The patient also has hypertension and hyperlipidemia. He drinks on average one alcoholic beverage every three days. He takes no medications.

On physical examination diffuse mild crackles are heard with 1+ lower extremity edema. The abdomen is soft and nontender.

Laboratory studies reveal an ALT of 107 U/L and an AST of 95 U/L. Serum bilirubin is 0.5 mg/dL. Serum alkaline phosphatase is 78 U/L. Hepatitis A, B, and C serologies are negative.

Which of the following is the most likely cause of his elevated liver functions?
A) Alcoholic hepatitis
B) Autoimmune hepatitis
C) Gallbladder inflammation
D) Liver cancer
E) Nonalcoholic fatty liver disease
F) Congestive heart failure

Answer: E

Nonalcoholic fatty liver disease(NAFLD) is the most common cause of elevated liver enzymes in American adults.

NAFLD liver disease affects 10 % to 24 % of adults, with a higher prevalence in individuals who have obesity and diabetes. OSA is associated with an increased prevalence of nonalcoholic steatohepatitis and fibrosis. Etiology of this association is thought to be related to the intermittent hypoxia that occurs during OSA, leading to liver damage. Diagnosis of NAFLD has historically been made based on abnormal hepatic histology, minimal alcohol consumption, and absence of viral hepatitis. Ultrasound is typically used because of its lack of radiation exposure and its cost-effectiveness. A liver biopsy may be performed to confirm the findings and to assess disease status and potential progression to NASH.

Reference

Fan JG, Jia JD, Li YM, Wang BY, Lu LG, Shi JP, Chan LY. Guidelines for the diagnosis and management of nonalcoholic fatty liver disease: update 2010. J Digestive Dis. 2011;12(1):38–44.

211. A 34-year-old female who is HIV positive is admitted with headache, fever, cough, chills, and weight loss during the past two weeks. The patient was released from jail three months ago. She was admitted to the hospital five weeks ago with cryptococcal meningitis. At that time, CD4 (T4) lymphocyte count was 41/μL, and HIV RNA viral load was greater than 700,000 copies/mL. She was treated with two weeks of amphotericin B. and discharged home. On follow-up care, two weeks ago, antiretroviral therapy was started. Additional medications are double-strength trimethoprim–sulfamethoxazole (800 mg/160 mg twice daily) and fluconazole (400 mg daily).

    The patient is thin and diaphoretic. Temperature is 38.9 C (101.8 F), pulse rate is 120 per minute, respirations are 22 per minute, and blood pressure is 128/74 mmHg. Mild neck stiffness is noted. Tachypnea and scattered crackles are noted on pulmonary examination. CD4 (T4) lymphocyte count is 206/μL, and HIV RNA viral load is 1275 copies/mL. Chest radiograph shows mild infiltrates in the lower lung fields.

    Which of the following is the most likely diagnosis?
    A) *Pseudomonas aeruginosa* pneumonia
    B) *Pneumocystis jirovecii* pneumonia
    C) Immune reconstitution inflammatory syndrome
    D) Cryptococcal pneumonia
    E) AIDS encephalopathy

Answer: C

Immune reconstitution inflammatory syndrome (IRIS) is an early complication of initiating antiretroviral therapy (ART) that involves rapid immune reconstitution in response to an uncovered or treated infection. IRIS is particularly problematic in cryptococcal meningitis. New neurologic symptoms can occur weeks or even months into cryptococcal treatment. This may present with a sudden onset of worsening meningitis symptoms.

This patient is less likely to have healthcare-associated pneumonia due to *Pseudomonas* because of the time course of symptoms. Pneumocystis jirovecii (carinii) pneumonia is less likely in a patient taking appropriate prophylaxis. Cryptococcal lung disease more commonly presents with nodules and patchy infiltrates.

Reference

Mientjes G, Scriven J, Marais S. Management of the immune reconstitution inflammatory syndrome. Curr HIV/AIDS Rep. 2012;9(3):238–250.

212. A 24-year-old man was initially unresponsive when he was rescued from a boating accident. He was given cardiopulmonary resuscitation (CPR) by the responding coast guard. Spontaneous respirations returned. On arrival in the emergency, the patient is afebrile. Blood pressure is 110/80 mmHg.

    Radiography of the chest reveals bilateral infiltrates. The toxicological investigation is ongoing.

    Which of the following is the most appropriate management?
    A) Monitor for fever, leukocytosis, and changes in infiltrates.
    B) Administer empirical antibiotics for community-acquired pneumonia.
    C) Administer empirical antibiotics for nosocomial pathogens.
    D) Administer steroids.

Answer: A

According to the World Health Organization (WHO), approximately 0.7 %, or 500,000, deaths each year are due to unintentional drowning. Initial management of near drowning should place emphasis on immediate resuscitation in the field and supportive treatment of respiratory failure. Frequent neurologic assessment should occur. All drowning victims should have 100 % oxygen during their initial evaluations. Early use of intubation CPAP/bilevel positive airway pressure (BiPAP) in the awake, cooperative, and mildly hypoxic individual is warranted if dyspnea persists.

The incidence of pneumonia is no greater than 12 %. It is best to monitor patients daily for definite fever, sustained leukocytosis, and persistent or new infiltrates prior to starting antibiotics.

References

Tadié JM, Heming N, Serve E, Weiss N, Day N, Imbert A, et al. Drowning associated pneumonia: a descriptive cohort. Resuscitation. 2012;83(3):399–401.

Wood C. Towards evidence-based emergency medicine: best BETs from the Manchester Royal Infirmary: BET 1: prophylactic antibiotics in near-drowning. Emerg Med J 2010;27:393–394.

213. A 68-year-old female is admitted to the hospital for symptoms of shock. She has a history of recurrent pyelonephritis and that is the presumed source of her sepsis. Other history is significant for hypertension.

Physical examination reveals pulse rate of 130 per minute and blood pressure of 62/45 mmHg. She is lethargic, and her extremities are cool.

Fluid resuscitation is started with 0.9 % sodium chloride and albumin. In addition, vasopressor therapy with norepinephrine is started because the patient's calculated mean arterial pressure (MAP) is only 48 mmHg.

Urine and blood cultures are pending. Intravenous antibiotic therapy is started.

Which of the following is the most likely result of increasing this patient's MAP to high blood pressure target of 75 mmHg as opposed to a low blood pressure target of 65 mmHg?
A) Reduced need for renal replacement therapy.
B) Decreased risk of a cardiac arrhythmia.
C) Mortality will be improved.
D) Increased need for renal replacement therapy.

Answer: A

The specific target blood pressure of a patient with septic shock is complex. All authorities recommend fluid resuscitation as the first form of therapy. The traditional pressure target is a (MAP) of 65–70 mmHg. A recent study has shown that the level of MAP targeted makes no difference in the outcomes of patients. There may be reasons to target a higher MAP in patients with preexisting hypertension since perfusion may decrease in these patients at a higher MAP.

In a recent study, MAP higher than 75 was associated with a reduced need for renal replacement therapy. This target also caused an increased incidence of atrial arrhythmias.

Reference

Asfar P, Meziani F, Hamel J-F, et al. High versus low blood-pressure target in patients with septic shock. N Engl J Med. 2014;370:1584–1593.

214. A 65-year-old man has a long-standing history of hypertension. His current medications are accupril (40 mg daily), amlodipine (10 mg daily), and metoprolol (100 mg twice daily).

On physical examination, his pulse rate is 62 per minute, and his blood pressure is 160/87 mmHg. Lung are clear and cardiac exam is normal.

His serum creatinine level is 1.3 mg/dL. Renal magnetic resonance angiography reveals a 65 % stenosis of the right renal artery.

Which of the following would provide the greatest benefit in managing this patient's hypertension?
A) Home BP telemonitoring and pharmacist case management
B) Stent placement for the renal-artery stenosis
C) Renal sympathetic nerve ablation
D) Renal-artery angioplasty

Answer: A

According to the Cardiovascular Outcomes in Renal Atherosclerotic Lesions Study (CORAL), renal-artery stenting in people with renal-artery stenosis offers no advantages over best medical therapy in reducing hard clinical events. A few studies have looked at the benefits of renal-artery stenting with mixed results. In general the use of renal-artery stents has declined. The CORAL study provides the most definitive evidence to date that renal-artery stents are of limited benefit. In the CORAL study, there were no differences in individual end points or in rates of all-cause mortality.

The most recent study, looking at renal sympathetic nerve ablation, showed no statistically significant difference between renal denervation and the sham procedure. Guidelines have recommended that it not be routinely used in clinical practice.

Reference

Cooper CJ, Murphy TP, Cutlip DE, et al.; for the CORAL Investigators. Stenting and medical therapy for atherosclerotic renal-artery stenosis. N Engl J Med. 2014;370(1):13–22.

215. A 22-year-old man presents to the emergency department after police found him wandering on the top of the hospital parking garage disoriented and combative state. His family arrives and believes he may have ingested "bath salts."

On physical exam, the patient is disoriented and is actively hallucinating. His temperature is 40 °C (104 °F). Pulse rate is 112 per minute, and blood pressure is 170/95 mmHg.

His BUN is 40 mg/dL], serum creatinine is 5.75 mg/dL, sodium128 mEq/L, potassium is 5 mEq, and chloride is 90 mEq/L.

Which of the following is the most likely cause of acute kidney injury in this patient?
A) Rhabdomyolysis
B) Renal arterial vasospasm
C) Acute renal venous thrombosis
D) Crystal-induced tubular obstruction
E) Acute urinary retention

Answer: A

Intoxication with "bath salts" and similar derivatives (synthetic cathinones) have been increasingly reported. Patients exhibit extreme agitation, hallucinations, and manic behavior that often leads to dehydration and excessive muscle breakdown. There have been reports of associated acute kidney injury, secondary to acute tubular necrosis due to rhabdomyolysis. Recommended treatment is aggressive volume repletion.

References

Adebamiro A, Perazella MA. Recurrent acute kidney injury following bath salts intoxication. Am J Kidney Dis. 2012;59(2):273–275.

Ross EA, Watson M, Goldberger B. "Bath salts" intoxication. NEJM. 2011;365:967–968.

216. A 78-year-old female with type I diabetes presents with a cellulitis and a chronic ulcer of her great toe. She reports the ulcer has been present for several weeks and lately her entire foot has become erythematous.

    On physical examination a 5 cm by 8 cm. Ulcer is observed on her right great toe. There is surrounding edema. On magnetic resonance imaging changes consistent with necrosis and osteomyelitis are noted in the first metatarsal. Podiatry is consulted. At this time, no surgical intervention is planned.

    What is the expected duration and route of antibiotics for this patient?

    A) Two weeks of parenteral antibiotics
    B) Six weeks of oral antibiotics
    C) Three months of parenteral and oral antibiotics
    D) Two months of parenteral antibiotics

Answer: C

The choice for diabetic foot infections (DFI) can be complex. The current practice that is beginning to emerge is that the role of parenteral antibiotics may be primarily to treat acute, severe soft tissue infection, which may be life- or limb-threatening, followed by transition to oral antibiotics. Treating chronic osteomyelitis is not an urgent matter, and the results may be just as good and more cost-effective with oral antibiotics as opposed to parenteral therapy. The recommended duration of antibiotic therapy for bone infections if identified has traditionally been six weeks.

The Infectious Diseases Society of America (ISDA) clinical practice guidelines for the diagnosis and treatment of DFIs are useful for estimating the length of therapy required based on the extent of the infection and viability of affected bone. Initial parenteral and then switching to oral for at least three months may be appropriate for a patient who will not undergo extensive resection of the infected bone. Current guidelines recommend at least three months or more of antibiotic therapy when diabetic foot osteomyelitis is not treated surgically or when residual dead bone remains after surgery.

A definitive plan cannot be established at time of diagnoses, and close follow-up must be arranged to modify therapy as needed based upon cultures and healing response..

Reference

Lipsky BA, Berendt AR, Deery HG et al. Infectious Diseases Society of America. Diagnosis and treatment of diabetic foot infections. Clin. Infect. Dis.2004 39, 885–910.

217. A 33-year-old male athlete who is in excellent health presents with headache, nausea, and cramping abdominal pain three hours into a triathlon being held in July. He reports drinking water at every station. He takes no medications and otherwise enjoys good health.

    On physical exam, the patient is anxious, diaphoretic, has a headache, and feels lightheaded. His temperature is 37.1 C (98.8 F). Heart rate is 90 bpm, respirations are 20 per minute, and blood pressure is 110/80 mmHg. Mucous membranes are dry, and skin is warm and clammy. Lungs are clear. No peripheral edema is noted.

    His sodium is 115 mEq/L; bicarbonate is 21 mEq/L.

    Which of the following is the most appropriate initial intravenous therapy for this patient?

    A) Infuse 0.9 % sodium chloride at 100 mL/h.
    B) Infuse 0.9 % sodium chloride at 200 mL/h.
    C) Administer 100-mL boluses of 3 % sodium chloride every 10 min for up to three boluses or until her symptoms resolve.
    D) Fluid restriction alone.

Answer: C

This patient has early signs of encephalopathy from exercise-associated hyponatremia (EAH). This is a dilutional hyponatremia due to excessive intake of hypotonic fluids. Rapid correction of the serum sodium with hypertonic saline is required to avoid further brain swelling, seizures, and death. The clinical manifestations of EAH-induced hyponatremia include dizziness, nausea, and vomiting to seizures, coma, and death. Hyponatremic patients with mild to moderate symptoms should be treated with fluid restriction and observed.

A study conducted on participants of the 2002 Boston Marathon found that thirteen percent finished the race with hyponatremia. Hyponatremia was just as likely to occur in runners who chose sports drinks as those who chose water.

References

Bennett BL, Hew-Butler T, Hoffman MD, Rogers IR, Rosner MH. Wilderness Medical Society practice guidelines for treatment of exercise-associated hyponatremia. Wilderness Environ Med. 2013;24(3):228–240.

Hew-Butler T, Ayus JC, Kipps C. Statement of the Second International Exercise-Associated Hyponatremia Consensus Development Conference, New Zealand, 2007. Clin J Sport Med 2008; 18: 111–2

218. A 55-year-old man is admitted to the hospital for, nausea, abdominal pain, and hematemesis. He is hemodynamically stable upon admission. He does not take nonsteroidal anti-inflammatory drugs and otherwise is healthy. He reports 1 to 2 alcoholic drinks per week.

Laboratory studies are significant for a serum total bilirubin

1.0 mg/dL and an INR of 1.0. Lipase is 205 units/L. Other liver functions are within normal limits.

On physical exam he has midepigastric pain, but otherwise it is normal. No ascites is present. An urgent EGD is performed which reveals an isolated fundic varix.

What is the appropriate next step in the management of this patient?
A) Prescribe beta-adrenergic blocking agent
B) Abdominal ultrasonography
C) Discharge home on proton-pump inhibitor
D) Perform endoscopic band ligation
E) Schedule transjugular liver biopsy

Answer: B

This patient presents with a variceal bleed from an isolated fundic varix. Variceal bleeding is often the first manifestation of splenic vein thrombosis (SVT). There is often no obvious underlying cause to SVT. In patients who have isolated fundal varices, splenic vein thrombosis should be ruled out. Ultrasonography is the test of choice.

In this case, the patient's laboratory tests history and physical exam are not consistent with cirrhosis or portal hypertension.

Splenectomy may considered as a therapeutic option and is considered by some as the definitive treatment for a bleeding varices due to SVT.

Reference

Valla DC, Condat B: Portal vein thrombosis in adults: pathophysiology, pathogenesis and management. J Hepatol 2000, 32:865–871

219. A 72-year-old man is admitted to the hospital with pneumonia. During a previous hospitalization for pyelonephritis three years ago, *Clostridium difficile* infection developed. This was treated with a two-week course of metronidazole.

Which of the following prophylactic therapies would be indicated in decreasing this patient's risk of *C. difficile* colitis?
A) Metronidazole
B) Low-dose vancomycin
C) Bifidobacterium and *Lactobacillus* strains
D) All of the above

Answer: C

Although metronidazole, fidaxomicin, and vancomycin have been effective in treating *Clostridium difficile* infection, there are little data on the effect of these agents as prophylaxis when used as co-therapy. However, a meta-analysis demonstrated that probiotics decrease the risk of *C. difficile* infection by more than 66 % when used prophylactically.

References

Johnston BC, Ma SS, Goldenberg JZ, et al. Probiotics for the prevention of Clostridium difficile-associated diarrhea: a systematic review and meta-analysis. Ann Intern Med. 2012;157(12):878–888.

Rodriguez S et al. Risk of Clostridium difficile infection in hospitalized patients receiving metronidazole for a non-C. difficile infection. Clin Gastroenterol Hepatol 2014 Mar 27

220. A 36-year-old woman is admitted for worsening abdominal pain. Her symptoms are chronic. This is her third presentation to the ER this year. She has had early satiety and episodes of postprandial vomiting for one year. She reports that eating one-half of a meal causes her to feel full.

Upper endoscopy is performed during this admission; biopsies of the duodenum and stomach and computed tomogram of the abdomen are normal. A gastric emptying scan shows 90 % emptying at two hours and 100 % emptying at four hours.

Which of the following medications will most likely relieve this patient's symptoms?
A) Bupropion
B) Buspirone
C) Omeprazole
D) Metoclopramide

Answer: A

Functional dyspepsia (FD) is the presence of gastroduodenal symptoms in the absence of organic, systemic, or metabolic disease. It has been described as a biopsychosocial disorder. It is one of the most common gastrointestinal disorders. Proton-pump inhibitors and prokinetic drugs have been used with limited results.

In one study, buspirone, possibly by initiating relaxation of the stomach, significantly reduced the overall severity of symptoms of dyspepsia, individual symptoms of post-prandial fullness, early satiation, and upper abdominal bloating.

Reference
Tack J, Janssen P, Masaoka T, et al. Efficacy of buspirone, a fundus-relaxing drug, in patients with functional dyspepsia. Clin Gastroenterol Hepatol. 2012;10:1239–1245.

221. A 55-year-old female presents with abdominal pain, nausea, and intermittent watery diarrhea for the past year. Prior workup has been negative. She denies fever, chills, or blood in her stool. Her appetite is normal. Her medical condition includes diet-controlled DM along with depression. She smokes a half a pack of cigarettes per day. The results of her CT scan of the abdomen and pelvis are normal. Her colonoscopy done during this admission is also normal. Mucosal biopsy shows a thickened subepithelial layer with collagen deposition.

    Which is likely the diagnosis?
    A) Irritable bowel syndrome
    B) Lymphocytic colitis
    C) Celiac sprue
    D) Ischemic colitis
    E) Collagenous colitis
    F) Crohn's disease

Answer: E
Microscopic or collagenous colitis occurs primarily in middle-aged to older-aged women. It may be associated with other autoimmune diseases, prescription drug use, and smoking. Microscopic colitis should be considered in any patient with unexplained nonbloody persistent diarrhea. The diagnosis is made solely by histology findings. Treatment should be initiated with the least toxic regimen or medication. Stronger medication should be used only if milder treatment fails. Treatment regimens should be switched cautiously with 4–6 weeks before deeming a particular medication as ineffective.

Reference
Pardi DS. After budesonide, what next for collagenous colitis?. Gut. 2009;58(1):3–4

222. A 75-year-old male with a past medical history of hypertension, coronary arterial disease, and dementia presents with worsening mild confusion from the nursing home. He currently takes aspirin and lasix. He has been getting more confused for the past two days. No recent history of head trauma.

On physical exam, his temperature is 37.4 °C (99.4 °F) and blood pressure is 120/78 mmHg. He has mild confusion but not much change from his baseline. Labs revealed normal serum electrolytes; urinalysis demonstrated positive nitrites, large WBC esterase, and microscopy reveled 30 WBC and 20 RBC. The plan is to discharge patient back to the nursing home with antibiotic treatment.

    Which of the following medications should be avoided?
    A) Amoxicillin
    B) Ciprofloxacin
    C) Cephalexin
    D) Nitrofurantoin
    E) Ceftriaxone

Answer: D
Medication-related problems are common, costly, and often preventable. Avoiding the use of inappropriate and high-risk drugs is an important, simple, and effective strategy in reducing medication-related problems and adverse drug reactions in older adults. A list of avoidable medicines was developed and published by Beers and colleagues for nursing home residents in 1991 and subsequently expanded and revised in 1997, 2003, and 2012. It includes a list of all medications that should be avoided in the elderly. This patient has a UTI, and nitrofurantoin, which is associated with renal failure in the elderly, should be avoided. The rest of the antibiotics mentioned are relatively safe in elderly.

Reference
Jano E, Aparasu RR. Healthcare outcomes associated with Beers' Criteria: A systematic review. Ann Pharmacother 2007;41:438–447.

223. A 58-year-old female is admitted for reduced urine output for the past two days. She has a history of osteoarthritis, hypertension, gout, and diabetes mellitus type 2. She is currently on insulin, allopurinol, and hydrochlorothiazide and takes ibuprofen and naproxen. She recently was seen by a primary care physician for sore throat and was prescribed a 10-day course of ampicillin, which she finished yesterday. Blood tests on admission reveal a serum creatinine of 3.4 mg/dl with a BUN of 42 mg/dl. Urinalysis showed numerous WBC and no RBC and no eosinophils. Due to her medicines and presentation, the diagnoses of interstitial nephritis is considered.

    What would be the most likely cause?
    A) Ampicillin
    B) Allopurinol
    C) Hydrochlorothiazide
    D) UTI
    E) Naproxen

Answer: E

Many drugs are implicated in interstitial nephritis, including antibiotics, proton-pump inhibitors, allopurinol, and NSAIDs. NSAID-induced interstitial nephritis presents with the absence of eosinophils on urine microscopy.

With the exceptions of interstitial nephritis induced by NSAIDs, patients commonly present with rash, fever, eosinophilia, eosinophiluria, and elevated immunoglobulin E (IgE) levels.

Recovery in renal function is usually observed after cessation of the offending agent. Implementing a short course of steroid therapy is generally recommended for patients that do not have a rapid recovery. No controlled studies exist on the effect of corticosteroids. Most practitioners recommend a relatively high dose with a rapidly tapering regimen within several weeks.

Reference

De Broe ME, Elseviers MM. Over-the-counter analgesic use. J Am Soc Nephrol. 7 2009

224. A 62-year-old female is evaluated for a 5-week history of nonproductive cough and fatigue over the past several months. The patient underwent resection of localized rectal carcinoma 16 months ago. This was followed by chemotherapy and radiation therapy. Chest radiograph at that time was normal.

Chest radiograph now shows multiple pulmonary nodules. Contrast-enhanced CT scan of the chest shows three nodules ranging from 1.6 to 1.9 cm in diameter. Two nodules are in the right lung, and one is in the left lower lobe.

What is the most appropriate next step in the management of this patient?

A) Bronchoscopy and biopsy
B) PET scan
C) Transthoracic needle aspiration of a nodule
D) Observe for now and repeat CT chest in 3 months
E) Video-assisted thoracoscopic surgery (VAT)

Answer: C

The reported yield for transthoracic needle aspiration is about 90 % for nodules of 1 to 2 cm compared to less than 50 % for bronchoscopy. The diagnostic yield of fiberoptic bronchoscopy depends on the lesion location and size. The diagnostic yield for lesions greater than 3 cm in diameter by bronchoscopy is 80 %. For lesions located in the lower lobe, basilar segments or in the apical segments of the upper lobes, yield is 58 %, compared with 83 % for other locations. CT-guided transthoracic needle biopsy would have significantly higher yield for nodules of this size than would bronchoscopy.

Reference

Lacasse Y, Wong E, Guyatt GH, Cook DJ. Transthoracic needle aspiration biopsy for the diagnosis of localized pulmonary lesions: a meta-analysis. Thorax. 1999;54(10):884–93.

225. You are called to see a patient on the cardiology service with right-sided weakness. He is a 75-year-old male who underwent cardiac catheterization procedure because of typical chest pain presentation. A coronary angiogram revealed significant in-stent restenosis, which was managed by balloon angioplasty. The patient was given 300 mg of Plavix in the catheterization lab.

On physical exam, his blood pressure is 180/95 mmHg, heart rate of 110 BPM, and his temperature was normal. Cardiac and chest examination are normal. On neurologic examination, the right side of the body is 3/5, while the left side is 5/5. The patient denies chest pain, no nausea, or vomiting.

What is your next step in management?

A) MRI of the head
B) CT angiogram of the chest
C) Start tissue plasminogen activator (TPA)
D) Carotid Doppler ultrasound
E) Transesophageal echocardiogram (TEE)

Answer: A

Ischemic stroke related to catheterization should be suspected in a patient who develops neurologic symptoms during or immediately post catheterization. MRI of the head would be appropriate to diagnose the stroke early as CT scan may miss early changes.

In most cases, the etiology is felt to be embolic due to atherosclerotic debris and not thrombus, and therefore acute therapy with systemic thrombolysis is not routinely performed.

CT angiogram of the chest will help in diagnosing aortic dissection, which may also complicate cardiac catheterization. This patient did not have chest pain to suggest dissection.

Reference

Lazar JM, Uretzky BF, Denys BG, et al. Predisposing risk factors and natural history of acute neurologic complications of left-sided cardiac catheterization. Am J Cardiol 1995;75:1056--1060.

226. You are the admitting hospital medicine physician in the emergency room. A previously healthy 25-year-old woman presents with a one-week history of polyuria, polydipsia, and 20-lb weight loss. On the day of presentation, she developed nausea and abdominal pain. Emergency room staff asks you to assess the patient.

On physical exam, she is severely dehydrated with decreased skin turgor; blood pressure is 80/palp mmHg and heart rate is 120. Finger stick blood sugar is 700 and urine dipstick indicates 3+ ketones and 3+ blood. Urine hCG is negative.

What is the most appropriate initial step in the treatment of this patient?
A) 10 units SC insulin
B) 10 units IV insulin
C) 1 l half normal saline at 200 cc/h
D) 1 l of normal saline bolus
E) 0.5 l half normal saline at 200 cc/h

Answer: D

In patients with evidence of diabetic ketoacidosis (DKA), volume resuscitation should be given prior to insulin. Fluid resuscitation is a critical component of treating patients with DKA. Insulin therapy will cause intracellular transport of glucose which may result in a significant fluid shift from the extracellular to the intracellular compartment. This may increase the risk of hypovolemic shock and thromboembolism. Insulin should be started after IV fluid replacement is started. Guidelines suggest one liter of fluid given before insulin is started.

Reference

Wallace TM, Matthews DR. Recent advances in the monitoring and management of diabetic ketoacidosis. QJM. 2004;97(12):773–80.

227. A 75-year-old woman with a history of coronary artery disease, diabetes, and cholelithiasis is admitted with RUQ pain. She is on daily aspirin and clopidogrel. An abdominal ultrasound reveals several stones in the gallbladder, a stone in the distal common bile duct without evidence of common bile duct dilation.

She is hemodynamically stable and afebrile. Her white blood cell count is normal. On admission her AST is 450 units/L . ALT is 434 units/L. Total bilirubin is 5.8 µmol/L. The next morning her AST is 400 units/L, ALT is 385 units/L, and total bilirubin is 5.0 µmol/L.

What is the most appropriate next step?
A) Biliary decompression via IR-guided cholecystostomy.
B) Hold clopidogrel, observe, and plan elective ERCP in 7 day.
C) ERCP now.
D) Proceed with laparoscopic cholecystectomy.
E) Hold clopidogrel and plan elective ERCP in 3–6 months.

Answer: B

This patient has choledocholithiasis with possible obstruction. At the current time there is no evidence of cholangitis. Her current laboratory workup reveals a decline in the degree of obstruction consistent with a passed stone. An emergent ERCP or cholecystostomy is not indicated at this time. The best plan for this patient would be to hold clopidogrel and proceed with an elective inpatient ERCP with sphincterotomy and stone extraction after seven days. An ERCP done while on clopidogrel would make sphincterotomy risky. In the interim, antibiotics may be started and observed for obstruction requiring urgent decompression or ERCP without sphincterotomy.

Reference

Cotton PB, Garrow DA, Gallagher J, Romagnuolo J. Risk factors for complications after ERCP: a multivariate analysis of 11,497 procedures over 12 years. Gastrointest Endosc. 2009;70(1):80–8.

228. An 82-year-old female presents with a chief complaint of shortness of breath. She states that two weeks prior, she describes a viral-type upper respiratory illness. On presentation, she is noted to have a multilobar loculated infiltrates. Blood cultures taken at the time of admission grow out methicillin-resistant *Staph. aureus* (MRSA). She reports a significant allergy to vancomycin.

Her temperature on presentation is 39 °C (102.2 °F), pulse rate is 120 per minute, respirations are 30 per minute, and blood pressure is 110/60. Diffuse crackles are noted throughout her left and right lung fields. Cardiac examination reveals tachycardia.

Which of the following is the most appropriate medications for this patient's presumed MRSA pneumonia?
A) Vancomycin
B) Daptomycin
C) Linezolid
D) Ceftriaxone and erythromycin
E) Clindamycin

Answer: C

United States guidelines recommend either linezolid or vancomycin as the first-line treatment for hospital-acquired (nosocomial) MRSA pneumonia. Some studies have suggested that linezolid is better than vancomycin against probable MRSA nosocomial pneumonia. This may be due to the fact that the penetration of linezolid into bronchial fluids is much higher than that of vancomycin. However this is debated.

Daptomycin is inhibited by pulmonary surfactant and this is not indicated here.

Reference
Vilhena C, Bettencourt A. Daptomycin: a review of properties, clinical use, drug delivery and resistance. Mini Rev Med Chem 2012;12:202–9.

229. A 47-year-old man is admitted to the hospital with an acute decompensation of his alcoholic-related cirrhosis. He presents to the emergency room confused with ascites.

On physical exam, he is clearly jaundiced with icteric sclera. Additionally, he has a distended abdomen with a fluid wave on physical exam. There is poor skin turgor. He has asterixis on extension of his hands. Preliminary workup reveals an ammonia level of 110 mg/dL, a total bilirubin of 7.1, an INR of 1.6, and a platelet count of 95,000. The potassium level is 3.1, BUN is 37, and creatinine is 1.5.

Which of the following is NOT likely to be contributing to this patient's confusion?
A) Bacterial infection of the ascites
B) Hypokalemia
C) Acute kidney injury
D) Volume depletion
E) Jaundice

Answer: E
The morbidity and mortality associated with elevated conjugated hyperbilirubinemia result from the underlying disease process. Conjugated bilirubin causes no direct toxicity to neural tissue in adults.

Bilirubin levels often correlate strongly with, but do not contribute to, short-term mortality.

Bacterial infections, including spontaneous bacterial peritonitis, dehydration, acute renal failure, electrolyte abnormalities, and metabolic acidosis are all very common causes of worsening hepatic encephalopathy.

Reference
Bustamante J, Rimola A, Ventura PJ, Navasa M, Cirera I, Reggiardo V, et al. Prognostic significance of hepatic encephalopathy in patients with cirrhosis. J Hepatol. 1999;30(5):890–5.

230. A 58-year-old male is admitted for worsening ascites. His past medical history is significant for chronic hepatitis C and hypertension. He denies nausea or vomiting.

On physical examination, he is afebrile, blood pressure is 110/70 mmHg, heart rate is 100 bpm, and respiratory rate is 22/min. There is ascites and bipedal pitting edema. Lung auscultation reveals minimal crackles in both lung bases. Laboratory test reveals a serum creatinine of 3.7 mg/dL. Furosemide was stopped. He was given 1.5 l of isotonic saline with no improvement of his renal function.

Which of the following is the most appropriate diagnostic test to perform next?
A) Paracentesis
B) Serum osmolality
C) Urine electrolytes and urine creatinine
D) ALT and AST
E) Renal ultrasound

Answer: C
This patient has possible hepatorenal syndrome. Urine electrolytes and urine creatinine should be performed to calculate the fractional excretion of sodium (FENa). A FENa value below 1 % would suggest prerenal causes, such as hepatorenal syndrome or hypovolemia. A repeat fluid challenge may help rule out hypovolemia as a cause.

Reference
Moreau R, Lebrec D. Diagnosis and treatment of acute renal failure in patients with cirrhosis. Best Pract Res Clin Gastroenterol. 2007;21(1):111–23.

231. A 64-year-old male with no prior medical history had a witnessed arrest and was found to have ventricular fibrillation. He was successfully resuscitated and was admitted to the hospital medicine service. All tests done on admission were within normal limits. Cardiac catheterization was performed and revealed nonobstructive coronary artery disease. He has no residual neurologic deficits.

What is the next step in management?
A) Discharge the patient on metoprolol.
B) Intracardiac defibrillator implantation.
C) Electrophysiology study.
D) Cardiac MRI.
E) 24-h home halter monitor.

Answer: B
The patient had survived a cardiac arrest with no obviously reversible cause of his ventricular fibrillation. According to American College of Cardiology (ACC) guidelines, intracardiac defibrillator implantation is indicated for secondary prevention. This is a class 1 recommendation.

Reference
Epstein AE, Dimarco JP, Ellenbogen KA, et al. ACC/AHA/HRS 2008 Guidelines for device-based therapy of cardiac rhythm abnormalities. Heart Rhythm. 2008;5(6):e1-62.473)

232. A 72-year-old female is admitted for a three-week rash not improving with topical steroids. He has a past medical history of hypertension and hyperlipidemia and has smoked at least one pack per day for the last 40 years. He is on lisinopril 20 mg daily and simvastatin 40 mg at and has been taking these medications for the last 5 years.

On physical exam, blood pressure is 128/82 mmHg. Heart rate is 86 bpm. He has bilateral periorbital purplish hue and erythematous flat rash on the chest and back and on shoulders. CXR is normal. All admission labs are within normal limits except a CPK of 475 units/L.

Which of the following is the next option?

A) Muscle biopsy
B) Electromyogram
C) Chest CT
D) Skin biopsy

Answer: C

This patient most likely has dermatomyositis secondary to small cell lung cancer. The most important step to take is a CT chest to evaluate for lung malignancy. Given the characteristic heliotrope rash and erythematous rash on torso, dermatomyositis is the most likely condition. Dermatomyositis has a 25 % association with malignancy. In this long-term smoker, greater than age 60, the rate of malignancy would be higher. Autoantibodies, muscle biopsy, EMG, and skin biopsy would all be considered once malignancy has been ruled out.

Reference
Callen JP. Dermatomyositis. Lancet. 1 2000;355(9197):53–7.

233. A 67-year-old female with history of hypertension, severe aortic stenosis, and diastolic congestive heart failure is admitted with one episode of bloody stool this morning. He has no prior history of lower gastrointestinal bleeding. He is currently on 81 mg. of aspirin. Last colonoscopy was three years ago and was normal with no diverticular disease.

On physical exam, his abdomen is nontender. A systolic ejection mummer is heard radiating to the carotids at the right second intercostal area. Vitals are stable. Labs revealed normal platelet count with hemoglobin of 12.9 g/dl. Colonoscopy done on this admission shows angiodysplasia seen in the descending colon.

What is the best step to treating this condition?

A) Aortic valve replacement
B) Colon resection
C) Mesenteric artery embolization
D) Mechanical hemostasis using endoscopic clips
E) Aortic valve replacement

Answer: A

This patient developed Heyde's syndrome, which is the occurrence of bleeding angiodysplasia in the colon in patients with severe aortic stenosis. A subtle form of von Willebrand disease present in Heyde's syndrome patients resolves rapidly after aortic valve replacement.

References
Heyde EC (1958). Gastrointestinal bleeding in aortic stenosis. N. Engl. J. Med.1958.259 (4): 19
Warkentin TE, Moore JC, Morgan DG (1992). "Aortic stenosis and bleeding gastrointestinal angiodysplasia: is acquired von Willebrand's disease the link?". Lancet 340 (8810): 35–7

234. A 71-year-old man with a history of congestive heart failure, EF 30 %, and hypertension was admitted five days ago for septic shock due to pneumonia. He was intubated but is now extubated. He is now hemodynamically stable.

The patient developed the new onset of persistent abdominal pain and bloody stool. Urgent C-scope revealed ischemic colitis. He is doing better, blood counts are stable but remains lethargic. No nutrition has been started yet.

Which of the following would be the most appropriate nutritional support?

A) No nutrition
B) Post-pyloric feedings
C) Peripheral parenteral nutrition
D) Intragastric tube feeding
E) Central parenteral nutrition

Answer: E

The patient has been on NPO for five days. His ability to have an adequate oral intake in the next few days is unlikely. Initiation of nutritional support is warranted. He has history of congestive heart failure and will not tolerate the large IV fluid volume that has to be given with peripheral parenteral nutrition to keep solution osmolality less than 900. Ischemic colitis will make enteral nutrition a poor option.

Although used with caution, the best option for this patient is central or total parenteral nutrition.

Reference
Stapelton RD, Jones NE, Heyland DK. Feeding critically ill patients: what is the optimum amount? Crit Care Med. 2007;35(9 suppl):S535-S540

235. A 57-year-old man was diagnosed three months ago with grade II astrocytoma. He is admitted for new onset seizure. While in the hospital the second day, he develops acute shortness of breath. CT angiogram reveals acute right-sided massive pulmonary embolism. Bedside echocardiogram by the on call cardiology fellow shows right ventricular dilatation and strain. The patient's blood pressure is 75/50 mmHg.

What is the best management option?
A) Thrombectomy
B) Low-molecular-weight heparin
C) Unfractionated heparin
D) Fondaparinux
E) Thrombolytics

Answer: A

Guidelines from the American Heart Association (AHA) advise that either catheter embolectomy and fragmentation or surgical embolectomy should be considered for patients with massive pulmonary embolism who have contraindications to fibrinolysis. Thrombolytics are relatively contraindicated for this patient with his recent diagnosis of intracranial neoplasm.

Reference

Jaff MR, McMurtry MS, Archer SL, Cushman M, Goldenberg N, Goldhaber SZ, et al. Management of Massive and Submassive Pulmonary Embolism, Iliofemoral Deep Vein Thrombosis, and Chronic Thromboembolic Pulmonary Hypertension: A Scientific Statement From the American Heart Association. Circulation. 26 2011;123(16):1788–1830.

236. A 55-year-old female with a past medical history of diabetes, hyperlipidemia, and coronary artery disease was admitted with septic shock from cellulitis. She was admitted to the ICU for respiratory failure and was subsequently intubated. On day three she was extubated and transferred to the floor. On day five she spiked a low-grade temperature and blood cultures from that day subsequently grew *Candida albicans*. Her vital signs are stable. She was started on intravenous fluconazole and vancomycin.

   What is the next appropriate step?
A) Remove all lines and start diflucan
B) Start double antifungal therapy
C) Start an echinocandin
D) Ophthalmology consult
E) A and D

Answer: E

In patients without neutropenia, fluconazole is the drug of choice in most cases of candidemia and disseminated candidiasis. An echinocandin is recommended for candidemia in most patients with neutropenia. A critical component in the management of candidemia and disseminated candidiasis is the removal of the possible focus of infection, such as intravenous and Foley catheters. Double antifungal therapy is not needed for management of candidemia.

A number of studies have shown that in the setting of candidemia, ocular problems such as endophthalmitis may develop in about 1 % of all patients with candidemia, and 2–9 % of patients might develop less serious eye diseases, including chorioretinitis. The 2009 Infectious Disease Society of America guidelines suggest getting an ophthalmologic consultation 1 week after the onset or detection of illness, evaluating for ocular involvement.

References
Oude Lashof AM, Rothova A, Sobel JD, et al. Ocular manifestations of candidemia. Clin Infect Dis. 2011;53:262–268.
Pappas PG, Rex JH, Lee J, et al. A prospective observational study of candidemia: epidemiology, therapy, and influences on mortality in hospitalized adult and pediatric patients. Clin Infect Dis. Sep 1 2003;37(5):634–43.

237. A 42-year-old woman is admitted to the hospital with confusion, disorientation, and ataxia. The patient feels weak and has memory loss. During the past three months, she has lost 105 lb after gastric banding.

   On physical exam, she appears confused. She has horizontal nystagmus. The tongue is slick. Examination revealed sensory and motor neuropathy in both lower extremities. Laboratory findings include Hb of 8.7 mg/dL and MCV of 102 fL.

   What is the most appropriate next step?
A) Intravenous thiamine
B) Intravenous immunoglobulin
C) B12 injection
D) Spinal tap
E) Lipid infusion

Answer: A

In recent years, acute Wernicke encephalopathy has been more frequently recognized in patients after bariatric surgeries. Thiamine (vitamin B1) deficiency can result in Wernicke encephalopathy (WE). It is typically a triad of acute mental confusion, ataxia, and ophthalmoplegia. Symptoms develop 4 to 12 weeks postoperatively. WE is a medical emergency and requires immediate administration of IV thiamine. Frequently unrecognized, WE is more prevalent than commonly considered.

Ocular abnormalities are the hallmarks of WE. The oculomotor manifestations are nystagmus and bilateral and lateral rectus palsies. The most common presenting symptoms of WE are mental status changes. Ataxia is due to a combination of polyneuropathy, cerebellar damage, and vestibular paresis. It is important to test for truncal ataxia with the patient sitting or standing.

T2-weighted MRI images typically demonstrate hyperintense signals in the midbrain, mammillary bodies, and thalamus, which may aid in diagnoses.

References

Aasheim ET. Wernicke encephalopathy after bariatric surgery: a systematic review. Ann Surg. 2008;248(5): 714–20.

Attard O, Dietemann JL, Diemunsch P, Pottecher T, Meyer A, Calon BL. Wernicke encephalopathy: a complication of parenteral nutrition diagnosed by magnetic resonance imaging. Anesthesiology. Oct 2006;105(4):847–8.

Donnino MW, Vega J, Miller J, et al. Myths and misconceptions of Wernicke's encephalopathy: what every emergency physician should know. Ann Emerg Med. Dec 2007;50(6):715–21.

238. A type 1 diabetic patient with chronic renal insufficiency is admitted with cellulitis. She has intermittent claudication and was found to have ABI of 0.4. Lower extremity angiogram will be performed. Her creatinine level 1.4 mg/dl.

    Which of the following pretreatments should be received to decrease the risk of contrast-induced nephropathy?
    A) Intravenous steroid
    B) N-acetylcysteine
    C) Intravenous hydration
    D) Intravenous magnesium
    E) No pretreatment is needed

Answer: C

Contrast medium-induced nephropathy (CIN) is the third leading cause of acute renal failure in hospitalized patients. Administration of fluids remains the cornerstone of preventive therapy to reduce the risk of CIN. It has proven to have renal protective effect even in patient with normal baseline renal function and is a reasonable option here.

If volume restriction is not an issue, the usual recommended infusion rate of intravenous 0.9 % sodium chloride is 1 ml/kg/h. This should be started 12 h before and continued for 12 h after the procedure. N-acetylcysteine may be of benefit in patients with baseline creatinine above 2 mg/dl.

Reference

Mueller C, Buerkle G, Buettner HJ, et al. Prevention of contrast media-associated nephropathy. Arch Intern Med 2002;162:329–36.

239. A 57-year-old male with a past medical history of diabetes, COPD was admitted for a severe exacerbation. He declined rapidly in the emergency room and was intubated.

    His current ventilator settings are a rate of 15, tidal volume of 700 ml, FiO2 of 60 %, and a PEEP of 15. His PCO2 on ABGs was 60 cm of H2O. His rate was increased to 20 breaths/min. Fifteen minutes later his blood pressure dropped from 126/78 mm of Hg to 98/62 mm of Hg and his tidal volume fell to 350 cc.

    Physical exam reveals engorged neck veins and slightly diminished breath sounds bilaterally. Stat chest X-Ray is negative for pneumothorax.

    What should be the next appropriate step?
    A) Increase the tidal volume and reduce the respiratory rate.
    B) Reduce the respiratory rate and PEEP.
    C) Increase the I: E ratio.
    D) Reduce the tidal volume, respiratory rate or I: E ratio.
    E) Increase PEEP.

Answer: D

This patient has air trapping commonly seen in COPD patients who are being ventilated. This has resulted in auto peep. Air trapping occurs due to repetitive breaths with high tidal volumes and higher rates with very minimal time for exhalation. This can lead to poor gas exchange and hemodynamic compromise. This can be treated by reducing rate and tidal volume and by increasing expiratory time.

Reference

Brenner B, Corbridge T, Kazzi A. Intubation and mechanical ventilation of the asthmatic patient in respiratory failure. J Emerg Med. 2009;37(2 Suppl):S23-34.

240. A 55-year-old male with long-standing alcohol abuse is admitted for acute upper gastrointestinal bleeding. The patient reports no other medical problems. He takes no medications. Six months ago he was seen in the emergency department for a spontaneous retroperitoneal bleeding.

    On physical exam the patient he is afebrile, blood pressure is 120/74 mmHg, heart rate is 78 bpm, respiratory rate is 16, and oxygen saturation is 97% on room air. Bleeding from his gingival membranes is noted. Otherwise, the rest of the exam is within normal limits. Laboratory findings reveal platelets of 250,000 and INR of 0.9.

    Which of the following deficiency is suspected?
    A) Vitamin K
    B) Vitamin C
    C) Folate
    D) Vitamin A
    E) Thiamine

Answer: A

Fat-soluble vitamin deficiencies occur in chronic alcoholics. One study found vitamin K deficiency in the majority of chronic alcoholics. Vitamin K plays an essential role in hemostasis. It is a fat-soluble vitamin that is absorbed in the small intestine and stored in the liver. Other causes of vitamin K deficiencies include poor dietary intake, liver disease, and intestinal malabsorption.

Reference

Martin J. Shearer, Xueyan Fu, Sarah L. Booth. Vitamin K Nutrition, Metabolism, and Requirement: Current Concept and Future Research. Martin J. Shearer, Xueyan Fu, Sarah L. Booth. Vitamin K Nutrition, Metabolism, and Requirement: Current Concept and Future Research. Advances in Nutrition. 2012;3: 182–195.2012;3:182–195.

241. A 43-year-old male is admitted for cellulitis. He reports that he works at a beef processing plant. On presentation, his symptoms are fever, headache, and bilaterally swollen erythematous hands.

On physical examination, his hands are noted to have small painless papules. Over the course of the next 24 h, the papules progress to central vesicles. The vesicles are painless and have a black eschar.

Which of the following is the most likely diagnosis?
A) Cutaneous anthrax
B) Bullous pemphigoid
C) Methicillin-sensitive Staph. aureus infection
D) Pasteurella infection

Answer: A

95 % of anthrax is cutaneous. The remaining cases are inhalational and gastrointestinal. Anthrax is primarily zoonotic. Exposure may be through agriculture or industrial handling of animals. Those at highest risk are farmers, and workers in facilities that use animal products, especially previously contaminated goat hair, wool, or bone. Cutaneous anthrax begins as a pruritic papule that enlarges within 24–48 h to form a vesicle. This subsequently becomes an ulcer surrounded progressing to a black eschar .

Gastrointestinal and cutaneous anthrax can be treated with ciprofloxacin or doxycycline for 60 days. Amoxicillin or amoxicillin clavulanate may be used to complete the course if the strain is susceptible.

Reference

Hicks CW, Sweeney DA, Cui X, Li Y, Eichacker PQ. An overview of anthrax infection including the recently identified form of disease in injection drug users. Intensive Care Med. Jul 2012;38(7):1092–104.

242. A 90-year-old man is admitted for nausea, vomiting, and dehydration. On the second day of his admission, he develops severe substernal chest pain, which began one hour prior to your evaluation. He has 2 mm ST segment depression in the inferior leads. Labs are pending.

Appropriate therapies at this time include:
A) Aspirin 325 mg (chewed)
B) Aspirin 325 mg (chewed), clopidogrel, and heparin
C) Glycoprotein IIb–IIIa inhibitor and clopidogrel
D) Aspirin 325 mg (chewed), glycoprotein IIb–IIIa inhibitor, and clopidogrel
E) Aspirin 325 mg (chewed), glycoprotein IIb–IIIa inhibitor, clopidogrel, and heparin

Answer: E

Elderly patients with acute myocardial infarction are at increased risk of developing complications, but treatment protocols primarily the same. Elderly patients have an increased risk of bleeding with thrombolytic therapy and should undergo primary angioplasty if otherwise the benefits of most treatment options remains the same.

Reference

Lim HS, Farouque O, Andrianopoulos N, et al. Survival of elderly patients undergoing percutaneous coronary intervention for acute myocardial infarction complicated by cardiogenic shock. J Am Coll Cardiol Cardiovasc Interv 2009; 2:146–152.

243. A 42-year-old man with sickle cell disease (SCD) is hospitalized for fever, bone pain, chest pain, and shortness of breath. His most recent blood transfusion was four weeks ago for symptomatic anemia.

On physical examination, the patient appears in acute pain and audibly wheezing. Temperature is 37.6 °C(99.7) °F. The remainder of the examination is unremarkable. CXR reveals multiple infiltrates, most of which are old.

What would be the most common cause of death for this patient?
A) Acute chest syndrome
B) Coronary artery disease
C) Cerebral aneurysm rupture
D) Anemia
E) Heart failure

Answer: A

Acute chest syndrome in adults is a common cause of death in sickle cell patients. This may be the result of infection, pain, or veno-occlusive disease. Early recognition is important. Treatment of acute chest syndrome consists of oxygen, antibiotics, incentive spirometry, transfusion, and bronchodilators. Some patients have repeat presentations of acute chest syndrome. Chronic transfusion reduces the recurrence and hydroxyurea reduces the rate of acute chest syndrome by about half.

Life expectancy continues to improve with SCD patients, and now in developed countries, it is approaching 50. As the population of patients with SCD grows older, new chronic complications are appearing. Pulmonary disease and in particular pulmonary hypertension is emerging as a relatively common complication.

There is no increase in cerebral aneurysm rupture in these patients. Coronary artery occlusion is not common in sickle cell patients, although valvular disease, pulmonary hypertension, and sudden arrhythmic death are.

Reference

Yawn BP, Buchanan GR, Afenyi-Annan AN, Ballas SK, Hassell KL, James AH, et al. Management of sickle cell disease: summary of the 2014 evidence-based report by expert panel members. JAMA. Sep 10 2014;312(10): 1033–48.

244. A 68-year-old female with a history of hypertension, hypercholesterolemia, and tobacco use is admitted with lightheadedness and mild associated dyspnea. The symptoms have been increasing in intensity over the past days. She denies any symptoms at rest. She denies any previous cardiac history. While you are evaluating her in the emergency room, she develops chest pain.

    Physical examination shows blood pressure of 100/64 mmHg and heart rate of 116/min. In general, she appears in moderate distress. Cardiac examination shows normal S1 and S2 and sinus tachycardia. Stat ECG shows 1 mm ST segment depression in leads V4 through V6.

    Laboratory data shows a troponin of 0.48 ng/mL, a WBC of 9,400/μL, and a hemoglobin of 6.8 g/dL.

    Which of the following is the most appropriate next step?
    A) Emergent cardiac catheterization
    B) Intravenous nitroglycerin, aspirin, and intravenous heparin
    C) Pharmacologic stress test with nuclear imaging
    D) Intravenous metoprolol
    E) Stool guaiac testing

Answer: E

The first and most important step for this patient with significant anemia is to determine the cause of her anemia and administer blood transfusion.

Before starting the urgent treatment for ischemia, which involves aggressive anticoagulants, it is important to determine the source of blood loss. Active bleeding can be worsened with anticoagulants and can actually cause further harm to a patient such as this.

The patient's symptoms and ECG may improve after transfusion, once the oxygen carrying capacity of her blood has been improved to normal levels, and stenting, which also involves the use of anticoagulants, can be detrimental in a patient such as this.

Reference

Rao SV, Sherwood MW. Isn't it about time we learned how to use blood transfusion in patients with ischemic heart disease? J Am Coll Cardiol. 2014

245. A 35-year-old woman is admitted with paresthesias that began in the left arm and spread to her left face over 30 min. She also reports a severe frontal headache. She has a limited past medical history but has a family history of migraine. She reports that she has had headaches in the past but not migraine headaches. Her only medication is a daily oral contraceptive pill.

    On physical examination, temperature is normal, blood pressure is 152/82 mmHg, pulse rate is 107/min, and respiration rate is 18/min. Her left arm feels heavy and numb, but focal deficits are hard to illicit. All other examination findings are normal.

    Results of laboratory studies and a CT scan of the head are also normal.

    Which of the following is the most likely diagnosis?
    A) Migraine with aura
    B) Multiple sclerosis
    C) Sensory seizure
    D) Transient ischemic attack
    E) Cluster headache

Answer: A

The migraine aura can present as a variety of neurologic symptoms that may precede or accompany the headache phase or may occur in isolation. It usually develops over 5–20 min and lasts less than 60 min. The aura can be a combination of visual, sensory, or motor symptoms. Motor symptoms may occur in up to 20 % of patients and usually are associated with sensory symptoms. Motor symptoms are often vague and described as a sense of heaviness of the limbs before a headache but without any true weakness.

Patients presenting with migraines with an aura have a strong risk factor for future stroke. In addition, they should also be counseled on the increased risk of stroke with smoking and oral contraceptive use. Patients should be screened for cardiovascular risk factors.

References

Allais G, Gabellari IC, De Lorenzo C, Mana O, Benedetto C. Oral contraceptives in migraine. Expert Rev Neurother. Mar 2009;9(3):381–93.

Headache Classification Committee of the International Headache Society. Classification and diagnostic criteria for headache disorders, cranial neuralgias and facial pain. Cephalalgia. 1988;8 Suppl 7:1–96.

246. A 21-year-old female presents to the ED in sickle cell crisis with severe leg and arm pain. She takes folic acid, hydroxyurea, and oxycodone IR at home. She is admitted and started with normal saline IV at 125 ml/h, oxycodone IR 10 mg PO every 4 h, and hydromorphone 0.5 mg IV every 3 h PRN for pain 7–10/10. In addition, her home medications, folic acid and hydroxyurea, will be resumed.

What other medication would this patient benefit from while in the hospital?
A) Morphine 2 mg IV every 2 h PRN for pain
B) Senna/docusate one tab PO BID
C) Acetaminophen 500 mg PO every 6 h PRN pain
D) Sodium bicarbonate 650 mg PO BID

Answer: B

Acetaminophen would not benefit this patient because it is indicated to treat mild to moderate pain, and the PRN indication is not consistent with the patient's current condition. Morphine is a good opioid analgesic for severe pain experienced in a sickle cell crisis but would represent a therapeutic duplication as hydromorphone is already on the patient's profile. Sodium bicarbonate has no indication in this setting. A common side effect of opioids such as hydromorphone and oxycodone is constipation. Bowel regimens are often neglected in the hospital which can lead to constipation and further discomfort. It should be considered in any patient receiving around the clock narcotics.

Reference
Yawn BP, Buchanan GR, Afenyi-Annan AN, Ballas SK, Hassell KL, James AH, et al. Management of sickle cell disease: summary of the 2014 evidence-based report by expert panel members. JAMA. 2014;312(10):1033–48.

247. A 65-year-old man with a history of insulin-dependent diabetes, coronary artery disease, and depression is admitted to the hospital for recurrent abdominal pain and hematochezia.

During his admission he required two units of packed red blood cells. He underwent colonoscopy by the colorectal surgeon and was found to have active oozing and mucosa consistent with ischemic colitis.

After one week of supportive care and rehydration, he is eating well, the bleeding has stopped, and he is ready for discharge. He is on an aspirin daily which will be restarted on discharge.

What is the most appropriate next step?
A) Refer to general surgery for colectomy.
B) Refer to interventional radiology for diagnostic angiography.
C) Recommend Holter monitor study for arrhythmia.
D) Refer for follow-up colonoscopy.
E) Observation alone.

Answer: D

It is recommended that patients with ischemic colitis have follow-up colonoscopy within 4–6 weeks of the inciting event to determine resolution of underlying colonic injury, development of stricture, and rule out possible proximal malignancy. Diagnostic angiograph is not indicated based solely on developing ischemic colitis nor is Holter monitoring.

Reference
Sreenarasimhaiah J. Diagnosis and management of intestinal ischaemic disorders. BMJ 2003;326:1372–1376.

248. A 35-year-old woman with a history of ulcerative colitis and primary sclerosing cholangitis is scheduled for an elective biliary dilation for recurrent biliary stricture. She is hemodynamically stable, afebrile, and without leukocytosis on laboratory workup.

What is the most appropriate step regarding pre-ERCP prophylaxis?
A) Ciprofloxacin starting before the procedure and continuing for 7 days
B) No antibiotics needed
C) Ciprofloxacin given once, one hour before the procedure
D) Hold the procedure until the patient receives a full course of ciprofloxacin
E) Ciprofloxacin given once following the procedure only if successful biliary dilation not achieved

Answer: C

According to guidelines on antibiotics in gastrointestinal endoscopy, patients with primary sclerosing cholangitis have a higher risk of incomplete biliary drainage during ERCP and therefore routine single dose pre-procedural ciprofloxacin is recommended. There is no requirement for a full course of antibiotics. ERCP for hilar cholangiocarcinoma also requires this regimen.

It is uncertain if antibiotic prophylaxis is beneficial for all patients undergoing ERCP. A meta-analysis of five randomized, placebo-controlled trials failed to show a decrease in the incidence of cholangitis and/or sepsis with routine antibiotic prophylaxis prior to ERCP in noncomplicated cases. However, this issue has not been resolved. More trials are required to prove the effectiveness of prophylactic antibiotics in this setting.

Reference
Banerjee S, Shen B, Baron TH, et al. Antibiotic prophylaxis for GI endoscopy. Gastrointest Endosc. May 2008;67(6):791–8

249. A 27-year-old female is admitted with complaints of intermittent abdominal discomfort. She has had several admissions over the last three years, but her status is getting worse. She has difficulty working and stays at home most of the time.

On physical exam, vital signs are within normal limits and abdominal exam is unremarkable. Laboratory values include WBC of 6,000, hematocrit of 30 %, normal electrolyte panel, and erythrocyte sedimentation rate of 57 mm/h. Stool studies show fecal leukocytes. Irritable bowel syndrome has been the diagnosis in the past and is suspected now.

Which intervention is most likely indicated at this time?
A) Reassurance
B) Fluoroquinolone antibiotic
C) Stool bulking agents
D) Selective serotonin reuptake inhibitor (antidepressant)
E) Colonoscopy

Answer: E
Although irritable bowel syndrome (IBS) is suspected, there are alarm features that warrant further investigation. The patient's low hematocrit, elevated erythrocyte sedimentation rate, and positive fecal leukocytes may suggest underlying gastrointestinal disorders. Colonoscopy would be warranted as the next step in management for a diagnosis.

The American College of Gastroenterologists (ACG) statement on the management of IBS does not recommend laboratory testing or diagnostic imaging in patients younger than 50 years with typical IBS symptoms and without alarm features. In addition to the above, alarm features include weight loss, iron-deficiency anemia, and a family history of colonic disease.

References
Brandt LJ, Chey WD, Foxx-Orenstein AE, Schiller LR, Schoenfeld PS, Spiegel BM, et al. An evidence-based position statement on the management of irritable bowel syndrome. Am J Gastroenterol. 2009;104 Suppl 1:S1-35.
Longstreth GF, Thompson WG, Chey WD, Houghton LA, Mearin F, Spiller RC. Functional bowel disorders. Gastroenterology. Apr 2006;130(5):1480–91.

250. A 78-year-old female is admitted with acute respiratory distress. Symptoms began abruptly 48 h ago with acute onset of fever muscle aches and cough. In the emergency room, she is placed on 100 % nonrebreather.

Her heart rate is 120 bpm, and blood pressure is 100/60 mmHg.

Her past medical history is significant for chronic obstructive pulmonary disease and hypertension. Chest radiograph reveals patchy diffuse infiltrates. Rapid influenza screen is positive.

In addition to resuscitative measures and broad-spectrum antibiotics, which antivirals should be given?
A) Oseltamivir
B) Zanamivir
C) Peramivir
D) No treatment

Answer: A
Much of our information concerning the treatment of severe influenza comes from the 2009 H1N1 epidemic. In those patients, therapy with oseltamivir reduced length of hospital stay, need for intensive care, and progression to severe disease or death. Ideally oseltamivir should be administered within 48 h of symptom onset. For critically ill patients with influenza infection, initiation of oseltamivir therapy up to 6–8 days from onset of symptoms may reduce mortality.

Adjuvant treatments are often considered for patients with life-threatening illnesses related to influenza. A study from Argentina described excellent outcomes in 13 patients with presumed H1N1 influenza A pneumonitis receiving a combination of oseltamivir and methylprednisolone (1 mg/kg/day) or hydrocortisone (300 mg/day). However, previous studies during earlier viral epidemics failed to demonstrate a beneficial effect of corticosteroids.

Severe and even fatal bronchospasm has been reported during treatment with zanamivir, and it should not be in individuals with underlying airway diseases.

Peramivir has not been extensively tested.. The drug was used on a compassionate and emergency basis during the H1N1 pandemic. It appeared to be relatively well tolerated but too few patients were enrolled to establish its efficacy. Its advantage is that it can be given intravenously.

References
Beigel JH, Farrar J, Han AM, Hayden FG, Hyer R, de Jong MD, et al. Avian influenza A (H5N1) infection in humans. N Engl J Med. Sep 29 2005;353(13):1374–85.
Domínguez-Cherit G, Lapinsky SE, Macias AE, Pinto R, Espinosa-Perez L, de la Torre A, et al. Critically Ill patients with 2009 influenza A(H1N1) in Mexico. JAMA. Nov 4 2009;302(17):1880–7.

251. A 37-year-old woman is admitted with moderate persistent epigastric abdominal pain. She reports drinking one-half liter of vodka per day. She rates the pain as 7/10. It is not associated with food intake. This is the

first time she had had these symptoms. She reports no other past medical history.

On physical exam, mild epigastric pain is noted. She is in moderate distress. Her WBC is 10,000 μL. Amylase is 330 units/L, and lipase is 300 units/L. An Abdominal radiograph is normal. She is admitted and placed on intravenous hydration.

What further imaging is needed?

A) CT of abdomen
B) EGD
C) None
D) MRCP
E) Abdominal ultrasound

Answer: E

Despite this patient's alcohol use, the first episode of pancreatitis warrants an abdominal ultrasound to assess the biliary tract. Ultrasonography of the abdomen is the most useful initial test in determining the etiology of pancreatitis. In Europe and other developed nations, patients tend to have gallstone pancreatitis, whereas in the United States, alcoholic pancreatitis is the most common.

CT is not indicated as this patient has moderate pancreatitis. There is a limited role in the first 48 h of admission. This patient has pancreatitis likely secondary to alcohol use. There are no current guidelines recommending CT scan in moderate cases of pancreatitis. Necrosis which may be found by CT scan usually takes several days to develop.

Reference

Tenner S, Baillie J, Dewitt J, et al. American College of Gastroenterology Guidelines: Management of Acute Pancreatitis. Am J Gastroenterol. 2013;

252. A 68-year-old male has been transferred from the intensive care unit to the floor. He has been in the hospital for 14 days due to community-acquired pneumonia. His hospital course has been complicated by sepsis, adrenal insufficiency, multiple organ failure, and mechanical intubation lasting eight days. He has received broad-spectrum antibiotics, steroids, and vasopressors.

On physical examination, he is alert, follows commands, and cooperates. Vital signs are stable. All cranial nerves are noticed to be intact. As his physical therapy is initiated, he is noted to have marked weakness of both the upper and lower extremities. The weakness is greater proximally more than distally. Areflexia is present.

CT scan of the head is normal. Electromyography reveals absent sensor responses in the legs and diffuse low amplitude throughout. Low amplitude motor units are consistent with myopathy. CPK is 2756.

Which of the following is the most likely diagnosis?

A) Critical illness myopathy
B) Guillain–Barré syndrome
C) Unmasked myasthenia gravis
D) Corticosteroid myopathy
E) Hospital-induced deconditioning

Answer: A

This patient has critical illness myopathy (CIM), which is seen in severely ill patients who often have a great than seven-day stay in the intensive care unit. Prolonged intubation is another risk factor. His profound weakness is out of proportion to what is expected from deconditioning. The difficulty with extubation and proximal limb weakness are classic findings as well. For uncertain reasons, creatinine kinase can be elevated.

The diagnosis of CIM is a clinical diagnosis, as there is no single laboratory, imaging, or nerve conduction test available to accurately make the diagnosis. Screening tools such as the Medical Research Council (MRC) score are primarily used in research but may gain acceptance as studies confirm their validity.

Prevention and treatment of CIM have focused on limiting vasopressors, sedation, corticosteroids, and other medications that may be a factor in disease progression. Early physical therapy, electrical muscle stimulation, and immunoglobulins are also being investigated as possible treatment options.

Little information exists on the long-term outcomes of patients with CIM. One limited study found that recovery from CIM was slow, with nearly all patients displaying abnormal clinical findings 1.5 years after the onset of this syndrome.

References

Tepper M, Rakic S, Haas JA, Woittiez AJJ. Incidence and onset of critical illness polyneuropathy in patients with septic shock. Neth J Med 2000;56:211–1

Zifko UA. Long-term outcome of critical illness polyneuropathy. Muscle Nerve 2000;(suppl 9):S49-52

253. A 35-year-old woman is admitted for an asthmatic exacerbation. Her medical history is significant only for asthma she has had since a child. Her medicines include beta-agonist inhalers and oral contraceptive pills.

On physical examination, vital signs are normal. She has diffuse wheezes. Examination of the skin discloses no petechiae or ecchymosis. The remainder of the examination is normal. The leukocyte count is 7000/μL with a normal differential, and the platelet count is 11,500/μL. Clumping of platelets is reported.

Which of the following is the most appropriate management?

A) Intravenous immune globulin
B) Prednisone
C) Platelet transfusion
D) Repeat complete blood count in a heparin or citrate anticoagulated tube

Answer: D

Unexpected lab results can occur due to mislabeling, automated testing machine problems, and interaction with preservatives. In this case, a repeat complete blood count in a heparin or citrate anticoagulated tube is needed. The patient's peripheral blood smear shows platelet clumping. This suggests pseudothrombocytopenia. Pseudothrombocytopenia is a laboratory artifact in which platelets drawn into an ethylenediaminetetraacetic acid (EDTA)-anticoagulated test tube clump and fail to be counted accurately by the automated counter, resulting in a spuriously low platelet count.

Reference

Cohen AM, Cycowitz Z, Mittelman M, Lewinski UH, Gardyn J: The incidence of pseudothrombocytopenia in automatic blood analyzers. Haematologia 2000, 30(2):117

Consultative and Comanagement

Ashley Casey and Kevin Conrad

254. A 66-year-old male presents to the emergency room with a chief complaint of a severe headache that developed approximately 10 h ago. He describes the headache as the worst headache of his life. He has a history of myelodysplasia for which he has been followed as an outpatient. He reports no history of spontaneous bleeds and denies any spontaneous bruising.

On physical examination, he is alert and oriented, and his speech is slightly slurred. The prothrombin time and activated partial thromboplastin time are within normal range. A CT scan is performed in the emergency room that shows an intracerebral bleed with a mild amount of extravasation of blood into the ventricular system.

Which of the following is the most appropriate minimum platelet threshold for this patient?

A) 40,000
B) 60,000
C) 100,000
D) 150,000

Answer: C

Thresholds for platelet transfusions are undergoing close examination. Some areas continue to provoke debate especially concerning the use of prophylactic platelet transfusions for the prevention of thrombocytopenic bleeding. Guidelines recommend maintaining platelet count at 100,000 after a central nervous system bleeding event. This would also be the case immediately prior to and after surgery performed on the central nervous system. This patient has a potentially life-threatening intracranial bleeding. The bleeding source is probably secondary to hypertensive disease and not thrombocytopenia. However, the patient is at continued risk for extension of the intracerebral bleeding because of her thrombocytopenia. Guidelines do not suggest additional benefits to maintaining platelet counts >100,000.

References
British Committee for Standards in Haematology, Blood Transfusion Task Force. Guidelines for the use of platelet transfusions. Br J Haematol. 2003;122:10–23.
Vavricka SR, Walter RB, Irani S et al. Safety of lumbar puncture for adults with acute leukemia and restrictive prophylactic platelet transfusion. Ann Hematol 2003;82:570–3.

255. A 44-year-old woman undergoes preoperative evaluation prior to surgery to repair a congenital defect of her pelvis. Her expected blood loss is 2.0 l. She has a prior history of severe anaphylactic reaction to a prior erythrocyte transfusion that she received for postpartum hemorrhage at age of 27 years. In addition she has a history of rheumatoid arthritis.

On physical examination, the temperature is 36.8 °C (98.5 °F), blood pressure is 140/70 mmHg, and heart rate is 76 bpm. Laboratory studies indicate a hemoglobin level of 12.0 g/dL, a leukocyte count of 6500 µL, and a platelet count of 150,000 µL.

Previous laboratory studies indicate an IgG level of 800 mg/dL and an IgM level of 65 mg/dL.

Which of the following is the most appropriate erythrocyte transfusion product for this patient?

A) Leuko-reduced blood
B) Cytomegalovirus-negative blood
C) Irradiated blood
D) Phenotypically matched blood
E) Washed blood

A. Casey, PharmD, BCPS, MT, ASCP
Department of Pharmacy, Ochsner Medical Center,
1514 Jefferson Hwy, New Orleans, LA 70121, USA
e-mail: acasey@ochsner.org

K. Conrad, MBA, MD (✉)
Department of Hospital Medicine, Ochsner Medical Center,
1514 Jefferson Hwy, New Orleans, LA 70121, USA
e-mail: kconrad@ochsner.org

© Springer International Publishing Switzerland 2016
K. Conrad (ed.), *Absolute Hospital Medicine Review: An Intensive Question & Answer Guide*,
DOI 10.1007/978-3-319-23748-0_2

Answer: E

This patient has IGA deficiency. The most appropriate product to minimize the risk of an anaphylactic transfusion reaction in this case is washed erythrocytes. Most patients with an IgA deficiency are asymptomatic. They are prone to gastrointestinal infections such as giardia. They also have an increased risk of autoimmune disorders such as rheumatoid arthritis and systemic lupus erythematosus. Some patients with IgA deficiency have anaphylactic reactions to blood products containing IgA. Fresh frozen plasma (FFP) is the main blood component containing IgA antibodies. Anaphylaxis may occur with a variety of transfusions including FFP, platelets, and erythrocytes. Washing erythrocytes and platelets removes plasma proteins and greatly decreases the incidence of anaphylaxis.

Reference

Wang N, Hammarström L. IgA deficiency: what is new?. Curr Opin Allergy Clin Immunol. 2012 Dec. 12(6):602–8.

256. A 34-year-old man with a history of superficial thrombophlebitis presents with bilateral foot pain of 3-days duration. Over the 6 months, he has had several distinct episodes of severe burning pain of the foot and several toes. The pain persists at rest and is debilitating. The patient smokes one to two packs of cigarettes a day.

    On physical examination, he is thin; his feet are erythematous and cold. There are ulcerations noted distally on both feet. The femoral pulses are strong and intact, and the dorsalis pedis and posterior tibialis pulses are absent bilaterally. No discoloration is noted on his leg and a normal hair pattern is noted on his legs. The pain is not worsened by deep palpation.

    What is the most likely diagnosis for this patient?
    A) Plantar fasciitis
    B) Spinal stenosis
    C) Thromboangiitis obliterans
    D) Raynaud phenomenon
    E) Atherosclerotic claudication

Answer: C

This patient has thromboangiitis obliterans, also called Buerger's disease. This results from inflammatory blockage of arterioles in the distal extremities and is usually seen in male smokers who are typically less than 40 years of age. Other typical features include a history of recurrent thrombophlebitis and rest pain. Distal pulses are often absent.

Plantar fasciitis is usually relieved with rest. Weight bearing and exercise exacerbate it. Spinal stenosis usually occurs in older patients. It is exacerbated by standing or walking and is relieved by rest. Atherosclerotic claudication is also seen in older patients. It has a steady progression. It starts with exercise-related pain and progresses slowly to pain at rest. Raynaud phenomenon is seen mostly in women. It is caused by vasospasm of small arterioles. It more commonly occurs in the hands but can be seen in the feet. The vasospasm is precipitated by cold, temperature change, or stress. Color changes, which can be profound, occur in the digits from white to blue to red. Pain is usually not severe and peripheral pulses remain intact even during episodes of vasospasm.

In Buerger's disease, among patients who stop smoking, 94 % avoid amputation. In contrast, among patients who continue using tobacco, there is an 8-year amputation rate of 43 %.

References

Espinoza LR. Buerger's disease: thromboangiitis obliterans 100 years after the initial description. Am J Med Sci. 2009;337(4):285–6.

Olin JW, Young JR, Graor RA, Ruschhaupt WF, Bartholomew JR. The changing clinical spectrum of thromboangiitis obliterans (Buerger's disease). Circulation. 1990;82 (5 Suppl):IV3–8.

257. Preoperative malnutrition is associated with which outcome in patients undergoing gastrointestinal surgery?
    A) Increased 30-day mortality
    B) Increased 60-day mortality
    C) Increased length of stay
    D) All of the above

Answer: D

Good nutritional status is an important factor in the outcome of gastrointestinal surgery. Several studies have confirmed this. Preoperative malnutrition is an independent predictor of length of hospital stay, 30-day, and 60-day mortality, as well as minor medical complications, in patients undergoing gastrointestinal surgery. Preoperative nutrition including total parenteral has been proven to be beneficial in malnourished patients undergoing gastrointestinal surgery.

Reference

Burden S, Todd C, Hill J, Lal S. Pre-operative nutrition support in patients undergoing gastrointestinal surgery. Cochrane Database Syst Rev. 2012;(11):CD008879.

258. A 52 year-old male presents with the chief complaint of daily seizures. He reports that he has had seizures weekly for the past several years since an automobile accident, but these have increased to nearly daily in the past few weeks. He states he takes levetiracetam, but is not certain of the dose. While in the emergency room, he has a generalized grand mal seizure and is given lorazepam. He has recently moved to the area and has no old records.

    He is admitted to the hospital medicine service and a 24 h EEG is instituted. On the first night of his admission, he has an apparent seizure but no seizure activity is noted on the EEG. The next morning he develops an inability to move the left side of his body and dysarthria. Urgent MRI of his head reveals no evidence of acute cerebrovascular accident.

The most likely cause of his paralysis is?

A) Early cerebral infarction
B) Todd's paralysis
C) Malingering
D) Migraine variant
E) Conversion disorder

Answer: C

This patient has several factors that suggest malingering. He presents with two relatively easy to mimic symptoms. First, he has a seizure with no eleptiform activity and then paralysis with a normal MRI. His recent travel from another area is also suggestive of the diagnosis.

Malingering is not considered a mental illness and its diagnosis and treatment can be difficult. Direct confrontation may not work best. Hostility, lawsuits, and occasionally violence may result. It may be best to confront the person indirectly by remarking that the objective findings do not meet the objective criteria for diagnosis. It is important to demonstrate to the patient that his abnormal behavior has been observed and will be documented. At the same time an attempt should be made to allow the patient who is malingering the opportunity to save face. Obviously this can be a challenge.

Invasive diagnostic maneuvers, consultations, and prolonged hospitalizations often do more harm than good and add fuel to the fire. People who malinger rarely accept psychiatric referral, and the success of such consultations is minimal. It may be considered to address a specific psychiatric complaint.

The most common goals of people who malinger in the emergency department are obtaining drugs and shelter. It may be beneficial to offer the patient some limited assistance in these areas. In the clinic or office, the most common goal is financial compensation.

References

McDermott BE, Feldman MD. Malingering in the medical setting. Psychiatr Clin North Am. 2007;30(4):645–62.
Purcell TB. The somatic patient. Emerg Med Clin North Am. 1991;9(1):137–59.

259. A 60-year-old male with chronic obstructive pulmonary disease is admitted for a hip fracture sustained after a fall. He undergoes surgery without complication. On the second day of hospitalization, he develops some mild dyspnea and nonproductive cough. He is currently on 2 l of oxygen at home and states that he will often get somewhat short of breath with any change in his living situation.

On physical exam, the patient appears comfortable. His temperature is 37.8 °C (100.1 °F), heart rate is 70 bpm, and respirations are 16 per minute. Oxygen saturation is 96 % on pulse oximetry with 2 l.

A chest X-ray shows no acute changes and white blood cell count is within normal limits.

Which of the following is the appropriate management of this patient?

A) Prednisone
B) Doxycycline plus prednisone
C) Levofloxacin
D) Azithromycin

Answer: A

American College of Chest Physician guidelines for chronic obstructive pulmonary disease exacerbation support inhaled beta agonists and steroids alone for mild flares. In this particular case, the patient is having a mild exacerbation of his typical chronic obstructive pulmonary disease. Antibiotics should be reserved for moderate to severe cases. The criteria for moderate disease exacerbation include cough, change in color of sputum, and increased shortness of breath.

References

Vollenweider DJ, Jarrett H, Steurer-Stey CA, Garcia-Aymerich J, Puhan MA. Antibiotics for exacerbations of chronic obstructive pulmonary disease. Cochrane Database Syst Rev. 2012;(12):CD010257.
Walters JA, Tan DJ, White CJ, Wood-Baker R. Different durations of corticosteroid therapy for exacerbations of chronic obstructive pulmonary disease. Cochrane Database Syst Rev. 2012;(12):CD006897.

260. A 74-year-old man is admitted for cough, dyspnea, and altered mental status. The patient is noted to be minimally responsive on arrival. Results of physical examination are as follows: temperature, 38.9 °C (102.1 °F); heart rate, 116 bpm; blood pressure, 96/60 mmHg; respiratory rate, 35 breaths/min; and O_2 saturation, 74 % on 100 % O_2 with a nonrebreather mask. The patient is intubated urgently and placed on mechanical ventilation.

On physical exam, coarse rhonchi are noted bilaterally. A portable chest X-ray reveals good placement of the endotracheal tube and lobar consolidation of the right lower lobe. Empirical broad-spectrum antimicrobial therapy is started.

Which is true concerning his nutritional management?

A) Enteral nutrition is less likely to cause infection than parenteral nutrition.
B) Parenteral nutrition has not consistently been shown to result in a decrease in mortality, compared with standard care.
C) The use of oral supplements in all hospitalized elderly patients has been shown to be beneficial.
D) Immune-modulating supplements are no better than standard high-protein formulas in critically ill patients.
E) All of the above

Answer: E

Comparisons of enteral nutrition with parenteral nutrition have consistently shown fewer infectious complications with enteral nutrition. Several studies have looked at specialized feeding formulas in the treatment of the critically ill. There is little evidence to support their use over standard high-protein formulas.

In one study among adult patients breathing with the aid of mechanical ventilation in the ICU, immune-modulating formulas compared with a standard high-protein formula did not improve infectious complications or other clinical end points.

Elderly patients require special consideration. A trial in 501 hospitalized elderly patients randomized to oral supplements or a regular diet showed that, irrespective of their initial nutritional status, the patients receiving oral supplements had lower mortality, better mobility, and a shorter hospital stay.

References

Langer G, Schloemer G, Knerr A, Kuss O, Behrens J. Nutritional interventions for preventing and treating pressure ulcers. Cochrane Database Syst Rev. 2003;(4):CD003216.

Zanten AR, Sztark F, Kaisers UX et al. High-protein enteral nutrition enriched with immune-modulating nutrients vs standard high-protein enteral nutrition and nosocomial infections in the ICU: a randomized clinical trial. JAMA. 2014;312:514–24.

261. You are called to see a patient urgently in the postpartum ward. She is a 32-year-old female who, 20 min prior, had an uneventful vaginal delivery. In the past 20 min, the patient has become abruptly short of breath, hypoxic, and severely hypotensive with a blood pressure of 72/palpation mm Hg. On physical exam, she is obtunded and in serve respiratory distress. She has no significant past medical history documented and has had an uneventful pregnancy. Mild wheezes with decreased breath sounds are heard. Chest radiograph and arterial blood gasses are pending.

    The most likely diagnosis is?
    A) Pulmonary embolism
    B) Sepsis
    C) Peripartum cardiomyopathy
    D) Amniotic fluid embolism
    E) Eclampsia

Answer: D

Amniotic fluid embolism is a rare complication of pregnancy. It presents acutely during and immediately after delivery, usually within 30 min. The exact mechanisms are unclear, but it is thought that amniotic fluid gains entry into the maternal circulation. This triggers an intensive inflammatory reaction, resulting in pulmonary vasoconstriction, pulmonary capillary leak, and myocardial depression. Patients present with acute hypoxemia, hypotension, and decreased mental status. Treatment is supportive but may be improved by early recognition and cardiopulmonary resuscitation. The other answers do occur in pregnancy, but the severity, rapid onset, and timing to delivery strongly suggest amniotic fluid embolism. The mortality rate may exceed 60 %. Immediate transfer to an intensive care unit with cardiovascular resuscitation is recommended.

Reference

Conde-Agudelo A, Romero R. Amniotic fluid embolism: an evidence-based review. Am J Obstet Gynecol. 2009;201(5):445.e441–3

262. You are asked to see a 64-year-old female for diarrhea. She was admitted to the hospital 4 days ago with acute abdominal findings and was found to have acute mesenteric ischemia. She underwent a small-bowel resection. 150 cm of small bowel is remaining. Her colon remained intact.

    Over the past 4 days since surgery, she has been on parenteral nutrition. Oral intake has been started gradually 2 days ago. Diarrhea has occurred both at night and day.

    Stool cultures and *Clostridium difficile* polymerase chain reaction are negative. Her current medications include low-molecular-weight heparin as well as loperamide two times daily.

    Which of the following is the most appropriate management?
    A) Increase loperamide.
    B) Initiate cholestyramine.
    C) Initiate omeprazole.
    D) Stop oral intake.
    E) Decrease lipids in parenteral nutrition.

Answer: C

Patients who have undergone significant bowel resection should receive acid suppression in the postoperative period with a proton pump inhibitor.

This patient has short-bowel syndrome. Any process that leaves less than 200 cm of viable small bowel or a loss of 50 % or more of the small intestine as compared to baseline places the patient at risk for developing short-bowel syndrome. In short-bowel syndrome, there is an increase in gastric acids in the postoperative period. This can lead to inactivation of pancreatic lipase, resulting in significant diarrhea. Stopping the patient's oral intake may lead to temporary improvement. It is important that the patient continues her oral feedings, as this will eventually allow the gut to adapt and hopefully resume normal function.

References

Howard L, Ament M, Fleming CR et al. Current use and clinical outcome of home parenteral and enteral nutrition therapies in the United States. Gastroenterology. 1995;109(2):355–65.

Lord LM, Schaffner R, DeCross AJ et al. Management of the patient with short bowel syndrome. AACN Clin Issues. 2000;11(4):604–18.

263. A 45-year-old female presents with left calf swelling. She states that she has been feeling well and reports no other constitutional symptoms. She has no family history of venous thromboembolism and has no personal history of venous thromboembolism as well. She denies recent travel, injury, or past medical problems. She currently takes no medications and has been on no medications in the past year. Physical examination reveals swelling of the left leg from mid-thigh to ankle. Doppler ultrasonography shows deep vein thrombosis in the femoral vein.

Prior to initiating heparin therapy, which of the following tests should be performed to determine the risk of reoccurrence and duration of treatment?
A) Factor V Leiden mutation
B) No further testing indicated
C) Prothrombin gene mutation
D) Factor V Leiden and prothrombin gene mutation
E) Erythrocyte sedimentation rate

Answer: B

This patient has an unexplained deep vein thrombosis. Current guidelines recommend treatment for 6 months. Recent studies have revealed that factor V Leiden and prothrombin mutation are not sufficiently predictive of future recurrence. They are currently not recommended unless the patient has a family history of thrombosis. Even with a family history, the utility of these tests is of uncertain benefit. Future studies may clarify the predictive value of these tests.

Reference

Kearon C, Crowther M, Hirsh J. Management of patients with hereditary hypercoagulable disorders. Annu Rev Med. 2000;51:169–85.

264. A 58-year-old female who underwent an elective cholecystectomy is noted to be in atrial fibrillation by telemetry. Her heart rate is 108 bpm. She has a history of hypertension. Her medications are verapamil and full-strength aspirin. She states that several years ago, she had palpitations after exercise, but that has since resolved, and she has noticed no problems. You are consulted by the surgical team for management of her heart rate in preparing her for discharge. On physical exam she appears in no distress and is not short of breath.

Which of the following is the appropriate management of the patient's atrial fibrillation?
A) Maintain her current dose of verapamil.
B) Increase her dose of verapamil with a target rate of 80 beats per minute.
C) Add digoxin to control her heart rate to a target of 80 beats per minute.
D) Consult cardiology for possible cardioversion.

Answer: A

A 2010 study compared lenient control of heart rate less than 110 beats per minute to more strict control of less than 80 beats per minute. The study found that achieving strict heart rate control resulted in multiple admissions with no perceivable benefit outcomes. In this particular case, a heart rate of 108 bpm is acceptable, and patient the can be discharged on her current medications. Follow-up with her primary care physician should be obtained to monitor heart rate.

Digoxin can be used in the acute setting but does little to control the ventricular rate in active patients. It is rarely used as monotherapy. Caution should be exercised in elderly patients with renal failure due to toxicity. Digoxin is indicated in patients with heart failure and reduced LV function.

Reference

Van Gelder IC, Groenveld HF, Crijns HJ et al. Lenient versus strict rate control in patients with atrial fibrillation. N Engl J Med. 2010;362:1363–73.

265. A 52-year-old, morbidly obese man is in the ICU for treatment of pneumonia, sepsis, and acute respiratory distress syndrome. Prior to this admission, he was receiving therapy for hypertension, type 2 diabetes mellitus, hyperlipidemia, obstructive sleep apnea, and chronic obstructive pulmonary.

He is on the ventilator for his second day and tube feeds are to be started. His BMI is 41.

What weight should be used to calculate his caloric needs?
A) Ideal body weight
B) Actual body weight
C) Adjusted body weight
D) None of the above

Answer: C

The use of actual body weight in determining the caloric needs of obese patients in the ICU routinely leads to overfeeding. The use of ideal body weight leads to underfeeding. Morbidly obese patients have, on average, 20 % to 30 % increased lean body mass compared with individuals of the same sex and similar height. Adjusted body weight would be the best starting point for determining caloric needs.

Judicious underfeeding such as using 22 kcal/kg, adjusted body weight of morbidly obese patients who are receiving mechanical ventilation may improve outcome. This may include reducing obesity-related hyperglycemia in the setting of critical illness, reducing infectious complications, decreasing ICU length of stay (LOS), ventilator days, and duration of antibiotic therapy.

References

Alberda C, Gamlich L, Jones N et al. The relationship between nutritional intake and clinical outcomes in critically ill patients: results of an international multicenter observational study. Intensive Care Med. 2009;35:1728.

Martindale RG, McClave SA, Vanek VW et al. Guidelines for the provision and assessment of nutrition support therapy in the adult critically ill patient: SCCM and ASPEN: executive summary. Crit Care Med. 2009;37:1757.

Port AM, Apovian C. Metabolic support of the obese intensive care unit patient: a current perspective. Curr Opin Clin Nutr Metab Care. 2010;13:184.

266. You are called to the floor to see a patient who has developed acute onset of shortness of breath. She is a 56-year-old female who was admitted for upper GI bleed. She is currently receiving her first unit of packed erythrocytes, which was started 1.5 h ago.

On physical examination, temperature is 38.9 °C(102 °F), blood pressure is 110/65, pulse rate is 115 beats per minute, and respirations are 22 per minute. Her current oxygenation is 83 %. She has been placed on 3 l by nasal cannula. No peripheral edema is noted. Mild wheezes and diffuse crackles are heard throughout her lung fields.

A stat X-ray is ordered which reveals diffuse bilateral infiltrates. On review of her records, type and screen reveal an A+ blood type with a negative antibody screen.

Which of the following is the most likely diagnosis?
A) Transfusion-related acute lung injury
B) Acute hemolytic transfusion reaction
C) Febrile nonhemolytic transfusion reaction
D) Transfusion-associated circulatory overload
E) Transfusion-related sepsis

Answer: A

This patient has likely developed transfusion-related acute lung injury (TRALI). The patient developed dyspnea, diffuse pulmonary infiltrates, and hypoxia acutely during the blood transfusion. It usually occurs shortly after the transfusion or can be delayed for several hours. Both the classic and delayed TRALI syndromes are among the most frequent complications following the transfusion of blood products. They are associated with significant morbidity and increased mortality.

Antileukocyte antibodies in the donor blood product directed against the recipient leukocytes cause this reaction. TRALI can occur with any blood product. Treatment of TRALI is supportive, with expected recovery within several days.

An acute hemolytic transfusion reaction is commonly caused by clinical error, leading to ABO incompatibility. This occurs early in the transfusion. Patients present with hypotension, disseminated intravascular coagulation, and hypoxia. This patient's symptoms are primarily shortness of breath, which does not suggest an acute hemolytic transfusion reaction. It can be difficult to distinguish TRALI from transfusion-related volume overload. In this particular case, the patient had only received a limited volume of one unit of packed blood cells. Per her history, there is no reason to believe she couldn't tolerate the volume given.

Reference

Curtis BR, McFarland JG. Mechanisms of transfusion-related acute lung injury (TRALI): anti-leukocyte antibodies. Crit Care Med. 2006;34:S118–23.

267. A patient with a new diagnosis of deep vein thrombosis is started on warfarin and enoxaparin. 48 h later the decision is made to switch to rivaroxaban.

When will it be appropriate to start the patient's new anticoagulant (weight=77 kg, CrCl=89 ml/min, INR=1.6)?
A) Ok to start now because INR <3.0
B) Ok to start now because INR <2.0
C) Not ok to start because INR >1.5
D) INR does not matter

Answer: A

Per package labeling by the pharmaceutical manufacture, discontinue warfarin and initiate rivaroxaban as soon as INR falls to <3.0. Answer B represents the correct conversion from warfarin to dabigatran.

INR is not used to monitor rivaroxaban; however, it's an indicator of warfarin's effectiveness, thus aiding in predicting a safe time to initiate a different anticoagulant. Rivaroxaban starts working in 2–4 h. Warfarin takes 3–5 days to start working and 3–5 days to be eliminated.

Reference

Garcia DA et al. CHEST guidelines – parenteral anticoagulants. Chest. 2012;141(2_suppl):e24S–43S.

268. Which vitamin deficiency occurs after bariatric surgery?
A) Iron.
B) Zinc.
C) B12.
D) Thiamine.
E) All of the answers are correct.
F) None of the answers is correct.

Answer: E

Vitamin and other nutritional deficiencies are common after bariatric procedures. This may be due to diet changes, change in gastric function, or malabsorption. In these patients, notable deficiencies occur with iron, zinc, and B12. Lifelong nutritional supplementation is essential.

Many patients often stop taking supplements after a few years after being lost to follow up. Despite improved surgical outcomes, complications from weight-loss surgery are frequent. A study of insurance claims of patients who had undergone bariatric surgery showed 21.9 % complications during the initial hospital stay. Over the next 6 months, 40 % developed complications. This occurred more often in those over 40. The rate of complications is reduced when the procedure is performed by an experienced, trained surgeon. Guidelines recommend that surgery be in a dedicated unit.

Reference

Chauhan V, Vaid M, Gupta M, Kalanuria A, Parashar A. Metabolic, renal, and nutritional consequences of bariatric surgery: implications for the clinician. South Med J. 2010;103(8):775–83; quiz 784–5.

269. A 52-year-old male presents for preop clearance for knee replacement surgery. He has hepatitis C cirrhosis. He has child A cirrhosis. He is suffering from disability due to his knee pain. He is a high school football coach and is considering retiring due to his knee-related issues.

    Which of the following should you tell this patient about his surgical risks?
    A) He should not have surgery because of the significant mortality risk.
    B) He has a slightly increased risk of death compared with patients who do not have cirrhosis.
    C) He should defer surgery until after he is successfully treated for hepatitis C.
    D) He should defer surgery until after he undergoes liver transplantation.
    E) He has no increased risk.

Answer: B

Patients with cirrhosis of all causes and stage are at an increased mortality risk from surgery. Even though this patient has a low MELD score and is a child A patient, there is clear evidence that he is at increased risk. Since he has severe morbidity, elective surgery is a reasonable option. He should be informed of the small but significant increased risk of death associated with surgery as compared to a someone without cirrhosis. Treatment for hepatitis C would not have an impact on surgical outcomes. Waiting for transplant, which is many years away, is not the best option.

Reference

Teh SH, Nagorney DM, Stevens SR et al. Risk factors for mortality after surgery in patients with cirrhosis. Gastroenterology. 2007;132(4):1261–9.

270. A 55-year-old, black woman undergoes a total colectomy for ruptured diverticulum. Her preoperative score on the Mini-Mental State Examination (MMSE) was 28 out of 30. Forty-eight hours after surgery, significant delirium develops. This is the first episode of delirium the patient has experienced. The patient's family members are concerned about whether she will regain cognitive function and in what time frame.

    Which of the following is most likely regarding cognitive function in patients such as this?
    A) Return to baseline in an average of 5 days
    B) Return to baseline in 2 weeks
    C) Return to baseline in an average of 30 days
    D) Return to baseline in an average of 6 months
    E) Permanent loss of cognitive function

Answer: A

Postoperative cognitive dysfunction (POCD) is common in adult patients of all ages, recovery in the younger age group is usually within 5 days, and complete recovery is the norm for patients less than 60 years old.

Patients older than 60 years of age are at significant risk for long-term cognitive problems, and in this group recovery from POCD may last as long as 6 months and may be permanent.

Patients with POCD in all age groups are at an increased risk of all-cause death in the first year after surgery.

Reference

Newfield P. Postoperative cognitive dysfunction. F1000 Med Rep. 2009;1(14):281.

271. A 48-year-old man is admitted with acute onset of dizziness. He describes it as a sensation that the room is spinning.

    All of the following would be consistent with a central cause of vertigo *EXCEPT*:
    A) Absence of tinnitus
    B) Gaze-evoked nystagmus
    C) Hiccups
    D) Inhibition of nystagmus by visual fixation
    E) Purely vertical nystagmus

Answer: D

Deafness, tinnitus, or hearing loss is typically absent with central lesions. Dizziness is a common complaint affecting approximately 20 % of the population over the course of the year. It results in many emergency room visits and hospitalizations.

Most dizziness is benign and is self-limited. Vertigo is often described as an external sensation such as the room is spinning. Vertigo is most commonly from peripheral causes which affect labyrinths of the inner ear.

Focal lesions of the brainstem and cerebellum can also lead to vertigo.

Vertical nystagmus with a downward fast phase and horizontal nystagmus that changes direction with gaze suggest central vertigo. Significant non-accommodating nystagmus is most often a sign of central vertigo but can occur with peripheral causes as well.

In peripheral vertigo, nystagmus typically is provoked by positional maneuvers. It can be inhibited by visual fixation. Central causes of nystagmus are more likely to be associated with hiccups, diplopia, cranial neuropathies, and dysarthria.

Reference

Kerber KA. Vertigo and dizziness in the emergency department. Emerg Med Clin North Am. 2009;27(1):39–50. doi:10.1016/j. emc.2008.09.002.

272. A 78-year-old male is admitted with weakness, failure to thrive, and nausea. He has a history of Parkinson's disease for the past 8 years for which he is on levodopa. His wife reports that he has occasional episodes of nausea that seem to last for a few days.

　　Which treatment strategy would be appropriate for his nausea?
　　A) Metoclopramide
　　B) Promethazine
　　C) Ondansetron
　　D) Prochlorperazine
　　E) All of the above

Answer: C

Gastrointestinal complaints are common with Parkinson's disease. Efforts should be made to minimize worsening of motor symptoms with pharmaceuticals. Prochlorperazine, metoclopramide, and promethazine are antidopaminergic medicines and can exacerbate or worsen Parkinson motor symptoms and should be avoided. Ondansetron has been used with minimal side effects.

References

Cooke CE, Mehra IV. Oral ondansetron for preventing nausea and vomiting. Am J Hosp Pharm. 1994;51(6):762–71.

Grimes DA, Lang AE. Treatment of early Parkinson's disease. Can J Neurol Sci. 1999;26 Suppl 2:S39–44.

273. The 6-month mortality for nursing home residents with documented advanced dementia is:
　　A) 54 %
　　B) 27 %
　　C) 83 %
　　D) 37 %

Answer: A

Mortality of patients diagnosed with end-stage dementia is significant. In a 2009 study, 323 nursing home residents with advanced dementia were followed. The patients were assessed at baseline and quarterly for 18 months through chart reviews, nursing interviews, and physical examinations. Mortality from all causes was greater than half at 54.8 %. In the last 3 months of life, 40.7 % of subjects underwent one or more intensive interventions that were defined as hospitalization, ED visit, parenteral therapy, or tube feeding.

Families and designated surrogate decision-makers were also followed and questioned on an understanding of the prognosis. Those families that demonstrated an understanding of the prognosis had fewer interventions.

Reference

Mitchell SL, Teno JM, Kiely DK et al. The clinical course of advanced dementia. N Engl J Med. 2009;361(16):1529–38.

274. You are called to see a 43-year-old female who is 3 days postpartum. She has had a non-complicated pregnancy. She has not been discharged due to feeding issues with her child. She had a normal spontaneous vaginal delivery. This is her fourth vaginal delivery.

　　On physical exam, she has nontender bilateral leg swelling, orthopnea, and a cough with frothy white sputum. Her blood pressure is 150/87 mmHg. Her temperature is 37.2 °C (99.0 °F). She has mild chest pain with inspiration. She has bilateral pulmonary crackles and pitting edema of her lower extremities. WBC is 16,000/μL. CXR is pending.

　　Which of the following is the most likely diagnosis?
　　A) Pulmonary embolism
　　B) Peripartum cardiomyopathy
　　C) Hospital-acquired pneumonia
　　D) Amniotic fluid embolism
　　E) Acute myocardial infarction

Answer: B

This patient has peripartum cardiomyopathy. This occurs in approximately 0.03 % of all pregnancies. Risk factors include greater maternal age, multiparity, and frequent pregnancies. Clinical management is the same as that of congestive heart failure due to dilated cardiomyopathy. Patients are at high risk of developing peripartum cardiomyopathy in subsequent pregnancies as well. This particular patient would warrant transfer to the cardiac care unit and aggressive fluid management.

The most recent studies indicate that the survival rate is very high at 98 %. In the United States, over 50 % of peripartum cardiomyopathy patients experience a complete recovery of heart function with conventional treatment protocols.

The cause of peripartum cardiomyopathy is unknown. Currently, researchers are investigating cardiotropic viruses, immune system dysfunction, trace mineral deficiencies, and genetics as possible causes.

References

Elkayam U, Akhter MW, Singh H et al. Pregnancy-associated cardiomyopathy: clinical characteristics and a comparison between early and late presentation. Circulation. 2005;111(16):2050–5.

Murali S, Baldisseri MR. Peripartum cardiomyopathy. Crit Care Med. 2005;33(10 Suppl):S340–6.

275. A 65-year-old male presents with progressive shortness of breath over the past month. He has a 40-pack-year history of smoking. CT scan of the chest reveals a right middle lobe mass for which he subsequently undergoes biopsy, which reveals adenocarcinoma. Magnetic resonance imaging of the brain reveals a 1-cm tumor in the left cerebral cortex, which is consistent with metastatic disease. The patient has no history of seizures or syncope. The patient is referred to outpatient therapy in the hematology/oncology service as well as follow-up with radiation oncology. The patient is ready for discharge.

    Which of the following would be the most appropriate therapy for primary seizure prevention?
    A) Seizure prophylaxis is not indicated.
    B) Valproate.
    C) Phenytoin.
    D) Phenobarbital.
    E) Oral prednisone 40 mg daily.

Answer: A

There is no indication for antiepileptic therapy for primary prevention in patients who have brain metastasis who have not undergone resection. Past studies have revealed no difference in seizure rates between placebo and antiepileptic therapy in patients who have brain tumors. Antiepileptic therapy has high rates of adverse reactions and caution should be used in their use.

Reference

Sirven JI, Wingerchuk DM, Drazkowski JF, Lyons MK, Zimmerman RS. Seizure prophylaxis in patients with brain tumors: a meta-analysis. Mayo Clin Proc. 2004;79(12):1489–94.

276. A 78-year-old male is admitted due to swelling over his chest wall. During discussion with the patient, he notes that he had an AICD implanted in the area of the swelling over 3 years ago. His postoperative course had been uneventful and he had never developed any wound dehiscence before.

    On physical examination, there are palpable swelling and fluctuance over the right upper chest wall at the site of a well-healed incision. The patient notes some fevers and chills on and off the last few weeks. You are very concerned for a cardiovascular implantable electronic device (CIED) infection.

Which of the following is appropriate in the care of your patient?
    A) Draw two sets of blood cultures before beginning initiation of antimicrobial therapy.
    B) Percutaneous aspiration of the generator pocket.
    C) Attempt to preserve the placement of this AICD via empiric antibiotics.
    D) Request removal of device and obtain gram stain and cultures of the tissue and lead tip.
    E) A and D.

Answer: E

A patient with a suspicion of a CIED infection should have two sets of peripheral blood cultures drawn before prompt initiation of antimicrobial therapy. The implantable device should be removed by an expert and the generator-pocket tissue and lead tip should be cultured on explanation. It is appropriate to obtain a transesophageal echocardiogram (TEE) to assess for CIED infection and valvular endocarditis. Percutaneous aspiration is not needed, as the device will be removed.

Reference

Baddour LM et al. Update on cardiovascular implantable electronic device infections and their management: a scientific statement from the American Heart Association. Circulation. 2010;121:458–77.

277. Which of the following occurs in the cognitive function following major cardiac surgery?
    A) All patients experience some transient cognitive decline.
    B) Return to baseline can take as long as 6 months.
    C) Greater declines will be seen in patients with postop delirium.
    D) Most return to baseline at 5 days.
    E) All of the above.

Answer: E

Postoperative confusion and delirium are common in cardiac surgery patients. A 2012 study revealed that all postoperative cardiac surgery patients experienced some degree of postoperative cognitive decline as measured by the Mini-Mental State Examination (MMSE). Most returned to baseline within 5 days with supportive care alone. For patients who had significant postop delirium, a return to baseline was delayed 6 months. Most non-delirious patients had a return to baseline in a few days. Risk factors for delirium include age, lower level of education, female, and having a history of stroke or transient ischemic attack.

References

Saczynski JS, Marcantonio ER, Quach L et al. Cognitive trajectories after postoperative delirium. N Engl J Med. 2012;367:30–9.

Tully P, Baune B, Baker R. Cognitive impairment before and 6 months after cardiac surgery increase mortality risk at median 11 year follow-up: a cohort study. Int J Cardiol. 2013;168(3):2796–802.

278. A 76-year-old man is scheduled to undergo an urgent colectomy for recurrent life-threatening diverticular bleeding. He denies any chest pain with exertion but is limited in his physical activity because of degenerative arthritis of his knees. This has left him unable to climb stairs. He has no history of coronary artery disease or congestive heart failure. He does have diabetes mellitus and hypertension. His current medications include aspirin 81 mg daily, enalapril 20 mg daily, and insulin glargine 32 units daily in combination with insulin lispro on a sliding scale. His blood pressure is 138/86 mmHg.

His physical examination findings are normal. His most recent hemoglobin A1C is 6.4 %, and his creatinine is 2.3 mg/dL. You elect to perform an electrocardiogram preoperatively, and it demonstrates no abnormalities.

What is his expected postoperative risk of a major cardiac event?
A) 0.5 %
B) 1 %
C) 5 %
D) 10 %
E) 20 %

Answer: D
One of the most widely used preoperative risk assessment tools is the Revised Cardiac Risk Index (RCRI). The RCRI scores patients on a scale from 0 to 6. The patient here has a RCRI score of 3. His score includes high-risk surgery, creatinine greater than 2 mg/dl, and diabetes mellitus requiring insulin. The six factors that comprise the RCRI are high-risk surgical procedures, known ischemic heart disease, congestive heart failure, cerebrovascular disease, diabetes mellitus requiring insulin, and chronic kidney disease with a creatinine greater than 2 mg/dL.
0 predictor = 0.4 %, 1 predictor = 0.9 %, 2 predictors = 6.6 %, ≥3 predictors = >11 %

References
Goldman L, Caldera DL, Nussbaum SR, Southwick FS, Krogstad D, Murray B, Burke DS, O'Malley TA, Goroll AH, Caplan CH, Nolan J, Carabello B, Slater EE. Multifactorial index of cardiac risk in noncardiac surgical procedures. N Engl J Med. 1977;297(16):845–50.
Lee TH, Marcantonio ER, Mangione CM, Thomas EJ, Polanczyk CA, Cook EF, Sugarbaker DJ, Donaldson MC, Poss R, Ho KK, Ludwig LE, Pedan A, Goldman L. Derivation and prospective validation of a simple index for prediction of cardiac risk of major noncardiac surgery. Circulation. 1999;100(10):1043–9.

279. A 24-year-old woman is admitted with significant fatigue, fever, and a sore throat. She reports due to throat pain she has been unable to swallow any liquids for the past 24 h.

On physical examination, she is found to have anterior cervical lymphadenopathy, erythematous throat, and mild hepatosplenomegaly. She remembers having mononucleosis in high school.

She has mild elevations of her transaminases. Her heterophile antibody test is positive.

Which of the following is true concerning the heterophile antibody test?
A) Heterophile antibody testing would not be helpful for this patient because the results may be positive owing to her previous episode of mononucleosis.
B) She has acute infectious mononucleosis from primary Epstein-Barr virus (EBV).
C) She has a mononucleosis-like CMV infection.
D) A positive result indicates moderate to severe clinical disease.
E) She has acute rheumatoid arthritis.

Answer: B
Despite a possible prior reported history of mononucleosis, this patient has acute infectious mononucleosis from EBV. This is confirmed by the positive heterophile test.
More than 90 % of patients with primary infectious mononucleosis test positive for heterophile antibodies. The monospot test is commonly used to test for heterophile antibodies. Patients may test positive for 3–4 months after the onset of illness, and heterophile antibodies may persist for up to 9 months. Patients with other forms of mononucleosis such as CMV or toxoplasmosis rarely test positive for heterophile antibodies.
Heterophile antibodies may be falsely positive. They are occasionally positive in patients with rheumatoid arthritis. The heterophile titer does not correlate with the severity of the illness.
Most patients with Epstein-Barr virus infectious mononucleosis are asymptomatic. Therefore, 90 % of adults show serological evidence of previous EBV infection.

Reference
Straus SE, Cohen JI, Tosato G et al. NIH conference. Epstein-Barr virus infections: biology, pathogenesis, and management. Ann Intern Med. 1993;118(1):45–58.

280. Which of the following surgeries would pose the greatest risk for postsurgical complications in the elderly?
A) Carotid endarterectomy
B) Nonemergent repair of a thoracic aortic aneurysm
C) Resection of a 5-cm lung cancer
D) Total colectomy for colon cancer
E) Total hip replacement

Answer: B

Hospitalists are often asked to provide guidance regarding the postoperative risk of complications after a variety of noncardiac surgical procedures. A "frailty score" for older patients may be more predictive than current models.

It is useful to categorize the surgical procedures into a low, intermediate, or higher risk category. Individuals who are at the highest risk include those undergoing an emergent major operation. This risk is amplified in elderly adults. High-risk procedures include aortic and other noncarotid major vascular surgery and surgeries with a prolonged operative time. Surgeries that are an intermediate risk include major thoracic surgery, major abdominal surgery, head and neck surgery, carotid endarterectomy, orthopedic surgery, and prostate surgery. Lower risk procedures include eye, skin, and endoscopy.

Reference

Seymour DG, Pringle R. Post-operative complications in the elderly surgical patient. Gerontology. 1983;29(4):262–70.

281. A 68-year-old female was admitted to the hospital 8 days ago for hernia repair. She was discharged without complications. Three days ago, the patient began to have progressive high-volume diarrhea. She presents to the emergency room with severe rigors and cramps to her lower abdomen.

    On physical exam, she has marked abdominal pain. Her temperature is 39.5 °C (103.0 °F), heart rate is 100 beats per minute, and respirations are 15 per minute. Her blood pressure is 100/62. She has marked hyperactive bowel sounds as well as significant abdominal distention. Laboratory studies include a leukocyte count of 28,000 and hematocrit of 25 %; and blood cultures are negative. Stools are sent for *Clostridium* toxin which is positive.

    Which of the following is the most appropriate treatment for the patient's diarrhea?
    A) Metronidazole orally
    B) Metronidazole intravenously
    C) Vancomycin oral
    D) Vancomycin intravenously

Answer: C

This patient has severe *Clostridium difficile*-associated diarrhea (CDI). For patients with severe CDI, suitable antibiotic regimens include vancomycin (125 mg four times daily for 10 days; may be increased to 500 mg four times daily) or fidaxomicin (200 mg twice daily for 10 days). Vancomycin has been shown to be superior to metronidazole in severe cases.

Fidaxomicin has been shown to be as good as vancomycin, for treating CDI. One study also reported significantly fewer recurrences of infection, a frequent problem with *C. difficile*.

Other considerations in this case may be to obtain a CT scan and possible colorectal surgery consultation.

References

Louie TJ, Miller MA, Mullane KM, Weiss K, Lentnek A, Golan Y et al. Fidaxomicin versus vancomycin for *Clostridium difficile* infection. N Engl J Med. 2011a;364(5):422–31.

Louie TJ, Miller MA, Mullane KM, Weiss K, Lentnek A, Golan Y, Gorbach S, Sears P, Shue Y-K, Opt-80-003 Clinical Study, Group. Fidaxomicin versus vancomycin for *Clostridium difficile* infection. N Engl J Med. 2011b;364(5):422–31.

282. A 67-year-old man was admitted with a cerebrovascular accident. He has done well during his hospitalization and is preparing for discharge to a skilled nursing facility. A catheter, which was placed in the emergency room, has been in for 3 days. He reports no prior incident of urinary retention. It is removed, and patient has difficulty voiding.

    Which of the following would be considered an abnormal post-void residual (PVR) amount?
    A) 15 ml
    B) 50 ml
    C) 100 ml
    D) 200 ml
    E) 300 ml

Answer: C

Abnormal residual bladder volumes have been defined in several ways. No particular definition is clinically superior. Some authorities consider volumes greater than 100 mL to be abnormal. Others use a value greater than 20 % of the voided volume to indicate a high residual. In normal adults, the post-void residual volume should be less than 50 ml. Over the age of 60, a range of 50 ml to 100 ml can be seen but is not known to cause significant issues. Post-void residual (PVR) volume increases with age but generally do not rise to above 100 ml unless there is some degree of obstruction or bladder dysfunction. Urinary retention is common after several days of catheter placement, particularly in males. Caution should be used when placing urinary catheters, as they are a significant cause of urinary retention. Whenever possible urinary catheters should be removed. Bladder training and time may improve the retention. Some consideration may be given to starting the male patient on medications to reduce benign prostatic hypertrophy as well.

Ultrasound can be used as a noninvasive means of obtaining PVR volume determinations, especially if a precise measurement is not required. The error using this formula, compared with the standard of post-void catheterization, is approximately 21 %. In patients with ascites bedside measurement by ultrasound of PVR can be inaccurate due to an inability to differentiate bladder fluid from ascitic fluid.

Reference
Lisenmeyer TA, Stone JM. Neurogenic bladder and bowel dysfunction. In: De Lisa J, editor. Rehabilitation medicine. Philadelphia: Lippincott-Raven; 1998. p. 1073–106.

283. A 37-year-old male has been admitted for alcohol-related pancreatitis. After six days, he continues with severe midepigastric pain that radiates to the back with nausea and vomiting. He has not been able eat or drink and has not had a bowel movement since being admitted.

On physical examination, the temperature is 37.6 °C (99.5 °F), the blood pressure is 120/76 mmHg, the pulse rate is 90 bpm, and the respiratory rate is 20 breaths/min. There is no scleral icterus or jaundice. The abdomen is distended and with hypoactive bowel sounds.

Laboratory studies show leukocyte count 12,400/μL, amylase 388 μ/L, and lipase 924 μ/L.

Repeat CT scan of the abdomen shows a diffusely edematous pancreas with multiple small peripancreatic fluid collections. Some improvement from the CT scan 3 days ago is noted. He is now afebrile.

Which of the following is the most appropriate next step in the management of this patient?
A) Enteral nutrition by nasojejual feeding tube
B) Intravenous imipenem
C) Pancreatic debridement
D) Parenteral nutrition
E) Continue with NPO status

Answer: A

This patient has ongoing moderate pancreatitis. With his possible underlying poor nutritional status due to alcoholism and expected inability to eat, the patient will need nutritional support. This patient will likely be unable to take in oral nutrition for several days.. Enteral nutrition is preferred over parenteral nutrition because of its lower complication rate and proven efficacy in pancreatitis.

Enteral nutrition is provided through a feeding tube ideally placed past the ligament of Treitz so as not to stimulate the pancreas.

Broad-spectrum antibiotics such as imipenem therapy are primarily of benefit in acute pancreatitis when there is evidence of pancreatic necrosis. Randomized, prospective trials have shown no benefit from antibiotic use in acute pancreatitis of mild to moderate severity without evidence of infection. Pancreatic debridement is undertaken with caution and is not indicated here.

References
Eatock FC, Chong P et al. A randomized study of early nasogastric vs. nasojejunal feeding in severe acute pancreatitis. Am J Gastroenterol. 2005;100:432–9.
Eckerwall GE, Axelsson JB, Andersson RG. Early nasogastric feeding in predicted severe acute pancreatitis: a clinical, randomized study. Ann Surg. 2006;244:959–65.

284. A 64-year-old female with a past medical history significant for type 2 diabetes mellitus is admitted with increasing shortness of breath. She is admitted for mild congestive heart failure and responds well to therapy.

Of note she reports increasing left knee pain. The pain is heightened when she tries to walk with physical therapy. Three months ago she had left knee arthroplasty, and postoperative course was uneventful. Her vital signs are stable. The patient's knee exam reveals a surgical scar but no joint effusion or redness.

What should be done next?
A) Orthopedics consult
B) Arthrocentesis
C) Discharged with mild opioid
D) Order a knee MRI
E) Discharged home with a trial of NSAIDs

Answer: A

At 3 months, new-onset pain signals a mechanical complication of the prosthesis. Orthopedics consult is indicated. Infection is certainly possible, but a prosthetic joint infection would have localized or systemic signs of infection.

Reference
Lentino JR. Prosthetic joint infections, bane of orthopedists, challenge for infectious disease specialists. Clin Infect Dis. 2003;36:1157–61.

285. A 82-year-old female is admitted to the hospital service with urinary tract infection and sepsis. On admission she is noted to be lethargic and unable to swallow medicines. She develops progressive respiratory failure and is intubated. A CXR is consistent with ARDS. An NG tube is placed for administration of medicines. You are considering starting tube feeds in this patient.

Which of the following is the most accurate statement regarding enteral tube feeds in this patient?
A) Early enteral tube feeds can be expected to reduce her mortality risk.
B) The use of omega-3 fatty acids will reduce her mortality risk.
C) Enteral tube feeds will increase the risk of infection.
D) The benefits of early nutrition can be achieved with trophic rates.

Answer: D

The benefits of early enteral tube feedings in the critically ill patient are uncertain. Studies have revealed inconsistent results. There is some suggestion that the incidences of infection can be reduced, but there is no data to suggest long-term mortality improvement. In patients with ARDS, trophic tube feedings at 10 ml/h seem to concur the same benefit as early full-enteral tube feedings.

References

Elpern EH, Stutz L, Peterson S, Gurka DP, Skipper A. Outcomes associated with enteral tube feedings in a medical intensive care unit. Am J Crit Care. 2004;13(3):221–7.

Gramlich L, Kichian K, Pinilla J, Rodych NJ, Dhaliwal R, Heyland DK. Does enteral nutrition compared to parenteral nutrition result in better outcomes in critically ill adult patients? A systematic review of the literature. Nutrition. 2004;20(10):843–8.

286. Which of the following is an acceptable indication for urinary catheter placement?
    A) A patient who has urinary incontinence and a stage II pressure ulcer
    B) A patient who is under hospice care and requests a catheter for comfort
    C) A patient who is delirious and has experienced several falls
    D) A patient who is admitted for congestive heart failure whose urine output is being closely monitored

Answer: B

Urinary tract infections (UTIs) are the most common hospital-acquired infections. Most attributed to the use of an indwelling catheter. There should always be a justifiable indication for placement of a urinary catheter, and whenever possible prompt removal should occur. This may be assisted by hospital protocols that trigger automatic reviews of catheter use.

Reference

Gould CV, Umscheid CA, Agarwal RK, Kuntz G, Pegues DA. Guideline for prevention of catheter-associated urinary tract infections 2009. Infect Control Hosp Epidemiol. 2010;31(4):319–26.

287. An 88-year-old man in hospice care is admitted for dyspnea. He has advanced dementia, severe COPD, and coronary artery disease. He has been in hospice for 2 months. He and his family would like to be discharged to home hospice as soon as possible. He is only on albuterol and ipratropium.

On physical examination, he is afebrile, and his blood pressure is 110/76 mmHg, pulse rate is 110 beats/min, and respiratory rate is 28 breaths/min. Oxygen saturation is 90 %. He is cachectic, tachypneic, and disoriented. He is in moderate respiratory distress. Chest examination reveals decreased breath sounds and fine inspiratory crackles.

In addition to continuing his bronchodilator therapy, which of the following is the most appropriate next step in the treatment of this patient?
    A) Ceftriaxone and azithromycin
    B) Morphine
    C) Methylprednisolone
    D) Haloperidol
    E) Lorazepam

Answer: B

This patient is enrolled in hospice. Every effort should be made to ensure comfort and limit unnecessary treatments. Dyspnea is one of the most common symptoms encountered in palliative care. Opioids are effective in reducing dyspnea in patients with chronic pulmonary disease. A 5-mg dose of oral morphine given four times daily has been shown to help relieve dyspnea in patients with end-stage heart failure. Extended-release morphine, starting at a 20 mg given daily has been used to relieve dyspnea in patients with advanced COPD.

Bronchodilator therapy should be continued to maintain comfort. Antibiotics and corticosteroids are not indicated. They would not provide immediate relief and would also be inconsistent with care focusing primarily on comfort measures.

Benzodiazepines have not demonstrated consistent benefit in treating dyspnea. They may be useful in specific patients who have significant anxiety associated with their dyspnea.

Reference

Currow DC, McDonald C, Oaten S, Kenny B, Allcroft P, Frith P et al. Once-daily opioids for chronic dyspnea: a dose increment and pharmacovigilance study. J Pain Symptom Manage. 2011;42(3):388–99.

288. A 59-year-old man presents with fever and a diffuse blistering skin rash. He is recently started on allopurinol for gout. The patient also complains of sore throat and painful watery eyes.

On physical examination, the patient is found to have blisters developing over a quarter of his body. Oral mucosal lesions are noted involvement. The estimated body surface area that is currently affected is 15 %.

Which of the following statements regarding this patient's diagnosis and treatment are TRUE?
    A) Immediate treatment with intravenous immunoglobulin has been proven to decrease the extent of the disease and improve mortality.
    B) Immediate treatment with glucocorticoids will improve mortality.
    C) The expected mortality rate from this syndrome is about 10 %.
    D) The most common drug to cause this syndrome is diltiazem.
    E) Younger individuals have a higher mortality than older individuals with this syndrome.

Answer: C

This patient has Stevens-Johnson syndrome (SJS). There is no definitive evidence that any initial therapy changes outcomes in SJS. Early data suggested that intravenous immunoglobulin (IVIG) was beneficial, and this traditionally has been the recommended treatment. However, more recent studies have not shown consistent benefit with IVIG. Immediate cessation of the offending agent or possible agents is necessary. Systemic corticosteroids may be useful for the short-term treatment of SJS, but these drugs increase long-term complications and may have a higher associated mortality. Therapy to prevent secondary infections is important. In principle, the symptomatic treatment of patients with Stevens-Johnson syndrome does not differ from the treatment of patients with extensive burns, and in many instances, these patients are often treated in burn wards.

Future studies are required to determine the role of IVIG in the treatment of SJS. The lesions typically begin with blisters developing over target lesions with mucosal involvement. In SJS, the amount of skin detachment is between 10 and 30 % . Mortality is directly related to the amount of skin detachment with a mortality of about 10 % in SJS. Other risk factors for mortality in SJS include older age and intestinal or pulmonary involvement. The most common drugs to cause SJS are sulfonamides, allopurinol, nevirapine, lamotrigine, and aromatic anticonvulsants.

References
Mockenhaupt M. The current understanding of Stevens–Johnson syndrome and toxic epidermal necrolysis. Expert Rev Clin Immunol. 2011;7(6):803–15.
Ward KE, Archambault R, Mersfelder TL. Severe adverse skin reactions to nonsteroidal antiinflammatory drugs: a review of the literature. Am J Health Syst Pharm. 2010;67(3):206–13.

289. A 57-year-old woman with a history of diabetes and familial history of breast cancer is admitted with malaise, an appetite decline, and new-onset ascites. She denies having fevers, chills, diarrhea, nausea, and vomiting.

On physical exam, there is no evidence of spider nevi or palmar erythema. Her serum albumin is 3.4 g/dL. On chest X-ray, a right-sided pleural effusion is noted. A diagnostic paracentesis reveals a glucose of 85 mg/dl, an albumin of 2.8 g/dL, and a WBC of 250/ul, of which 45 % are neutrophils.

Based on the data provided, what is the most likely cause of her ascites?
A) Cirrhosis
B) Metastatic disease
C) Pelvic mass
D) Spontaneous bacterial peritonitis
E) Tuberculous peritonitis

Answer: C
Meigs' syndrome is the triad of benign ovarian tumor with ascites and pleural effusion that resolves after resection of the tumor. Typical diagnostic paracentesis reveals a serum-ascites albumin gradient < 1.1 suggesting a non-portal hypertension-mediated process. Of the possibilities for that, ovarian mass is the most likely here. Transdiaphragmatic lymphatic channels are larger in diameter on the right. This results in the pleural effusion being typically classically located on the right side. The etiologies of the ascites and pleural effusion are poorly understood. Further imaging is indicated.

Reference
Riker D, Goba D. Ovarian mass, pleural effusion, and ascites: revisiting Meigs syndrome. J Bronchology Interv Pulmonol. 2013;20(1):48–51.

290. A 77-year-old female patient presents with dizziness, headache, nausea, and vomiting for the past 48 h. She states that the floor feels like it is moving when she walks. The patient is alert, and she tells you she suffered from no recent trauma.

On physical exam you note the patient's speech is slightly abnormal. During the neurological examination, the patient is able to understand your questions, respond appropriately, and repeat words, but her words are poorly articulated. She has a great deal of difficulty walking across the room without assistance.

What is your next step in the management of this patient?
A) Administer unfractionated heparin
B) Epley maneuver
C) CT scan without contrast
D) Emergent MRI or MRA
E) Observation alone

Answer: D
This patient has central vertigo possibly due to a cerebellar infarction. Multiple cerebellar signs are noted which help distinguish this from benign peripheral vertigo. Due to obstruction by a posterior fossa bone artifact, CT scan may not be of benefit. Emergent MRI and MRA if available are the tests of choice. This should be done to confirm the diagnosis and followed for the development of an obstructing hydrocephalus, which can occur with cerebellar infarction.

Since the posterior fossa is a relatively small and nonexpandable space, hemorrhage or edema can lead to rapid compression. Early neurosurgical consultation should be considered.

Reference
Schneider JI, Olshaker JS. Vertigo, vertebrobasilar disease, and posterior circulation ischemic stroke. Emerg Med Clin North Am. 2012;30(3):681–93.

291. A 72-year-old female is admitted to the hospital for an elective right hip replacement. She has a 31-year history of type 1 diabetes mellitus. Prior to admission, the patient's diabetes was managed with a premixed 70/30 insulin. She took 25 units of this preparation before breakfast and 10 units before his evening meal. She reports that she has had good glycemic control in the past.

On physical examination, temperature is normal. Blood pressure is 147/83, pulse rate is 70 beats/min, and respiratory rate is 12 breaths/min. Other physical examination findings are within normal limits.

Which of the following is the most appropriate insulin therapy after surgery?
A) Continuous intravenous insulin infusion
B) Previous schedule of 70/30 insulin
C) Subcutaneous insulin infusion
D) Insulin glargine once daily and insulin aspart before each meal
E) Sliding-scale insulin alone
F) Insulin aspart before each meal alone

Answer: D

This patient should receive basal insulin as well as scheduled insulin before each meal. This should be adjusted for conditions that occur in the hospital. A patient with long-standing type 1 diabetes makes no endogenous insulin and requires a maintenance dose of insulin postoperatively.

It is expected that her PO intake would be markedly decreased, and subsequently her insulin dose should be decreased. One-half of her usual insulin dose would be a reasonable approach. Continuous infusions of insulin, either intravenous or subcutaneous, are not necessary in this patient, but should be considered if glycemic control becomes erratic. Both would increase nursing services and possibly require transfer to the intensive care unit. A sliding scale that does not include basal insulin will cause wide swings from hyperglycemia to hypoglycemia.

Reference
ACE/ADA Task Force on Inpatient Diabetes. American College of Endocrinology and American Diabetes Association consensus statement on inpatient diabetes and glycemic control. Endocr Pract. 2006;12:458–68.

292. A 65-year-old male with hypertension, dyslipidemia, and osteoarthritis of the knees is admitted for evaluation of chest pain. The chest pain is intermittent, occasionally occurring at rest and not worsened by exertion. He is pain-free on arrival to the floor. The patient's home medications include aspirin 81 mg daily and lisinopril 20 mg daily. His vital signs show blood pressure 146/70 mmHg and heart rate 60 beats/min.

Physical examination is unremarkable. He has no further chest pains during his stay in the hospital. Serial troponins are normal. EKG shows normal sinus rhythm with a left bundle branch block (LBBB).

Which of the following is the most appropriate next step in management?
A) Exercise stress test without imaging
B) Exercise stress test with nuclear imaging
C) Pharmacologic stress test with nuclear imaging
D) Exercise stress with echocardiography
E) Cardiology consultation for catheterization
F) Discharge home

Answer: C

This patient has atypical chest pain. It is not certain that coronary angiography is needed. He is however at high risk for coronary artery disease and risk stratification is needed. Stress testing is indicated here prior to possible cardiac catheterization.

Exercising imaging tests in patients with LBBB can produce false-positive test results. The LBBB causes artifacts with both nuclear images and echocardiograms when done with exercise testing. Pharmacologic stress test with nuclear imaging can be used in this circumstance.

Reference
Botvinick EH. Current methods of pharmacologic stress testing and the potential advantages of new agents. J Nucl Med Technol. 2009;37(1):14–25.

293. You are urgently called to see in consultation of a 36-year-old woman who is in postop recovery. She has a sudden elevation of her temperature and is thought to be septic. Her laparoscopic cholecystectomy was completed 45 min ago without complication.

On physical exam her temperature is 40.5 °C (105 °F). She has respiratory rate of 28 breaths per minute. She is tachycardic, shaking, and confused. There is diffuse muscular rigidity noted.

Which of the following drugs should be administered immediately?
A) Acetaminophen
B) Haloperidol
C) Hydrocortisone
D) Ibuprofen
E) Dantrolene

Answer: E

The patient has malignant hyperthermia. Dantrolene should be given. Physical cooling in addition to dantrolene with cooling blanket or IV fluids should be used as well. Dantrolene may be used in other central causes of extreme hyperthermic such as neuroleptic malignant syndrome. In this case, the episode was probably caused by succinyl-choline and/or inhalational anesthetic.

This syndrome occurs in individuals with inherited abnormality of skeletal muscle sarcoplasmic reticulum. More than 30 mutations account for human malignant hyperthermia. Genetic testing is available to establish a diagnosis. The caffeine halothane contracture test remains the criterion standard. This is a muscle biopsy and performed at a designated center.

The syndrome presents with hyperthermia or a rapid increase in body temperature that exceeds the ability of the body to lose heat. Muscular rigidity, acidosis, cardiovascular instability, and rhabdomyolysis also occur. Antipyretics such as acetaminophen, ibuprofen, and corticosteroids are of little use.

The dantrolene dose is 2.5 mg/kg rapid IV bolus and may be repeated PRN.

Occasionally a dose up to 30 mg/kg is necessary.

References

MacLennan DH. The genetic basis of malignant hyperthermia. Trends Pharmacol Sci. 1992;13(8):330–4.

Schneiderbanger D, Johannsen S, Roewer N, Schuster F. Management of malignant hyperthermia: diagnosis and treatment. Ther Clin Risk Manag. 2014;10:355–62.

294. A 70-year-old female is seen for preoperative evaluation for elective total knee replacement. She has a mechanical bileaflet aortic valve and takes warfarin. She has no history of stroke. On physical examination, there is a regular rhythm with a noted mechanical click. Recent echocardiography of the heart is normal. Lungs are clear to auscultation. INR is 2.1.

Which of the following is the most appropriate perioperative recommendation regarding anticoagulation in this patient?

A) Discontinue warfarin 5 days before surgery and bridge with full-dose IV heparin before and after surgery.

B) Discontinue warfarin 5 days before surgery and restart on the evening of the surgery.

C) Continue with warfarin.

D) Reverse anticoagulation with fresh frozen plasma transfusion 1 h before surgery and restart warfarin on the evening of the surgery.

Answer: B

In patients with mechanical valves and at low risk for thromboembolism, low-dose low-molecular-weight heparin or no bridging is recommended. The short-term risk of anticoagulant discontinuation in this patient is small. The current recommendation is to stop warfarin 5 days before the procedure. The INR goal is 1.5. Warfarin should be restarted within 24 h after the procedure.

In patients with a mechanical valve and an increased risk of a thromboembolic event, it is recommended that unfractionated heparin be begun intravenously when the INR falls below 2.0. This should be stopped 4–5 h before the procedure and restarted after surgery. In patients with a mechanical heart valve who require emergent surgery, reversal with fresh frozen plasma may be performed.

Reference

Douketis JD, Berger PB, Dunn AS et al. The perioperative management of antithrombotic therapy: American College of Chest Physicians Evidence-Based Clinical Practice Guidelines (8th Edition). Chest J. 2008;133 (6 suppl):299S–339S.

295. Initiating non-hospice palliative care early in the diagnosis of nonoperative cancer results in what outcomes?

A) Lived longer

B) Better quality of life

C) Less depression

D) Less aggressive care

E) All of the above

Answer: E

Patients randomized to the palliative care early live longer as well as achieve other desirable endpoints. This is according to a trial with patients with small cell lung cancer.

Palliative care does not limit the use of chemotherapy. This differs from hospice care, which occurs in the patient's last 6 months of life.

Reference

Saito AM, Landrum MB, Neville BA, Ayanian JZ, Weeks JC, Earle CC. Hospice Care and Survival among Elderly Patients with Lung Cancer. Journal of Palliative Medicine. 2011;14(8):929–939. doi:10.1089/jpm.2010.0522.

296. A 57-year-old female with a history of endocarditis has had a peripherally inserted central catheter (PICC) line for intravenous antibiotics. She presents 3 weeks after line removal with persistent, dull, aching pain in her right shoulder and swelling of her right hand. The pain worsens with exercise. The swelling is relieved with elevation. The physical exam reveals diffuse nonpitting edema of her hand. The ultrasound shows a right subclavian vein thrombosis.

What is the best approach to treating her upper extremity deep venous thrombosis (UEDVT)?

A) Serial ultrasound alone to assess resolution of DVT

B) Low-molecular-weight heparin and 1 month of warfarin, INR goal 2–3

C) Low-molecular-weight heparin and 3 months of warfarin, INR goal 2–3

D) Initiate warfarin therapy alone

E) Aspirin 325 mg for 6 months

Answer: C

UEDVT is common secondary to increased interventions in the upper extremity. It has become more easily recognized due to improvement and availability of noninvasive ultrasound technology. UEDVT accounts for up to 10 % of all DVT.

American College of Chest Physicians guidelines recommend treating UEDVT patients with unfractionated heparin or low-molecular-weight heparin with the addition of warfarin, with an INR goal of 2–3 for at least 3 months depending upon the overall clinical scenario.

Two previous small studies evaluating catheter-related thrombosis reported no subsequent embolic phenomenon. However, since UEDVT has been more widely recognized, most authors are recommending three months of treatment until further studies define the correct duration of treatment.

Reference

Margey R, Schainfeld RM. Upper extremity deep vein thrombosis: the oft-forgotten cousin of venous thromboembolic disease. Curr Treat Options Cardiovasc Med. 2011;13(2):146–58.

297. An 88-year-old female who was admitted to the hip fracture service for a right hip fracture has currently become agitated and confused. She underwent hip fracture repair two days prior. She has a history of osteoporosis, dementia, and type 2 diabetes.

    Her postoperative medicines include oxycodone 5 mg every 4 h as needed for pain as well as IV morphine 1–2 mg/h as needed for the pain. During the patient's first night, she was calm and relatively free of pain. However, on her second night, she has become acutely agitated and is reported by the nurse to be screaming and pulling out lines and drains. Her temperature is 99.1 °F. Her pulse rate is 100 beats/min. Her respirations are 20 per minute. Her oxygenation is 92 % on room air. Her hematocrit and hemoglobin are within normal limits as well as the rest of her electrolytes.

    Which of the following is the appropriate response/treatment for this patient's delirium?
    A) Four-point restraints
    B) One 2 mg dose of intravenous lorazepam
    C) One 5 mg dose of oral haloperidol
    D) One 0.5 mg dose of oral haloperidol
    E) One 5 mg dose of intravenous haloperidol

Answer: D

Treatment of postoperative-induced delirium is a common issue confronted in the hospital setting. Delirium that causes injury to the patient or others should be treated with medications. This can be a difficult management issue. No medication is currently approved by the Food and Drug Administration for the treatment of delirium. Current guidelines recommend using low-dose antipsychotics such as haloperidol. The use of benzodiazepines should be limited, unless concurrent alcohol withdrawal is present.

A specific FDA warning has been issued for intravenous haloperidol due to the risk of torsades de pointes in 2007. Low-dose haloperidol, less than 2 mg, has a low incidence of extrapyramidal side effects. QTc prolongation monitoring is recommended for patients. If feasible, this patient should have had a baseline EKG as well as a follow-up EKG. Haloperidol at doses greater than 4.5 mg increases the incidence of extrapyramidal side effects and should be avoided.

Reference

Inouye SK. The dilemma of delirium: clinical and research controversies regarding diagnosis and evaluation of delirium in hospitalized elderly medical patients. Am J Med. 1994;97(3):278–88.

298. A 65-year-old male is contemplating undergoing elective hernia repair. The hernia site is painful at times but does not inhibit physical activity. He has a history of coronary artery disease, but no prior surgery. His most recent ejection fraction 2 years previously was 45 %. He also has a 30-pack-year history of tobacco. He quit 5 years ago. You ask him about his current exercise capacity.

    Which of the following would NOT be considered poor exercise tolerance and increase his risk of perioperative complications?
    A) Inability to achieve four metabolic equivalents during an exercise test
    B) Inability to carry 15–20 lb
    C) Inability to climb two flights of stairs at a normal pace
    D) Inability to walk four blocks at a normal pace
    E) Inability to play singles tennis
    F) Inability to play golf

Answer: E

One metabolic equivalent (MET) is sitting quietly. Exercise tolerance is an easy and important predictor of postoperative complications. General guidelines are available that attempt to categorize the risk of complications according to functional status. The risk of postoperative complications increases when an individual cannot meet a metabolic equivalent (MET) level of 4.

Activities that require a MET level of 4 include carrying 15–20 lb, playing golf, and playing doubles tennis. Individuals experience increased risk of postoperative complications if they are unable to walk four blocks or climb two flights of stairs when walking at a normal pace. Singles tennis is 7 METS.

References

Girish M, Trayner E Jr, Dammann O et al. Symptom-limited stair climbing as a predictor of postoperative cardiopulmonary complications after high-risk surgery. Chest. 2001;120:1147.

Reilly DF, McNeely MJ, Doerner D et al. Self-reported exercise tolerance and the risk of serious perioperative complications. Arch Intern Med. 1999;159:2185.

299. A 74-year-old female was admitted for emergent colectomy to treat a presumed diverticular bleed. The patient also has breast cancer treated with hormonal therapy. She had been started on warfarin 3 weeks ago as therapy for a deep venous thrombus of the left femoral vein.

Prior to the colectomy, her INR was 3.4. She was treated with intravenous vitamin K and fresh frozen plasma prior to surgery.

The surgery was uneventful. On hospital day 2, she has a sudden onset of tachypnea and hypoxemia. A computed tomography pulmonary angiogram reveals a thrombus in the pulmonary artery to the right lower lobe. Her INR is 1.0.

What is the most likely cause of her thrombosis?

A) Surgery-induced thrombosis
B) Depletion of thrombin due to the surgical acute-phase response
C) Thrombogenesis due to postoperative hypovolemia
D) Undetected prior thrombus
E) Rebound hypercoagulability and subsequent thromboembolism

Answer: E

Rebound hypercoagulability is the most likely cause. This may occur after abrupt cessation of warfarin. In addition, surgery increases the risk of thromboembolic events. Following an abrupt withdrawal of warfarin, thrombin and fibrin formation increase and very high levels of thrombin activation are seen. If possible, warfarin withdrawal should be gradual which would not have been feasible in the current case. Safely resuming anticoagulation after surgery should be a goal as well.

References

Garcia DA et al. Risk of thromboembolism with short-term interruption of warfarin therapy. Arch Intern Med. 2008;168:63.

Malato A et al. Patients requiring interruption of long-term oral anticoagulant therapy: the use of fixed sub-therapeutic doses of low-molecular-weight heparin. J Thromb Haemost. 2010;8:107.

300. A 40-year-old female with no significant past medical history is admitted with radiating flank pain. She believes she may have passed a small renal stone. She is admitted for IV pain control and intravenous fluids. She never passed a stone before. She has no dysuria, abdominal pain, nausea, or fever. She is on no medications.

What should NOT be considered in the management plan for this patient?

A) CT scan of the abdomen and pelvis without contrast
B) Ultrasound of the kidneys
C) Urinalysis to rule out UTI
D) 24-h urinalysis

Answer: D

Most guidelines recommend diagnostic imaging to confirm the diagnosis in first-time episodes of ureterolithiasis. Noncontrast computed tomography (CT) scans of the abdomen and pelvis have become the imaging modality of choice. Renal ultrasonography or a contrast study such as intravenous pyelography (IVP) may be preferred in ceratin circumstances.

Initial workup should also include microscopic examination of the urine for evidence of hematuria and infection. Measurements of serum electrolyte, creatinine, calcium, and uric acid are required. Serum WBC may indicate infection.

For first episodes of renal colic, 24-h urine and stone analysis are not usually recommended.

Reference

Cooper JT, Stack GM, Cooper TP. Intensive medical management of ureteral calculi. Urology. 2000;56(4):575–8.

301. A 60-year-old man who has metastatic lung cancer and painful bone metastases reports severe pruritus that started when he began to take morphine for his pain. Pain in his chest wall and legs has been successfully treated with sustained-release morphine (80 mg every 12 h) and short-acting morphine (15 mg orally every 2 h as needed for breakthrough pain) which he uses two or three times daily, depending on his level of activity.

On physical examination, the temperature is 37 °C (98.6 °F), pulse rate is 80 beats per minute, respirations are 16 per minute, and blood pressure is 115/70 mmHg. Oxygen saturation by pulse oximetry is 95 % on room air. The patient is alert and oriented. His pupils are 4 mm initially and constrict to 2 mm with a light stimulus. The lungs are clear. Cardiac examination shows a normal rate and regular rhythm. No rash is seen. Examination of the abdomen is significant for suprapubic dullness and sensitivity. Neurological examination is nonfocal.

Which of the following should be done next?

A) Change to oxycodone, 40 mg every 12 h, and oxycodone, 5–10 mg every 2 h as needed
B) Lower the dosage of sustained-release morphine to 30 mg every 12 h

C) Continue with same morphine dose
D) Change to oxycodone, 60 mg every 12 h, and oxycodone, 15 mg every 2 h as needed

Answer: A

Oxycodone may cause somewhat less nausea, hallucinations, and pruritus than morphine. Mild to moderate morphine-induced puritis may be managed by small-dose reductions or antihistamines. This patient has severe puritis which may be relieved by changing to oxycodone.

The patient's baseline long-acting morphine daily dose was 160 mg, with a minimum short-acting morphine dose of 30 mg daily, which yields a total daily dose of 190 mg. The morphine-to-oxycodone ratio is 1.5:1. This patient's morphine-equivalent daily dose of oxycodone would be 120 mg. The daily dose of oxycodone would be 60 mg. Thus, the every-12-h dose of long-acting oxycodone would be 40 mg.

Reference

Pergolizzi J, Boger RH, Budd K et al. Opioids and the management of chronic severe pain in the elderly: consensus statement of an International Expert Panel with focus on the six clinically most often used World Health Organization Step III opioids (buprenorphine, fentanyl, hydromorphone, methadone, morphine, oxycodone). Pain Pract. 2008;8(4):287–313.

302. A 68-year-old female who has metastatic small cell lung cancer presents to the emergency room with shortness of breath. She is noted to be in marked respiratory distress and is intubated by emergency room personnel. She is admitted to the intensive care unit.

On review of the medical records, you find that the patient has an advanced directive, which indicates that the patient did not want to be intubated. This is noted both in a signed advanced directive as well as in the hospital records. You arrange a family meeting to discuss goals of care. The patient's daughter has recently quit her job and has moved in with her mother to provide care. You discuss the case with her, and she states that her mother has changed her mind recently and would like to be on the ventilator at all costs.

Which of the following is the correct course of action?
A) Follow the patient's written documentations and extubate the patient and provide comfort care.
B) Follow the daughter's instructions and have patient remain intubated.
C) Request an ethics consultation.
D) Consult the hospital's legal affairs department.

Answer: C

It is of primary importance to follow the patient's wishes. In this particular case, there is some difficulty in determining if the patient has recently changed her mind, as is suggested by the daughter. She has clearly documented her advance directives, and it would be appropriate to withdraw life support if the daughter did not provide the conflicting statement.

Financial conflicts of interest often interfere with the surrogates ability to act in the best interest of the patient. In this particular case, there are circumstances that suggest that financial considerations may be influencing the statement. It would be difficult for an individual practitioner to make this determination, without the potential of liability. Subsequently, an ethics consultation would be the correct course of action. As there are several factors, ethics and clinical, involved, an attorney alone would not be in a position to resolve the issue.

References

Luce JM. Physicians do not have a responsibility to provide futile or unreasonable care if a patient or family insists. Crit Care Med. 1995;23:760–6.

Sulmasy DP, Terry PB, Weisman CS et al. The accuracy of substituted judgments in patients with terminal diagnoses. Ann Intern Med. 1998;128:621–9.

303. An 83-year-old female is admitted from a nursing home to the hospital for shortness of breath. On chest X-ray, she has a new-onset pleural effusion for which thoracentesis is indicated. On her medical record, it is reported that she has a history of dementia.

On physical exam she is awake and alert. She knows that she is in the hospital, knows her name and address, but is confused about the current date. On review of her medical records, you discover that she has neither family members nor a durable power of attorney.

In attempting to obtain consent for the procedure, which of the following is the next best step?
A) Proceed without consent.
B) Assign guardianship.
C) Determine capacity yourself.
D) Psychiatric consultation for competency.
E) Ethics consultation.

Answer: C

There are four components of determining capacity in decision-making concerning a particular treatment or test: (1) an understanding of relevant information about proposed diagnostic tests or treatment, (2) appreciation of their medical situation, (3) using reason to make decisions, (and 4) ability to communicate their choice. In most instances, the primary physician should possess the ability to determine capacity.

Capacity is not the same measurement as competence. Competence is determined by a court of law and uses issues of capacity in evaluating the legal ability to contract.

A psychiatric consultation can determine competency but is usually not needed to determine capacity. Assigning guardianship or an ethics consultation can be a lengthy process and should be reserved for cases with significant issues to be resolve.

Reference

Sessums LL, Zembrzuska H, Jackson JL. Does this patient have medical decision-making capacity? JAMA. 2011;306:420–7.

304. What are the primary benefits so far demonstrated in studies on surgical services comanaged by hospitalists?
    A) Improvement in all-cause mortality
    B) Reduced length of stay
    C) Improvement in patient satisfaction
    D) Decreased costs
    E) All of the above

Answer: B

Several studies have looked at the impact of hospitalists on comanaging surgical services. There had been conflicting results. While most studies have demonstrated an overall positive effect on most parameters, the primary statistically significant benefit has been in length of stay reductions.

Reference

Batsis JA, Phy MP, Melton LJ 3rd, Schleck CD, Larson DR, Huddleston PM, Huddleston JMA. Effects of a hospitalist care model on mortality of elderly patients with hip fractures. Hosp Med. 2007;2(4):219–25.

305. A 65-year-old male is admitted to the hospital for elective total knee arthroplasty. He has a history of type 2 diabetes mellitus and is treated with metformin. He reports fair glucose control with diet and oral agents. He has never been on insulin.

    On physical examination he has mild edema of his lower extremities but otherwise is within normal range.

    Preoperative laboratory studies have been done 1 week prior. His hemoglobin A1c revealed a concentration of 6.8 %. Plasma glucose level measured on the day of surgery is 210 mg/L.

    Which of the following is the most appropriate treatment for patients with elevated blood sugars preoperatively and postoperatively?
    A) Metformin
    B) Sliding-scale insulin
    C) IV hydration
    D) Basal and sliding-scale insulin
    E) Diet control alone

Answer: D

The goal of glycemic control in the hospitalized patient is balancing the risks of hypoglycemia against the known benefits in morbidity and mortality. Although tight control has been advocated in the past, current consensus guidelines recommend less stringent glycemic goals, typically between 80 and 150 mg/dL. The ultimate goal in the management of diabetic patients (DM) is to achieve outcomes equivalent to those in patients without DM.

A meta-analysis of 15 studies reports that hyperglycemia increased both in-hospital mortality and incidence of heart failure in patients admitted for acute myocardial infarction. Several other studies have also demonstrated the benefits of glycemic control in the perioperative area.

Type 2 diabetes mellitus often requires insulin while in the hospital. The requirements may be unpredictable. This may be due to the stress of hospitalization, dietary changes, glucose added to IV fluids, and medicine interactions.

Sliding scale alone has often been traditionally used in the past. However, this method of control often results in wide fluctuations in glycemic control. The optimal plasma glucose level postoperatively is not known, and certainly tight control has its risks.

References

Clement S, Braithwaite SS, Magee MF et al. Management of diabetes and hyperglycemia in hospitals. Diabetes Care. 2004;27(2):553–91.

Lazar HL, Chipkin SR, Fitzgerald CA et al. Tight glycemic control in diabetic coronary artery bypass graft patients improves perioperative outcomes and decreases recurrent ischemic events. Circulation. 2004;109(12):1497–502.

306. A 55-year-old female has been admitted for cellulitis. She has responded well to antibiotics and is ready for discharge. On admission she was noted to be in atrial fibrillation. She has been treated with low-molecular-weight heparin in the hospital. She first noted the irregular heartbeat 4 weeks ago. She denies chest pain, shortness of breath, nausea, or gastrointestinal symptoms. Past medical history is unremarkable. There is no history of hypertension, diabetes, or tobacco use. Her medications include metoprolol.

    On physical examination, she has a blood pressure of 124/76 mmHg and a pulse of 70 beats/min. An echocardiogram shows a left atrial size of 3.5 cm. Left ventricular ejection fraction is 63 %. There are no valvular or structural abnormalities.

    Which of the following would be the appropriate treatment of her atrial fibrillation?
    A) She requires no antiplatelet therapy or anticoagulation because the risk of embolism is low.
    B) Lifetime warfarin therapy is indicated for atrial fibrillation in this situation to reduce the risk of stroke.
    C) She should be started on IV heparin and undergo electrical cardioversion.

D) She should continue on SC low-molecular-weight heparin and transitioned to warfarin.

E) Her risk of an embolic stroke is less than 1 %, and she should take a daily aspirin.

Answer: E

Patients younger than 60 years of age without structural heart disease or without risk factors have a very low annual risk of cardioembolism of less than 0.5 %. Therefore, it is recommended that these patients only take aspirin daily for stroke prevention.

The risk of stroke can be estimated by calculating the CHADS2 score. Older patients with numerous risk factors may have annual stroke risks of 10–15 % and must take a vitamin K antagonist or alternate indefinitely. Cardioversion may be indicated for symptomatic patients who want an initial opportunity to remain in sinus rhythm.

Reference

Cairns JA, Connolly S, McMurtry S, Stephenson M, Talajic M, CCS Atrial Fibrillation Guidelines Committee. Canadian Cardiovascular Society atrial fibrillation guidelines 2010: prevention of stroke and systemic thromboembolism in atrial fibrillation and flutter. Can J Cardiol. 2011;27(1):74–90.

307. In a recent patient survey demonstrating that patients receiving chemotherapy for incurable cancers may not understand that chemotherapy is unlikely to be curative, how often did patients with lung cancer report inaccurate beliefs about chemotherapy?
A) 25 %
B) 51 %
C) 69 %
D) 81 %
E) 85 %

Answer: C

Many patients receiving chemotherapy for incurable cancers may not understand that chemotherapy is unlikely to be curative. The hospitalist is often the one to provide conflicting news about survival to patients and family. In the reported study of 1193 patients participating in the Cancer Care Outcomes Research and Surveillance (CanCORS) study of those patients alive 4 months after diagnosis and chemotherapy for newly diagnosed metastatic (stage IV) lung cancer, 69 % of patients with lung cancer reported not understanding that chemotherapy was not at all likely to cure their cancer.

References

Smith TJ, Longo DL. Talking with patients about dying. N Engl J Med. 2012;367:1651–2.
Weeks JC et al. Patients' expectations about effects of chemotherapy for advanced cancer. N Engl J Med. 2012;367:1616–25.

308. Which of the following have not been shown to prevent atelectasis in the postoperative patient?
A) Albuterol inhaler
B) Continuous positive airway pressure
C) Incentive spirometry
D) Deep breathing exercises

Answer: A

Bronchodilators may be needed to treat reactive airway disease. However they have not been shown to prevent atelectasis in postoperative patients. Several lung expansion modalities including incentive spirometry, deep breathing exercises, and positive airway pressure have been shown to be of benefit. Patients who are too weak for incentive spirometry may benefit from CPAP. This may be of benefit even in the absence of obstructive sleep apnea. The duration per day of CPAP therapy to prevent atelectasis is not known. Several hours per day may be a reasonable approach.

Reference

McCool FD, Rosen MJ. No pharmacologic airway clearance therapies: ACCP evidence-based clinical practice guidelines. Chest. 2006;129(1 Suppl):250S–9S.

309. A 82-year-old man who has bone metastases due to bronchogenic lung cancer is admitted to the hospital for failure to thrive. After a family meeting it was decided that the patient will be discharged to home hospice. The family is at the bedside. Each night, despite aggressive suctioning, the patient has developed harsh, gurgling sounds. His family is distressed by the sounds.
What is best option to reduce the difficulty with nocturnal breathing?
A) Repositioning
B) Transdermal scopolamine
C) Nebulized saline
D) Deep suctioning
E) Morphine

Answer: A

Repositioning can decrease the secretions without adverse effects. Several antimuscarinic agents have been used, but they have not been shown to be superior to placebo and can result in distressing symptoms such as urinary retention and dry mouth. Suctioning, and certainly deep suctioning, disrupts sleep and causes more physical discomfort. Nebulized saline is labor intensive and will not decrease the secretions.

Repositioning is an easy and effective maneuver which can be continued at home.

Reference

Wee B, Hillier R. Interventions for noisy breathing in patients near to death. Cochrane Database Syst Rev. 2008;(1): CD005177.

310. What body mass index in males is considered a probable mortality endpoint in males?
   A) 20.5 kg/m
   B) 16 kg/m
   C) 13 kg/m
   D) 11 kg/m

Answer: C

It is important to understand the thresholds of body mass index (BMI) that indicate end-stage malnutrition. Normal BMI ranges between 20 and 25 kg/m², and a patient is considered underweight with likely moderate malnutrition at a BMI of 18.5 kg/m². Severe malnutrition is expected with a BMI of less than 16 kg/m². In men, a BMI of less than 13 kg/m² is near end stage.

Reference

Romero-Corral A, Montori VM, Somers VK, Korinek J, Thomas RJ, Allison TG, Mookadam F, Lopez-Jimenez F. Association of bodyweight with total mortality and with cardiovascular events in coronary artery disease: a systematic review of cohort studies. Lancet. 2006; 368(9536):666–78.

311. Which of the following statements is true concerning percutaneous esophageal gastrostomy tubes (PEG)?
   A) PEG tubes reduce aspiration as opposed to nasogastric tubes.
   B) In end-stage advanced malignancy with cachexia, PEG tubes have been proven to improve survival and reduce morbidity.
   C) PEG tubes have been proven to improve survival in end-stage dementia.
   D) Mean survival after PEG tube placement for failure to thrive is 6 months.

Answer: D

The physician is often faced with this decision in a variety of end-of-life situations to consider placement of a PEG tube. Survival benefits of PEG tube placement are often minimal at best. There is a wide range of cultural expectations in reference to this issue. It is important to understand the facts concerning the possible benefits or lack of benefits of PEG tube placement when counseling the patient and family. As noted in this question, survival benefits for PEG tube placement in a patient with failure to thrive to variety of conditions are modest at best.

312. A 29-year-old woman develops left leg swelling during week 18 of her pregnancy. Left lower extremity ultrasonogram reveals a left iliac vein deep venous thrombosis (DVT).
   Proper management includes:
   A) Bedrest
   B) Catheter-directed thrombolysis
   C) Enoxaparin
   D) Inferior vena cava filter placement
   E) Warfarin

Answer: C

Pregnancy causes a hypercoagulable state and may result in deep venous thrombosis (DVT). DVT occurs in 1 in 2000 pregnancies. DVT occurs more commonly in the left leg than the right leg during pregnancy because of compression of the left iliac vein by the gravid uterus.

Approximately 25 % of pregnant women with DVT have a factor V Leiden mutation, which also predisposes to pre-eclampsia. Warfarin is contraindicated because of a risk of fetal abnormality. Low-molecular-weight heparin (LMWH) is appropriate therapy at this point in pregnancy. This is typically switched to unfractionated heparin 4 weeks before anticipated delivery. Ambulation, rather than bedrest, should be encouraged. There is no proven role for local thrombolytic therapy or an inferior vena cava filter in pregnancy. This would be considered only when anticoagulation is not possible.

References

Dulitzki M, Pauzner R, Langevitz P et al. Low molecular weight heparin during pregnancy and delivery: a preliminary experience with 41 pregnancies. Obstet Gynecol. 1996;87:830.

James AH, Jamison MG, Brancazio LR, Myers ER. Venous thromboembolism during pregnancy and the postpartum period: incidence, risk factors, and mortality. Am J Obstet Gynecol. 2006;194(5):1311–5.

313. A 59-year-old man has been admitted for congestive heart failure. His symptoms have resolved. Prior to discharge the cardiology service would like him to undergo placement of an automatic implantable cardiac converter defibrillator (AICD).

   He is on warfarin with an INR of 2.9. His other problems include rate-controlled atrial fibrillation and coronary artery disease. An echocardiogram performed 2 weeks ago showed a left ventricular ejection fraction of 25 % and a well-functioning mechanical mitral valve. Trace edema is noted in the extremities.

   How should his warfarin be managed prior to placement of his AICD?
   A) Continue warfarin, with a target INR of 3.5 or less on the day of the procedure.
   B) Discontinue warfarin 5 days before the procedure and resume the day after the procedure.
   C) Discontinue warfarin 5 days before the procedure and bridge with an unfractionated heparin infusion.
   D) Discontinue warfarin 5 days before the procedure and bridge with low-molecular-weight heparin.

Answer: A

Not all procedures require warfarin to be stopped. In some cases, there is data to support continuing warfarin as opposed to bridging therapy. A randomized, controlled trial found that patients at high risk for thromboembolic events on warfarin who need a pacemaker or implantable cardioverter defibrillator (ICD) can safely continue warfarin without bridging anticoagulation. Continuing warfarin treatment at the time of pacemaker in patients with high thrombotic risk was associated with a lower incidence of clinically significant device-pocket hematoma, as opposed to bridging with heparin.

Reference

Birnie DH, Healey JS, Wells GA et al. Pacemaker or defibrillator surgery without interruption of anticoagulation. N Engl J Med. 2013;368:2084–93.

314. A 56-year-old male is admitted to the hospital with fever and cough. He was well until 1 week before admission when he noted progressive shortness of breath, cough, and productive sputum. On the day of admission, the patient's wife noted him to be lethargic. The past medical history is notable for alcohol abuse and hypertension.

On examination, the patient is lethargic. Temperature is 38.9 °C (102 °F), blood pressure is 110/85 mmHg, and oxygen saturation is 86 % on room air. There are decreased breath sounds at the right lung base. Heart sounds are normal. The abdomen is soft. There is no peripheral edema. Chest radiography shows a right lower lobe infiltrate with a moderate pleural effusion.

The white blood cell count is 15,000/μL and 6 % bands. He is admitted and started on broad-spectrum antibiotics. On hospital day 3 he is not eating due to lethargy. A nasogastric tube is inserted, and tube feedings are started. The next day, plasma phosphate is found to be 1.2 mg/dL and calcium is 9.2 mg/dL.

What is the most appropriate approach to correcting the hypophosphatemia?

A) Administer IV calcium gluconate 1 g followed by infusion of IV phosphate at a rate of 8 mmol/h for 6 h.
B) Administer IV phosphate alone at a rate of 4 mmol/h for 6 h.
C) Administer IV phosphate alone at a rate of 8 mmol/h for 6 h.
D) Stop tube feedings, phosphate is expected to normalize over the course of the next 24–48 h.
E) Initiate oral phosphate replacement at a dose of 1750 mg/day.

Answer: C

Severe hypophosphatemia occurs when the serum concentration falls below 2 mg/dL . In this circumstance, IV replacement is recommended. In this patient with a level of 1.2 mg/dL, the recommended infusion rate is 8 mmol/h over 6 h for a total dose of 48 mmol. Levels should be checked every 6 h as well.

Malnutrition from fasting or starvation may result in depletion of phosphate. When nutrition is initiated, redistribution of phosphate into cells occurs. This is common in alcoholics.

It is generally recommended to use oral phosphate repletion when the serum phosphate levels are greater than 1.5–2.5 mg/dL. The dose of oral phosphate is 750–2000 mg daily of elemental phosphate given in divided doses. Until the underlying hypophosphatemia is corrected, one should measure phosphate and calcium levels every 6 h. The infusion should be stopped if the calcium phosphate product rises to higher than 50 to decrease the risk of heterotopic calcification.

If hypocalcemia is present with the hypophosphatemia, it is important to correct the calcium prior to administering phosphate. It may be best to restart feedings slowly in the malnourished patient while following electrolytes closely.

Reference

Camp MA, Allon M. Severe hypophosphatemia in hospitalized patients. Miner Electrolyte Metab. 1990;16:365–8.

315. A 58-year-old male is admitted to the hospital for elective hip replacement therapy. He has a history of chronic pulmonary disease and takes inhaled steroids as well as albuterol inhalers. He was admitted to the hospital 2 weeks ago for a moderate exacerbation of COPD for which he recently completed a 10-day course of prednisone.

He is currently asymptomatic, and his breathing is back to baseline. He states that he has not taken steroids within the past year other than his recent admission. You are asked to provide clearance for the orthopedic service of this patient. Which of the following is the most appropriate treatment?

A) Obtain a Cortrosyn stimulation test and begin steroids if there is evidence of cortisol deficiency.
B) Administer intravenous hydrocortisone 50 mg on the morning of surgery.
C) Administer intravenous hydrocortisone 100 mg preoperatively and then 50 mg every 8 h for 2 days after surgery.
D) Proceed with surgery.
E) Postpone surgery for 2 weeks.

Answer: D

Patients who have received oral steroids for less than 3 weeks have no suppression of their hypothalamic pituitary axis, nor do they require evaluation of their axis for stress dose steroids. A Cortrosyn stimulation test should be done when a patient's status of the hypothalamic pituitary adrenal axis is uncertain. It is usually not needed in the preoperative evaluation. Without any evidence of overt adrenal insufficiency, perioperative steroids are not recommended. In this particular case, the patient may proceed with surgery without the need for supplemental steroids.

Reference

Marik PE, Pastores SM, Annane D et al. Recommendations for the diagnosis and management of corticosteroid insufficiency in critically ill adult patients: consensus statements from an international task force by the American College of Critical Care Medicine. Crit Care Med. 2008;36(6):1937–49.

316. An 86-year-old male is admitted for cough, dyspnea, and dysphagia. He has a known large non-small cell cancer in the upper lobe of the right lung and is on week 4 of palliative irradiation. He reports anorexia, difficulty swallowing solid food, and right shoulder pain. His wife and family are concerned about dehydration. They request IV fluids and nutrition.

On physical examination, the patient is thin and appears weak but alert. Pulse rate is 120 beats per minute, respirations are 24 per minute, and blood pressure is 150/70 mmHg. There are temporal wasting and a dry oropharynx. The patient's breathing is shallow, with mild tachypnea. Breath sounds are diminished in the upper lobe of the right lung. You convene a family meeting to discuss options.

Which of the following would be the most likely outcome of intravenous hydration or nutrition in this patient?

A) Reduced BUN/serum creatinine ratio
B) Prolonged survival
C) Increased albumin level
D) Improved quality of life

Answer: A

Families feel an important obligation to provide nutrition and hydration to the dying patient. A randomized controlled trial found that parenteral hydration did not improve quality of life in advanced cancer. The intravenous fluids would likely reduce this patient's prerenal azotemic state in the short term but would not have a beneficial impact on his quality of life. These facts can guide counseling of patients and families in seeking noninvasive measures for this stage of advanced cancer.

Reference

Medically assisted hydration for adult palliative care patients. Cochrane Database Syst Rev. 2014 Apr 23 ;4:CD006273. doi: 10.1002/14651858.CD006273.pub3.

317. You are consulted to see a 33-year-old woman with diabetes mellitus and hypertension. She is in her 38th week of pregnancy. Her blood pressure is 160/92 mmHg. She has 4+ proteinuria. Two hours prior to the consult, she had a generalized grand mal seizure.

Management should include all of the following EXCEPT:

A) Emergent delivery
B) Intravenous labetalol
C) Intravenous magnesium sulfate
D) Intravenous phenytoin

Answer: D

This patient has severe eclampsia. Delivery should be performed as rapidly as possible. Eclampsia is commonly defined as new onset of grand mal seizure activity or unexplained coma during pregnancy or postpartum in a woman with signs or symptoms of preeclampsia.

Delivery in a mother with severe eclampsia before 37 weeks' gestation decreases maternal morbidity and mortality. This must be weighed against the increased fetal risks of complications of prematurity. Aggressive management of blood pressure, usually with labetalol or hydralazine intravenously, decreases the maternal risk of stroke. Similar to a nonpregnancy-related hypertensive crisis, the decrease in blood pressure should be achieved slowly to avoid hypotension and risk of decreased blood flow to the fetus.

Eclamptic seizures should be controlled with magnesium sulfate. It has been shown to be superior to phenytoin and diazepam in large randomized clinical trials

Reference

Lucas MJ, Leveno KJ, Cunningham FG. A comparison of magnesium sulfate with phenytoin for the prevention of eclampsia. N Engl J Med. 1995;333(4):201–5.

318. A 26-year-old woman is evaluated in the emergency department for abdominal pain. She reports a vague loss of appetite for the past day and has had progressively severe abdominal pain at her umbilicus. The pain is collicky. She reports that she is otherwise healthy and has had no sick contacts. Surgery has been consulted and recommends observation. You are consulted for admission.

On physical exam her temperature is 38.2 °C (100.8 °F), heart rate 110 bpm, and otherwise normal vital signs. Her abdomen is tender in the right lower quadrant and pelvic examination performed in the emergency room is normal. Urine pregnancy test is negative.

Which of the following imaging modalities would you do next?

A) Colonoscopy
B) Pelvic ultrasound

C) CT of the abdomen without contrast

D) Ultrasound of the abdomen

E) Transvaginal ultrasound

F) Plain film of the abdomen

Answer: C

CT scan is indicated for the diagnoses of acute appendicitis. It has been shown to be superior to ultrasound or plain radiograph in the diagnosis of acute appendicitis, The appendix is not always visualized on CT, but nonvisualization of the appendix on CT scan is associated with surgical findings of a normal appendix 98 % of the time.

This patient presented with classic findings for acute appendicitis. Initial anorexia progressed to vague periumbilical pain. This was followed by localization to the right lower quadrant. Low-grade fever and leukocytosis may be present. Acute appendicitis is primarily a clinical diagnosis. However, imaging modalities are frequently employed as the symptoms are not always classic and take time to evolve. Plain radiographs are rarely helpful. Ultrasound may demonstrate an enlarged appendix with a thick wall, but is most useful to rule out gynecological disease such as ovarian pathology, tuboovarian abscess, or ectopic pregnancy, which can mimic appendicitis.

References

Graffeo CS, Counselman FL. Appendicitis. Emerg Med Clin North Am. 1996;14(4):653–71.

Terasawa T, Blackmore CC, Bent S, Kohlwes RJ. Systematic review: computed tomography and ultrasonography to detect acute appendicitis in adults and adolescents. Ann Intern Med. 2004;141(7):537–46.

319. A 38-year-old obese woman is admitted to the hospital for elective cholecystectomy. The surgery is uncomplicated, but postoperatively her urine output is 6 L/day . She complains of severe thirst. On the second postoperative day, her BUN and creatinine are noted to be elevated, and you are consulted.

On your questioning, she reports a 1-year history of extreme thirst and urinary frequency. Aside from oral contraceptives, she takes no medications and reports no past medical history.

Which of the following is the most appropriate first step to confirm her diagnosis?

A) 24-h urine volume and osmolarity measurement

B) Fasting morning plasma osmolarity

C) Fluid deprivation test

D) MRI of the brain

E) Fasting morning glucose

Answer: A

The patient has idiopathic diabetes insipidus. This may present with long-standing urinary frequency and thirst. The symptoms may have a gradual onset and the patient may not perceive it as abnormal. It may go undiagnosed for some time. Diabetes insipidus may be unmasked when the patient is unable to have free access to water as occurred here. Diabetes insipidus may be nephrogenic or central insipidus. It is confirmed by measurement of 24-h urine volume, which is more than 50 mg/kg per day (3500 mL in a 70-kg male), and urine osmolarity of greater than 300 mosmol/L.

Reference

Crowley RK, Sherlock M, Agha A, Smith D, Thompson CJ. Clinical insights into adipsic diabetes insipidus: a large case series. Clin Endocrinol. 2007;66(4):475–82.

320. A 82-year-old female is admitted with abdominal distension. She has a history of metastatic breast cancer and has been taking extended-release morphine, 60 mg every 12 h, and one or two 15-mg morphine tablets daily for breakthrough right upper quadrant pain from her enlarged liver. Her pain has been well controlled, but he has had decreased bowel movements.

On physical exam, temperature is 36.3 °C (97.3 °F), pulse rate is 90 beats per minute, respirations are 16 per minute, and blood pressure is 120/80 mmHg. Physical examination shows a slightly protuberant but nontender abdomen. Bowel sounds are normal.

An abdominal and pelvic computed tomography scan shows a large amount of stool but no bowel obstruction.

Which of the following is the correct treatment for this patient's ongoing constipation?

A) Add lactulose.

B) Add N-methylnaltrexone.

C) Add docusate.

D) Place a nasogastric tube for bowel decompression.

E) Request a colorectal surgery consult for manual disimpaction.

Answer: A

Constipation is the most frequent side effect associated with long-term opioid therapy. Osmotic laxatives, such as mannitol, lactulose, and sorbitol, are effective in the palliation of opioid-induced constipation. Although expert consensus supports the use of prophylactic bowel regimens in all patients taking opioids, little evidence demonstrates the efficacy of one regimen over another.

Bulk-forming laxatives increase stool volume but should be used with caution in patients with advanced cancer because they require adequate fluid intake and physical activity to prevent exacerbation of constipation.

Docusate has very little effect when given alone for opioid-induced constipation. Gastric motility is decreased in these patients and softening of the stool alone may not alleviate the symptom. In many situations, its efficacy has been questioned.

N-methylnaltrexone is used for the treatment of opioid-induced constipation in patients with advanced illness who are receiving palliative care, when response to laxative therapy has been insufficient.

In this patient adding, starting and continuing with lactulose is the next step. In addition a bowel diary may be beneficial to review on her follow-up appointment.

Reference

Pappagallo M. Incidence, prevalence, and management of opioid bowel dysfunction. Am J Surg. 2001;182 (suppl 5A):11S–8S.

321. A 53-year-old woman who has hepatitis C cirrhosis is admitted for worsening ascites. In addition to complaints of abdominal pain, she complains of severe puritis. She has been on cholestyramine for several months for the itching.

On physical exam multiple excoriations of her skin are noted and she is unable to stop scratching. She is very anxious and fatigued.

Her serum laboratory results are stable from last admission, including a stable total bilirubin. Ultrasonography shows no evidence of biliary ductal dilatation or changes in her liver.

Which of the following should you now recommend?
A) Ursodeoxycholic acid at 30 mg/kg daily
B) Diphenhydramine 50 mg every 6 h
C) Naltrexone 25 mg daily
D) Morphine 5 mg BID
E) Hydroxyzine 10 mg BID

Answer: C

Refractory itching is a common in end-stage liver disease patients. It may be severe leading to significant excoriations. Cholestyramine has been the mainstay of treatment. Patients who do not respond to continued doses of cholestyramine probably will not respond to an antihistamine. Naltrexone is tolerated well and is a reasonable option in these cases. Patients started on naltrexone should be followed for signs of withdrawal.

Reference

Wolfhaqen FH, Sternieri E, Hop WC et al. Oral naltrexone therapy for cholestatic pruritus: a double-blind, placebo-controlled study. Gastroenterology. 1997;113:1264–9.

322. A 69-year-old female with osteoarthritis of the knees for many years and has been advised by her orthopedist that the timing is now right to undergo knee arthroplasty. She has a history of diabetes, high cholesterol, hypertension, and coronary artery disease.

Nine months ago, she underwent a drug-eluting stent placement for worsening angina, which she tolerated well. She has been angina-free since that time and is able to walk up several flights of stairs without angina.

Current medications are aspirin, clopidogrel, losartan, and metoprolol. Your recommendations concerning surgery are the following:
A) Surgery can proceed as planned.
B) Surgery should wait for 2 months.
C) Surgery can occur in 3 months.
D) Surgery can occur in 9 months.

Answer: C

Elective surgery should be delayed at least 1 year after the placement of a drug-eluting stent. Rapid thrombosis of a drug-eluting stent (DES) is a catastrophic complication. The risk of stent thrombosis is increased in the perioperative setting and is strongly associated with the cessation of antiplatelet therapy. To avoid thrombosis with DES, aspirin and antiplatelet agents should be continued throughout surgery. In spite of the increased risk of bleeding, this strategy is acceptable in many types of invasive surgical procedures with no change in outcome.

In situations where surgery may be needed on a semi-urgent basis in patients who have received a drug-eluding stent within 1 year and the risk of bleeding is high. In these situations, consultation with cardiology is recommended.

Elective surgery with bare metal stents should be delayed for 30–90 days.

Reference

Abualsaud AO, Eisenberg MJ. Perioperative management of patients with drug-eluting stents. J Am Coll Cardiol Intv. 2010;3(2):131–42.

323. A 74-year-old female was transferred to the intensive care unit after an in-hospital cardiac arrest. She has a history of near end-stage congestive heart failure. Return of spontaneous circulation occurred after a prolonged code at the 25-min mark of ACLS.

On physical examination, the patient's respiratory rate is greater than the rate set on the ventilator. The doll's eye reflex is negative, as are the corneal reflexes and pupillary light reflexes. The only muscle movements are myoclonus.

A family meeting is arranged to discuss prognosis and treatment. At this point they want all resuscitative measures to be continued. They want to know if she will regain consciousness and what is the time frame for her possible recovery.

At what point after this patient's brain injury can you most accurately give the family a prognosis about the risk of death or persistent unconsciousness?
A) 24 h
B) 48 h
C) 72 h
D) 96 h

Answer: C

Several prospective studies showed that absent corneal reflexes and absent motor responses to noxious stimuli at 72 h are highly predictive of no cognitive function return. Caution should be used to ensure the patient is under limited sedation or other underlying reversible conditions when these exam findings are made.

References

Labelle A, Juang P, Reichley R et al. The determinants of hospital mortality among patients with septic shock receiving appropriate initial antibiotic treatment. Crit Care Med. 2012;40:2016–21.

Tweed WA, Thomassen A, Wernberg M. Prognosis after cardiac arrest based on age and duration of coma. Can Med Assoc J. 1982;126(9):1058–60.

324. A patient with severe dementia is admitted for worsening anorexia and nausea over the past 6 weeks. She lives at home with her family. The family would like to continue palliative care but are looking to improve her appetite and diminish her nausea. You and the family meet and agree on a conservative course of action.

    Which of the following statements accurately characterizes the treatment of these complications of severe dementia?
    A) Haloperidol has minimal effects against nausea.
    B) Even though this patient has severe dementia, it would be unethical to withhold nutrition and hydration.
    C) A feeding tube will reduce the risk of aspiration pneumonia.
    D) A trial of antidepressants is indicated.
    E) Impaction may explain all the symptoms.
    F) A trial of megestrol acetate.

Answer: E

Anorexia and gastrointestinal symptoms are common near the end of life. Despite a nonaggressive approach, some simple measures may improve symptoms. Haloperidol may be highly effective against nausea and may be less sedating than many commonly used agents, such as prochlorperazine. Impactions are common and can present with a variety of symptoms. Treatment can be relatively easy and can improve comfort.

Because of the terminal and irreversible nature of end-stage dementia and the substantial burden that continued life-prolonging care may pose, initiating aggressive hydration and nutrition would not be indicated.

Appetite stimulants such as megestrol acetate have not been shown to be of any benefit in the anorexia of end-stage dementia.

Reference

Hanson LC, Ersek M, Gilliam R, Carey TS. Oral feeding options for patients with dementia: a systematic review. J Am Geriatr Soc. 2011;59(3):463–72.

325. A 23-year-old female is admitted with a new deep venous thrombosis (DVT). She is pregnant and in her late second trimester. You are consulted for management of her DVT. In review of her labs, it is noticed that her liver functions are elevated. Her AST is 120 units/L; her ALT is 140 units/L. T. bili is 1.6 mg/dL.

    Which of the following is the likely diagnosis?
    A) Hyperemesis gravidarum
    B) HELLP
    C) Cholestasis of pregnancy
    D) Acute fatty liver of pregnancy
    E) None of the above

Answer: C

Gestational age of the pregnancy is a great guide to the differential of liver disease in the pregnant woman. Cholestasis of pregnancy is common and most typically presents in the late second trimester. Approximately 1 % of pregnancies in the United States are affected by this condition. Some hepatic diseases of pregnancy are mild, and some require urgent and definitive treatment. A common condition of the first trimester is hyperemesis gravidarum and may result in elevated AST and ALT; however this usually resolves by week 20 of gestation. Acute fatty liver of pregnancy is a cause of acute liver failure that can develop in the late second or third trimester. Elevated LFTs and bilirubin are most commonly seen. Although symptoms and signs are similar to those of preeclampsia and HELLP syndrome, aminotransferase levels tend to be much higher.

Reference

Riely CA. Liver disease in the pregnant patient. Am J Gastroenterol. 1999;94:1728–32.

326. A 66-year-old male is admitted with acute onset of left hemiplegia. He has a history of hypertension, nonvalvular atrial fibrillation, and thyroid disease. He has been lost to medical follow-up in recent years and has been on no anticoagulation.

    On physical exam, motor strength is 1/5 in the left arm and 2/5 in the left leg. Electrocardiogram reveals atrial fibrillation with a heart rate of 70 beats per minute. MRI performed on presentation reveals a right middle cerebral artery infarction.

    Which of the following is appropriate treatment for stroke prevention?
    A) Aspirin 350 mg daily alone
    B) Clopidogrel 25 mg daily
    C) Warfarin, adjusted to achieve an INR of 2–3
    D) Unfractionated heparin bolus, followed by infusion
    E) Enoxaparin

Answer: C

Guidelines do not support the routine use of anticoagulation for acute ischemic stroke. In this particular case with a large territory middle cerebral artery infarct, any urgent anticoagulation may increase the risk of conversion to hemorrhage.

Several randomized, controlled trials that used heparin early after ischemic stroke failed to show a significant overall benefit of treatment over controls. An exception may be in patients with acute ischemic stroke ipsilateral to a severe stenosis or occlusion of the internal carotid artery.

Stroke prevention treatment for atrial fibrillation is most often determined according to the CHADS2/CHADS2VAS system. Warfarin continues to be the most commonly used agent, although a number of newer agents including dabigatran are increasingly being prescribed.

Current recommendation is that warfarin be started during the hospitalization. Bridging with low-molecular-weight heparin is not usually needed but may be considered in certain circumstances.

References

Fiorelli M, Bastianello S, von Kummer R et al. Hemorrhagic transformation within 36 hours of a cerebral infarct: relationships with early clinical deterioration and 3-month outcome in the European Cooperative Acute Stroke Study I (ECASS I) cohort. Stroke. 1999;30(11):2280–4.

Paciaroni M, Agnelli G, Micheli S, Caso V. Efficacy and safety of anticoagulant treatment in acute cardioembolic stroke: a meta-analysis of randomized controlled trials. Stroke. 2007;38(2):423–30.

327. A 37-year-old male with a history of intravenous drug abuse is admitted with fever and hypertension. A diagnosis of mitral valve endocarditis is made by echocardiogram. He is noted to have a large lesion on his mitral valve with moderate regurgitation. He is started on broad-spectrum antibiotics and has a clinically good response.

When is surgery indicated in the presence of endocarditis?
    A) Heart failure
    B) After several embolic events
    C) Myocardial abscess
    D) Confirmed fungal endocarditis
    E) All of the above

Answer: E

Fifteen to twenty percent of the patients who have endocarditis will ultimately require surgical intervention. Congestive heart failure in a patient with native valve endocarditis is the primary indication for surgery.

The decision to proceed with surgery is often difficult due to patient comorbidities. Traditional criteria include those listed above. It is suggested that surgery may be considered in patients with large lesions and significant valvular disease. Early surgery reduces the risk of embolic events, although this has not been proven to change overall mortality. Failure of medical treatment is another indication for surgery, although guidelines are not specific. In addition surgery should be considered in patients with multiresistant organisms. Endocarditis in many circumstances warrants early cardiothoracic surgery consultation.

References

Kang DH, Kim YJ, Kim SH et al. Early surgery versus conventional treatment for infective endocarditis. N Engl J Med. 2012;366(26):2466–73.

Thuny F, Grisoli D, Collart F, Habib G, Raoult D. Management of infective endocarditis: challenges and perspectives. Lancet. 2012;379(9819):965–75.

328. Which of the following patients with metastatic disease is potentially curable by surgical resection?
    A) A 22-year-old man with a history of osteosarcoma of the left femur with a 1-cm metastasis to his right lower lobe
    B) A 63-year-old woman with a history of colon cancer with one metastases to the left lobe of the liver
    C) Operable non-small cell lung cancer with a single brain metastasis
    D) All of the above
    E) None of the above

Answer: D

In colon, non-small cell lung and osteosarcoma cancer cures have been reported with resection of solitary metastatic lesions. Metastases typically represent widespread systemic dissemination of disease and are associated with poor prognosis. Palliative chemotherapy is generally the accepted method of treatment. Over the last several years, numerous reports and studies have demonstrated long-term survival after resection of isolated metastasis. After extensive investigation for further metastatic sites, isolated metastasis should be considered for reaction in select cases.

Reference

Manfredi S, Bouvier AM, Lepage C et al. Incidence and patterns of recurrence after resection for cure of colonic cancer in a well defined population. Br J Surg. 2006;93:1115–22.

329. A 56-year-old white male with known clinical atherosclerotic disease is admitted with severe leg cramps. His past medical history is significant for a myocardial infarction (MI) 4 years ago requiring stent placement. At the time of his MI, he was initiated on a high-intensity statin; since then he has developed severe leg cramps.

What would be the next best alternative in lipid therapy for this patient?

A) Start atorvastatin 20 mg PO daily.
B) No longer a need for statin therapy since his MI was 4 years ago.
C) Start rosuvastatin 20 mg PO QHS.
D) Start pravastatin 10 mg PO QHS.

Answer: A

He should be on a high-intensity statin, but he was unable to tolerate the side effects. According to American College of Cardiology guidelines, patients with known clinical atherosclerotic disease should be on a moderate-intensity statin if not a candidate or cannot tolerate the high-intensity regimen. Atorvastatin 20 mg is a moderate-intensity statin. The moderate-intensity daily dose will lower LDL-C by approximately 30 to <50 %, whereas the high-intensity therapy lowers LDL-C by approximately ≥50 %. Lastly, pravastatin 10 mg is a low-intensity statin.

Reference

Stone NJ, Robinson J, Lichtenstein AH et al. 2013 ACC/AHA guideline on the treatment of blood cholesterol to reduce atherosclerotic cardiovascular risk in adults: a report of the American College of Cardiology/American Heart Association Task Force on Practice Guidelines. J Am Coll Cardiol. 2013. pii: S0735-1097(13)06028-2.

330. A 62-year-old man is admitted for dehydration. He also reports severe nausea and vomiting that began 24 h ago. He recently started chemotherapy for non-small cell lung cancer. His last dose was 48 h ago.

On physical examination his abdomen is soft and nontender. Bowel sounds are present. He is admitted and started in intravenous fluids. Despite several doses of ondansetron, he continues to have near constant nausea.

What would be the next appropriate treatment for his nausea and vomiting?
A) Dexamethasone
B) Haloperidol
C) Lorazepam
D) Octreotide

Answer: A

Dexamethasone is recommended for the management of delayed chemotherapy-induced nausea and vomiting. Delayed nausea and vomiting are any nausea and vomiting that occurred after the day that chemotherapy is infused. Nausea and vomiting are two of the most feared cancer treatment-related side effects for cancer patients.

Dexamethasone has synergistic action with many antiemetic medications. Its specific antiemetic mechanism of action is not fully understood. It is generally started at 8 mg once or twice daily. Corticosteroids may be effective as monotherapy as well.

Reference

Kris MG, Hesketh PJ, Somerfield MR et al. American Society of Clinical Oncology guideline for antiemetics in oncology: update 2006. J Clin Oncol. 2006;24(18):2932–47.

331. A 63-year-old man is admitted to the hospital because of hematemesis. He has gastroesophageal reflux disease and atrial fibrillation; he takes warfarin. He had felt well until this morning when nausea developed after eating. He vomited blood once and was brought to the hospital.

On physical exam, the temperature is normal. Pulse rate is 84 beats per minute and irregular, and blood pressure is 112/74 mmHg. Abdominal examination is normal. Hemoglobin is 11.8 g/dL, serum creatinine is 0.9 mg/dL, and eGFR is greater than 60 mL/min/1.73 m^2.

Intravenous isotonic saline is given, and nasogastric lavage is subsequently performed. Upper endoscopy reveals a duodenal ulcer, which is successfully cauterized. Warfarin is discontinued, and intravenous pantoprazole is begun. No additional bleeding is noted after 48 h, and the patient is prepared for discharge.

How long after the bleeding episode can this patient's warfarin be safely restarted?
A) One week.
B) One month.
C) Six weeks.
D) Three months.
E) Warfarin should not be restarted.

Answer: A

Gastrointestinal (GI) bleeding affects an estimated 4.5 % of warfarin-treated patients annually and is associated with a significant risk of death. These patients present a dilemma for clinicians regarding when to restart warfarin. A recent study examined patients who had GI bleeds when on warfarin. They found that warfarin therapy resumption within 1 week after a GI bleed was, after 90 days, associated with a lower adjusted risk for thrombosis and death without significantly increasing the risk for recurrent GI bleeding compared to those who did not resume warfarin. The median time to restart warfarin was 4 days. From this study, a reasonable period of 7 days is suggested.

References

Lee JK, Kang HW, Kim SG, Kim JS, Jung HC. Risks related with withholding and resuming anticoagulation in patients with non-variceal upper gastrointestinal bleeding while on warfarin therapy. Int J Clin Pract. 2012;66:64–8.

Qureshi W, Mittal C, Patsias I et al. Restarting anticoagulation and outcomes after major gastrointestinal bleeding in atrial fibrillation. Am J Cardiol. 2014;113:662–8.

332. An 82-year-old male is admitted for community-acquired pneumonia. During the first 24 h of admission, he undergoes cardiopulmonary arrest. He was subsequently successfully coded on the floor. The family cannot be contacted, and full resuscitation measures are taken. He is transferred to the ICU.

Which of the following will characterize the patient's post-arrest clinical course?
A) Increased intracranial pressure
B) Intact cerebrovascular autoregulation
C) Myocardial dysfunction
D) Minimal inflammatory response

Answer: C

The post-cardiac arrest syndrome (PCAS) is an inflammatory syndrome that best resembles sepsis. Inflammatory mediators are released, resulting in activation of the coagulation cascade. Cerebral edema, ischemic degeneration, and impaired autoregulation characterize the brain injury pattern in the PCAS. Brain injury alone contributes greatly to overall morbidity and mortality in the resuscitated cardiac arrest patient. There is impaired autoregulation as well as impaired oxidative metabolism. There is predictable myocardial dysfunction. Myocardial dysfunction in the PCAS seems to be reversible and is characterized largely by global hypokinesis.

Elevations of intracranial pressure are not prominent. Treatment during this period involves hemodynamic support and the use of inotropic and vasopressor agents if warranted. Hyperthermia should be avoided at all costs in patients with the PCAS. If aggressive therapy is pursued, consider sedation with hypothermia to improve neurological outcome in the ICU setting.

References

Benson DW, Williams GR Jr, Spencer FC, Yates AJ. The use of hypothermia after cardiac arrest. Anesth Analg. 1959;38:423–8.

Wright WL, Geocadin RG. Postresuscitative intensive care: neuroprotective strategies after cardiac arrest. Semin Neurol. 2006;26(4):396–402.

333. A 72-year-old female is admitted with abdominal distension. She has history of colon cancer. Her last bowel movement was 4 days ago despite her taking scheduled polyethylene glycol. Her cancer was diagnosed 2 years ago and has been treated with chemotherapy after her disease was determined to be surgically unresectable.

On physical exam the bowel is distended with absent bowel sounds. Lungs are normal. A nasogastric tube is placed with some mild improvement of distension.

CT scan shows dilated loops of small bowel and colon with a transition point in the mid-descending colon.

Which of the following will most likely improve this patient's ability to eat and ensure adequate caloric intake and fluids?
A) Referral for radiation
B) Placement of a colonic stent across the single site of obstruction
C) Fleet enema
D) Exploratory surgery
E) Placement of a venting percutaneous endoscopic gastrostomy (PEG) tube

Answer: B

A single-site bowel obstruction can be successfully palliated with colonic stent placement. Most self-expandable metal stent (SEMS) placement is a minimally invasive option for achieving acute colonic decompression in obstructed colorectal cancer. This would be a reasonable approach in this patient as opposed to surgery.

When performed by experienced endoscopists, the technical success rate is high with a low procedural complication rate.

Reference

Dalal KM, Gollub MJ, Miner TJ et al. Management of patients with malignant bowel obstruction and stage IV colorectal cancer. J Palliat Med. 2011;14:822.

334. Which of the following is least likely to decrease the risk of central line-associated bloodstream infection (CLABSI)?
A) Internal jugular compared to femoral vein site selection
B) Correct hand hygiene
C) Correct gowning and gloving pre-procedure
D) Pre-procedure preparation of chlorhexidine
E) Daily review with nursing staff of line necessity with removal and rotation of unnecessary lines
F) Subclavian compared to femoral vein site selection

Answer: A

Evidence suggests that all of the above measures reduce line infection rates except the use of internal jugular site as opposed to the femoral site. The subclavian site is associated with the lowest risk of infection.

Several studies have demonstrated that the use of maximal barrier precautions including a cap, mask, sterile gown, gloves, and a sterile full-body drape when inserting central lines reduces CLABSI.

Hand hygiene is an important practice in the prevention of CLABSI. Hand decontamination with either antiseptic-containing soaps, alcohol-based gels, or a combination has consistently been shown to reduce CLABSI rates.

Skin antisepsis with chlorhexidine was found to be associated with a 50 % reduction in the subsequent risk of CLABSI compared with povidone iodine.

Reference

Maki DG, Stolz SM, Wheeler S, Mermel LA. Prevention of central venous catheter-related bloodstream infection by use of an antiseptic-impregnated catheter. A randomized, controlled trial. Ann Intern Med. 1997;127(4):257–66.

335. A 32-year-old female is admitted with multiple sclerosis. She initially undergoes intravenous steroid therapy with little clinical response. On day 4 of her hospitalization, plasma exchange/plasmapheresis are initiated.
    Which of the following electrolytes should be followed closely during her hospitalization?
    A) Potassium
    B) Calcium
    C) Sodium
    D) Phosphorous

Answer: B

Patients undergoing plasmapheresis can experience symptoms of hypocalcemia and/or hypomagnesemia during and after the procedure. Current plasmapheresis regimens often include prophylactic replacement of calcium. Hypocalcemia has also been reported following massive transfusions due to the binding citrate agent. However, this is transient, and there is no evidence that calcium supplementation will be of benefit. Septic shock and severe sepsis are also associated with hypocalcemia. This is due to abnormalities of vitamin D and parathyroid hormone. There is no evidence that septic patients benefit from calcium repletion.

References

Drew MJ. Plasmapheresis in the dysproteinemias. Ther Apher. 2002;6(1):45–52.

Mokrzycki MH, Kaplan AA. Therapeutic plasma exchange: complications and management. Am J Kidney Dis. 1994;23(6):817–27.

336. A 65-year-old male with metastatic non-small cell lung cancer is admitted for increasing pain and exhaustion. The patient has metastasis to his spine. He states the pain has become unbearable and is unable to sleep. He describes the pain in his legs as episodic, shooting and burning. The pain is worse at night than during daytime. He has been taking escalating doses of hydromorphone. The initial hydromorphone dosage of 4 mg several times daily was not very effective, and he tells you that he is now taking 8-mg hydromorphone tablets four or five times daily. He states that the hydromorphone provides brief relief.

Which of the following should you prescribe now to help reduce this patient's pain?
    A) Topiramate
    B) Dexamethasone
    C) Lorazepam
    D) Gabapentin
    E) Methadone

Answer: D

Pain is moderate to severe in about 40–50 % of advanced cancer patients. It is severe or excruciating in 25–30 % of cases. A stepwise approach to pain in cancer management has been well established and continues to evolve. Specific patterns of pain on cancer management should be recognized and treated appropriately.

Patients with spinal metastasis commonly have neuropathic pain. Gabapentin is frequently used to treat neuropathic pain and is well tolerated. Several drugs in addition to opioid narcotics have been proven to be of benefit in neuropathic pain due to malignancy.

The analgesic doses of gabapentin reported to relieve pain in non-end-of-life pain conditions ranged from 900 mg/day to 3600 mg/day in divided doses. A common reason for inadequate relief is failure to titrate upward after prescribing the usual starting dose of 100 mg by mouth three times daily.

References

Coderre TJ, Kumar N, Lefebvre CD, Yu JSC. Evidence that gabapentin reduces neuropathic pain by inhibiting the spinal release of glutamate. J Neurochem. 2005;94:1131–9.

Wiffen PJ, McQuay HJ, Edwards JE, Moore RA. Gabapentin for acute and chronic pain. Cochrane Database Syst Rev. 2005;(3):CD005452.

337. What nutritional supplements have been proven to assist in the healing of decubitus ulcers?
    A) Protein
    B) Zinc
    C) Ascorbic acid
    D) Increased caloric intake
    E) All of the above

Answer: A

One of the most important reversible host factors contributing to wound healing is nutritional status. Several studies suggest that dietary intake, especially of protein, is important in healing pressure ulcers. Most of these studies have been observational and are limited. Current guidelines strongly suggest that nutrition is important in the healing of decubitus ulcers but the exact components of the nutrition remain uncertain.

The optimum dietary protein intake in patients with pressure ulcers is unknown, but may be much higher than the current adult recommendation of 0.8 g/kg/day. Increasing protein intake beyond 1.5 g/kg/day may not increase protein synthesis and may cause dehydration. It has been suggested that a reasonable protein requirement is therefore between 1.0 and 1.5 g/kg/day.

Zinc and vitamin C are often included in supplements but have not been shown to improve healing in decubitus ulcers.

References

Sandstead SH, Henrikson LK, Greger JL et al. Zinc nutriture in the elderly in relation to taste acuity, immune response, and wound healing. Am J Clin Nutr. 1982; 36:1046–59.

Thomas DR. The role of nutrition in prevention and healing of pressure ulcers. Med Clin North Am. 1997;13:497–511.

Vilter RW. Nutritional aspects of ascorbic acid: uses and abuses. West J Med. 1980;133:485–92.

338. A 35-year-old female is admitted with severe pain to her left foot. She states that she had a fracture of her ankle due to a fall 2 months ago. Since that time, she has had limited mobility and has infrequently gotten out of bed. She has had a follow-up appointment with her orthopedist who reports the ankle is healing well. She states that for the past 2 weeks, she has been completely unable to ambulate and has been bed bound. She reports a past medical history of anxiety and fibromyalgia.

On physical exam, the ankle is noted to be painful to mild touch. She states that the pain has a burning quality. The affected area is also noted to have an increased temperature, but no erythema is noted. X-rays are negative for fracture or any other noted pathology.

What test would be most likely to make the diagnosis?

A) Magnetic resonance imaging.
B) Computed tomography
C) Triple-phase bone scan
D) Electromyography
E) Depression screen

Answer: C

This patient's symptoms are consistent with a complex regional pain syndrome. This was formerly known as reflex sympathetic dystrophy. This condition often occurs following trauma or surgery that results in a extended immobilization of the affected limb. Attempts have been made to quantify this syndrome. Criteria have been established to make the diagnosis. This includes pain due to mild stimuli and burning quality as well as changes in temperature, hair, and color of the affected extremity. Bone scan has been shown to reveal a typical pattern and

can be a useful adjunct in confirming the diagnosis. Diffuse increased perfusion to the entire extremity is usually noted.

Therapy is directed toward nonnarcotic alternative medications that address neuropathic pain and increasing mobility to the affected area. Prevention focuses on early physical therapy.

Reference

Bruehl S, Harden RN, Galer BS et al. External validation of IASP diagnostic criteria for Complex Regional Pain Syndrome and proposed research diagnostic criteria. International Association for the Study of Pain. Pain. 1999;81(1–2):147–54.

339. A 78-year-old woman tripped while walking her dog. She presents with severe pain in her left hip. She had no chest pain, shortness of breath, or loss of consciousness. The patient is admitted to the hospital for perioperative management for probable open reduction and internal fixation of the left hip fracture.

She has a history of hypertension, osteoarthritis, and osteoporosis. She currently smokes on half a pack of cigarettes per day.

On exam, her temperature is 37.1 °C (98.8 °F), pulse rate is 90 beats per minute, respirations are 18 per minute, and blood pressure is 158/74 mmHg. Oxygen saturation by pulse oximetry is 96 %. The cardiopulmonary examination is normal. No edema is noted, but the left leg is shortened and externally rotated. Complete blood count and basic metabolic panel are normal. Chest radiograph is normal. Electrocardiogram shows sinus rhythm.

Which of the following interventions is most likely to increase mortality in the postoperative period?

A) Proceeding to surgery urgently in the next 48 h
B) Prescribing a beta-adrenergic blocking agent within 24 h before surgery
C) Postoperative venous thromboembolism prophylaxis
D) Early postoperative mobilization
E) Nicotine patch

Answer: B

A recent meta-analysis demonstrated that, despite a reduction in nonfatal myocardial infarction, perioperative beta-blockers started less than one day prior to noncardiac surgery were associated with an increased risk of death 30 days after surgery. Proceeding to surgery within 48 h has been shown to be beneficial in hip fracture patients.

Reference

Bouri S, Shun-Shin MJ, Cole GD, Mayet J, Francis DP. Meta-analysis of secure randomised controlled trials of beta-blockade to prevent perioperative death in non-cardiac surgery. Heart. 2014;100(6):456–64.

340. You are consulted to see a 36-year-old woman that has been admitted for shortness of breath to the obstetrics service. She is 4 months pregnant and has a prior history of asthma.

She uses her albuterol inhaler several times per week to achieve symptomatic relief, but this has proven to be inadequate. History includes mild persistent asthma that was well controlled before her pregnancy with an as-needed short-acting β2-agonist and medium-dose inhaled glucocorticoids.

On physical examination, vital signs are normal. The lungs have diffuse wheezes. She appears in minimal distress. Cardiac examination shows normal S1 and S2 with no gallops or murmurs. No leg edema is noted.

What is the correct treatment?
A) Prednisone.
B) Add a long-acting β2-agonist.
C) Add theophylline.
D) Double the dose of inhaled glucocorticoid.
E) A and B.

Answer: E

Approximately one-third of patients with asthma experience worsening of symptoms during pregnancy. Patients who present with mild exacerbations of asthma may be treated with bronchodilator therapy and steroids.

Severe asthma exacerbations warrant intensive observation. Close monitoring of oxygen levels should be undertaken.

Inhaled beta2-agonists are the mainstay of treatment. In particular, beta-adrenergic blocking agents should be avoided due to a possible increased bronchospastic effect.

The early use of systemic steroids has not been shown to be detrimental and should be given when indicated.

Intense follow-up care should occur. This may include referral to an asthma specialist.

Reference
Rey E, Boulet LP. Asthma in pregnancy. BMJ. 2007;334(7593):582–5.

341. A 32-year-old male is evaluated in the emergency department for diffuse muscle aches. He reports starting an extremely intense "boot camp" exercise routine 3 days ago.

On physical examination, the patient is diffusely tender to touch. He appears uncomfortable. Arms and legs display moderate diffuse swelling. Temperature is normal, blood pressure is 92/50 mmHg, pulse rate is 120 beats/min, and respiratory rate is 20 breaths/min. Oxygen saturation is 97 %. Skin is mottled on the posterior back. Neurological examination findings are nonfocal.

Creatinine is 2.2 units/L, bicarbonate is 17 meq/L, and creatinine kinase (CPK) is 36,000 units/L.

Which of the following is the most appropriate treatment for this patient?
A) Hemodialysis
B) Intravenous mannitol
C) Rapid infusion of intravenous 0.9 % saline
D) Rapid infusion of 5 % dextrose in water
E) Surgical consultation

Answer: C

Rhabdomyolysis is a syndrome caused by extensive injury to skeletal muscle. It involves leakage of potentially toxic intracellular contents into plasma. This can occur in both the trained and non-trained athlete. This often occurs with the initiation of a new intense exercise regimen. The most severe complication is acute kidney injury (AKI). Etiologies of AKI may be related to hypovolemia, vasoconstriction, and myoglobin toxicity. Compartment syndrome of inflamed muscles may be either a complication of or the inciting cause of rhabdomyolysis. Mild diffuse swelling of muscle groups is common. Recommendations for the treatment of rhabdomyolysis include fluid resuscitation first and subsequent prevention of end-organ complications. This is best achieved with 0.9 % saline. Other measures to preserve kidney function may be considered after adequate volume has been given.

Other supportive measures include correction of electrolyte imbalances. Fluids may be started at a rate of approximately 400 mL/h and then titrated to maintain a urine output of at least 200 mL/h. Treatment should continue until CPK displays a marked reduction or until the urine is negative for myoglobin.

Reference
Bosch X, Poch E, Grau JM. Rhabdomyolysis and acute kidney injury. N Engl J Med. 2009;361(1):62–72.

342. A 34-year-old woman is admitted overnight for the acute onset of pain after 10 days of bloody diarrhea. The diarrhea has escalated to 15 times per day. She has ulcerative colitis that was diagnosed 5 years ago. She currently takes azathioprine.

On physical examination, she appears ill. Following aggressive fluid resuscitation overnight, temperature is 38.6 °C (101.5 °F), blood pressure is 68/45 mmHg, pulse rate is 120 beats/min, and respiratory rate is 35 breaths/min. Abdominal examination discloses absent bowel sounds, distention, and diffuse marked tenderness with mild palpation. Radiographs on admissions reveal colonic distension of 5 cm. This am repeat radiographs reveal colonic distension of 8 cm.

Which of the following is the most appropriate management?
A) CT scan
B) Immediate surgery
C) Start infliximab
D) Start intravenous hydrocortisone
E) Immediate gastroenterology consult

Answer: B

Early surgical consultation is essential for cases of toxic megacolon (TM). Indications for urgent operative intervention include free perforation, massive hemorrhage increasing toxicity, and progression of colonic dilatation which is the case here. Most guidelines recommend colectomy if persistent dilatation is present or if no improvement is observed on maximal medical therapy after 24–72 h.

The rationale for early intervention is based on a marked increase in mortality after free perforation. The mortality rate for perforated, acute toxic colitis is approximately 20 %.

Some recommend providing up to 7 days of medical therapy if the patient demonstrates clinical improvement despite persistent colonic dilatation. TM was first thought to be the only complication of ulcerative colitis. It has been described in a number of conditions, including inflammatory, ischemic, infectious, radiation, and pseudomembranous colitis.

References
Marshak RH, Lester LJ. Megacolon a complication of ulcerative colitis. Gastroenterology. 1950;16(4):768–72.
Strong SA. Management of acute colitis and toxic megacolon. Clin Colon Rectal Surg. 2010;23(4):274–84.

343. A 62-year-old woman with a history of stage III colorectal cancer resected 2 years prior is admitted for cellulitis. She responds well to antibiotics. Her routine follow-up for colorectal cancer requires a follow-up CT scan of the chest and abdomen.

A contrast-enhanced CT scan of the chest, abdomen, and pelvis was performed and it reveals a new 1.6-cm liver mass suspicious for malignancy and a large left main pulmonary artery filling defect.

Which of the following is the correct treatment?
A) Low-molecular-weight heparin (LMWH) treatment dose injections
B) LMWH treatment dose followed by warfarin
C) LMWH 40 mg daily
D) Observation alone

Answer: A

Pulmonary embolism (PE) is often incidentally found on computed tomography scans performed for various indications. Treatment protocols have not been established.

Current guidelines recommend using the same approach as is used for patients with suspected PE. This is in accordance with American College of Chest Physicians and American Society of Clinical Oncology consensus recommendations. The recommended duration of anticoagulation for patients with cancer-related PE is 3–6 months and indefinitely if the malignancy persists. LMWH is still the treatment of choice in this group as there are less bleeding and less recurrence than with oral vitamin K antagonists. Convenience, life expectancy and patient preference often indicate therapeutic options.

References
Aviram G, Levy G, Fishman JE, Blank A, Graif M. Pitfalls in the diagnosis of acute pulmonary embolism on spiral computer tomography. Curr Probl Diagn Radiol. 2004;33(2):74–84.
O'Connell CL, Boswell WD, Duddalwar V et al. Unsuspected pulmonary emboli in cancer patients: clinical correlates and relevance. J Clin Oncol. 2006;24(30):4928–32.

344. A 32-year-old woman is admitted for a 4-day history of sore throat, fever, and neck pain. She has severe pain on the left side of her neck with swallowing. She is currently unable to swallow solid foods. She has had fevers for the last week, with rigors starting today. Over the last 3 days, she has had increasing cough. She is otherwise healthy and takes no medications.

On physical examination, the temperature is 39.0 °C (102.1 °F), blood pressure is 140/76 mmHg, pulse rate is 110 beats/min, and respiratory rate is 28 breaths/min. The neck is tender to palpation along the left side, without lymphadenopathy. Poor dentition is noted. The pharynx is erythematous. The chest is clear to auscultation. The remainder of the examination is normal. Chest radiograph reveals multiple punctate densities.

Which of the following tests is most likely to establish the diagnosis?
A) Computed tomography (CT) of the chest with contrast
B) CT of the neck with contrast
C) Radiography of the pharyngeal soft tissues
D) Transthoracic echocardiography
E) Rapid strep test

Answer: B

Lemierre's syndrome generally occurs in young adults. The infection usually begins with a sore throat, fever, septicemia, thrombosis, and metastatic abscesses. Poor dentition can be causative as well. This patient should undergo computed tomography (CT) of the neck with contrast. The diagnosis should be suspected in anyone with pharyngitis, persistent fever, neck pain, and septic pulmonary emboli. CT of the affected vessel with contrast would confirm the diagnosis. Ultrasonography can also confirm internal jugular vein thrombosis, showing localized echogenic regions within a dilated vessel.

Treatment includes intravenous antibiotics that cover streptococci, anaerobes, and β-lactamase-producing organisms. Penicillin with a β-lactamase inhibitor and carbapenem are both reasonable choices. In the preantibiotic era, Lemierre's syndrome was often fatal.

Vascular surgery consultation is reasonable as ligation or excision of the internal jugular vein may be required, and drainage of other abscesses near vascular tissue may be necessary.

Reference

Golpe R, Marin B, Alonso M. Lemierre's syndrome (necrobacillosis). Postgrad Med J. 1999;75:141–4.

345. An 85-year-old man with very poor functional status is admitted from the nursing home with severe shortness of breath. He has a history of a prior cerebrovascular accident that has resulted in right hemiparesis and aphasia.

Chest X-ray shows that he has severe pneumonia. Before the entire family arrives, the patient is intubated immediately and transferred to the ICU. After a joint conference, the family decides to remove life support. Which of the following statements accurately characterizes ventilator withdrawal in this situation?
A) You should suggest 24 more hours of observation.
B) Limit family interaction while the patient is extubated.
C) Pulse oximetry should be followed to help guide the family through the dying process.
D) You should demonstrate that the patient is comfortable receiving a lower fraction of inspired oxygen (FIO2) before withdrawing the endotracheal tube.
E) Such patients generally die within 30 min to an hour after the endotracheal tube is removed.

Answer: D

The family should be given the opportunity to be with the patient when the endotracheal tube is removed. The decision should be theirs to make and be a part of hospital protocol. All monitors including oxygen saturation should be turned off. The patient's comfort should guide therapy. FIO2 should be diminished to 20 %. The patient should be observed for respiratory distress before removing the endotracheal tube. Distress and air hunger can be treated with opioids and benzodiazepines prior to endotracheal tube removal.

The family often expects an immediate response when the ventilator is turned off. It is important to inform them that the patient may live for hours to days. Also it is important to explain that you and staff will continue to follow and provide comfort during this period.

End-of-life care is increasingly seen not as medical failure but a special time to assist the patient, family, and staff with the physical and emotional needs that occur with the dying of a patient. Resources, protocols, and education should be provided to staff to enhance these efforts.

References

Torkelson DJ, Dobal MT. Constant observation in medical-surgical settings: a multihospital study. Nurs Econ. 1999;17(3):149–55.

Wiegand DL. In their own time: the family experience during the process of withdrawal of life-sustaining therapy. J Palliat Med. 2008;11(8):1115–21.

346. A 75-year-old woman is admitted with an ischemic cerebrovascular accident. She is dysarthric and fails a bedside swallow study. On day 3 she is started on tube feeds at 40 ml/h. Her goal rate is 70 ml h. Four hours after her tube feeds are started, gastric residuals are measured to be 375 ml.

Which of the following should you recommend now?
A) Withhold the feeding for 2 h, and then restart at 20 mL/h.
B) Decrease the feeding rate to 20 mL/h.
C) Continuing the feeding at the current rate.
D) Advancing the feedings toward the patient's goal rate.
E) Start motility agent.

Answer: D

In this patient, the feedings should be increased toward the goal rate. There is no correlation between gastric residual volume and the incidence of aspiration. Evidence shows that checking gastric residuals doesn't provide reliable information on tube-feeding tolerance, aspiration risk, or gastric emptying. Current guidelines recommend withholding feedings for gastric residual volumes greater than 500 mL.

Reference

McClave S et al. Poor validity of residual volumes as a marker for risk of aspiration in critically ill patients. Crit Care Med. 2005;33:324–30.

What is the best method for assessing pain in the nonverbal patient?
A) Monitoring vital signs
B) Eliciting information from patient surrogates
C) Observing behaviors
D) Analgesic trials
E) B, C, and D

Answer: E

In nonverbal patients, pain assessment relies less on vital-sign changes and more on observing behaviors. Pain assessment in nonverbal and dementia patients can be challenging. Information should be elicited from multiple sources including the patient's surrogates who may have better insight into the patient's nonverbal communication. Analgesic trials may be helpful when pain is suspected but not confirmed. A series of validated tools for physicians and nurses can be used to develop hospital-wide programs.

Reference

Lukas A, Barber JB, Johnson P, Gibson SJ. Observer-rated pain assessment instruments improve both the detection of pain and the evaluation of pain intensity in people with dementia. Eur J Pain. 2013;17(10):1558–68.

347. A 48-year-old female is transferred to your hospital after an automobile accident where she sustained an open fracture to her femur. An open reduction is planned. 48 h after admission she develops the acute onset of shortness of breath. Over the next hour she develops mild confusion and a petechial rash in her axilla.

What is NOT true concerning her diagnosis and treatment?
A) Respiratory changes are often the first clinical feature to present.
B) Neurological changes occur in up to 80 % of cases.
C) Mortality is estimated to be 5–15 %.
D) Supportive care is the mainstay of therapy.
E) Steroids have no role in the treatment.

Answer: E

The fat embolism syndrome typically presents 24–72 h after the initial injury.

Dyspnea, tachypnea, and hypoxemia are the earliest findings. This may progress to respiratory failure and a syndrome indistinguishable from acute respiratory distress syndrome (ARDS) may develop. Cerebral emboli produce neurological signs in up to 80 % of cases. This is often the second symptom to appear. The characteristic petechial rash may be the third component of the triad to occur.

There is no specific therapy for fat embolism syndrome. Early immobilization of fractures has been shown to reduce the incidence of fat embolism syndrome and should be of primary importance with extensive long bone fractures. The risk is reduced by operative correction rather than conservative management. The use of steroids has been extensively studied for both prevention and treatment. It is recommended by some, for the management of the fat embolism syndrome. However, there have been no prospective, randomized, and controlled clinical studies that have demonstrated a significant benefit with their use.

References
Kaplan RP, Grant JN, Kaufman AJ. Dermatologic features of the fat embolism syndrome. Cutis. 1986;38:52–5.
Lindeque B, Schoeman H, Dommisse G, Boeyens MC, Vlok AL. Fat embolism and the fat embolism syndrome. J Bone Joint Surg. 1987;69B:128–31.

348. A 75-year-old woman who lives in a nursing facility fell and fractured her hip. She is admitted to the combined medicine orthopedic service for open reduction and internal fixation of the hip. She was admitted for an acute myocardial infarction 5 months prior to the current admission, which was treated with angioplasty and a drug-eluting stent. Outpatient medications are omeprazole, alendronate, weekly methotrexate, aspirin (325 mg daily), clopidogrel (75 mg daily), and paroxetine.

The patient's outpatient medications are continued perioperatively. The patient is placed empirically on ceftriaxone for a possible urinary tract infection. On day 3 she develops incisional bleeding at the site of her hip fracture repair site.

On physical exam, temperature is 38.0 °C (100.4 °F), pulse rate is 90 beats/per minute, respirations are 22 per minute, and blood pressure is 120/80 mmHg. A large hematoma with serosanguinous drainage is noted along the right hip.

Which of the following medications is most likely to increase the risk of bleeding in this patient?
A) Omeprazole
B) Ceftriaxone
C) Methotrexate
D) Paroxetine

Answer: D

Perioperative use of selective serotonin reuptake inhibitors (SSRIs) has been linked to an increased risk of bleeding, transfusion, hospital readmission, and death.

Despite this, stopping SSRIs preoperatively may not be warranted.

In the preoperative setting, abruptly stopping an SSRI before surgery could precipitate an SSRI withdrawal syndrome. In addition worsening of depression or other underlying conditions being treated by the drug could occur. It is important for clinicians to be aware of the risk for SSRI-associated bleeding complications.

Reference
Labos A. Risk of bleeding associated with combined use of selective serotonin reuptake inhibitors and antiplatelet therapy following acute myocardial infarction. CMAJ. 2011;183(16):1835.

349. A 62-year-old female is admitted for facial and neck cellulitis. Computed tomography of the neck in the

emergency department reveals soft tissue swelling and an incidental 1.2-cm nodule on the thyroid gland, which was nonpalpable on physical examination. She responds well to antibiotics and is ready for discharge. All thyroid functions are within normal limits.

Which of the following is the most appropriate management for this patient?

A) No further evaluation is needed.
B) Repeat computed tomography of the neck in 6 months.
C) Repeat computed tomography of the neck in 1 year.
D) Ultrasonography of the thyroid gland.
E) Thyroid uptake scan.

Answer: D

Current guidelines currently recommend that incidentally discovered thyroid nodules found by CT scan have the same follow-up as clinically evident nodules. Based on this patient having a greater than 1-cm thyroid nodule, the next step in the evaluation should be a diagnostic thyroid ultrasound. This can occur in the outpatient setting as it is not related to the reason for presentation.

Reference

Thyroid Association (ATA) Guidelines Taskforce on Thyroid Nodules and Differentiated Thyroid Cancer, Cooper DS et al. Revised American Thyroid Association management guidelines for patients with thyroid nodules and differentiated thyroid cancer. Thyroid. 2009;19:1167–214.

350. Which of the following is the percentage of surrogate decision-makers for critically ill patients experienced bereavement in addition to the normal grieving process several months after the event?

A) Less than 5 %
B) Approximately 33 %
C) Approximately 70 %
D) Greater than 85 %

Answer: B

Surrogate decision-making can place a great deal of stress on caregivers. Approximately 33 % of people who serve as surrogate decision-makers for critically ill patients experience ongoing stress that can last for months and sometimes years. A proactive and formalized approach to treating surrogate decision-makers is needed. In one pilot study, brief counseling and a brochure on bereavement significantly decreased post-traumatic stress disorder (PTSD)-related symptoms and symptoms of anxiety and depression among family members.

Reference

Wendler D, Rid A. Systematic review: the effect on surrogates of making treatment decisions for others. Ann Intern Med. 2011;154:336–46.

351. Which of the following potential risk factors is associated with severe postextubation dysphagia?

A) Age
B) Weight
C) Sex
D) Intubation in the ED
E) Reintubation
F) C and E

Answer: F

Severe postextubation dysphagia requiring dietary modification is associated with reintubation, male gender, and ventilator days. Age, weight, and place of intubation are not correlated with dysphagia.

Reference

Macht M et al. Postextubation dysphagia is persistent and associated with poor outcomes in survivors of critical illness. Crit Care. 2011;15:R231.

352. A 45-year-old attorney presents with midepigastric pain, nausea, and vomiting. He has no prior medical history. He denied any alcohol intake and takes no over the counter medicines.

On physical exam, blood pressure is 140/70 mmHg, and heart rate is 70 bpm. Mild midepigastric tenderness is appreciated.

On admission amylase is 235 units/L, lipase is 175 unit/L, and alkaline phospatase is 52 g/dl. He is started in intravenous fluids and has a rapid resolution of his symptoms the following day. Amylase on the second day is 38 units/L and lipase is 86 units/L. Ultrasound of the abdomen reveals a gallbladder with several stones. No gallbladder wall thickening is appreciated.

What is the correct management of this patient?

A) Discharge home with no further intervention.
B) Surgical follow-up for cholecystectomy
C) Cholecystectomy prior to discharge
D) HIDA scan

Answer: C

If possible, patients admitted with gallstone pancreatitis should undergo cholecystectomy before discharge, rather than being scheduled as an outpatient. Patients discharged without a cholecystectomy are at high risk for recurrent bouts of pancreatitis. Recurrent episodes may be more severe than the original presentation.

In one study, patients with mild gallstone pancreatitis who underwent laparoscopic cholecystectomy within 48 h of admission resulted in a shorter hospital stay. There was no apparent impact on the technical difficulty of the procedure or the perioperative complication rate.

In cases of severe pancreatitis, it may be appropriate to delay surgery in order to allow time for systemic and pancreatic inflammation to resolve.

Reference
Aboulian A, Chan T, Yaghoubian A, Kaji AH, Putnam B, Neville A et al. Early cholecystectomy safely decreases hospital stay in patients with mild gallstone pancreatitis: a randomized prospective study. Ann Surg. 2010;251(4):615–9.

353. Which of the following will provide the best bowel preparation for a morning colonoscopy?
    A) 4 L polyethylene glycol-based preparation plus citric acid taken the evening before the procedure
    B) 2 L polyethylene glycol-based preparation taken the evening before the procedure
    C) 2 L of polyethylene glycol-based preparation on the evening before and 2 L of the same preparation on the morning of the procedure
    D) 1 L of polyethylene glycol-based preparation n the evening before and 1 L of the same preparation on the morning of the procedure

Answer: C
Significant evidence exists that better colon preparation is associated with increased detection of colon polyps. Split-dose bowel preparation remains an essential concept for enhancing the quality of colonoscopy. This limits the amount of agent remaining in the colon prior to examination.

Many bowel preparations for colonoscopy are available. No preparation has been shown to be superior to 4 L of a polyethylene glycol-based preparation split into two 2-L doses that are given the evening prior to and the morning of the procedure.

References
Enestvedt BK, Tofani C, Laine LA et al. 4-Liter split-dose polyethylene glycol is superior to other bowel preparations, based on systematic review and meta-analysis. Clin Gastroenterol Hepatol. 2012;10(11):1225–31.
Hassan C, Fuccio L, Bruno M et al. A predictive model identifies patients most likely to have inadequate bowel preparation for colonoscopy. Clin Gastroenterol Hepatol. 2012;10(5):501–6.

354. A 67-year-old man with metastatic lung cancer is admitted for failure to thrive. During this admission, several end-of-life issues are addressed. He has chosen not to consider additional chemotherapy or radiation therapy. His cancer is unlikely to respond to such treatment.

He and his family are focused on upcoming visits with his 4 children and 14 grandchildren over the next several weeks. However, the family reports that his lethargy, poor appetite, and depression will make this difficult. You estimate the patient's life expectancy to be weeks to several months.

Which of the following would be the best management of this patient's symptoms?
    A) Initiation of a trial of a methylphenidate
    B) Referral of the patient to a psychologist
    C) Trial of a selective serotonin reuptake inhibitor
    D) Initiation of enteral feedings through a nasogastric tube
    E) Initiation of oral morphine

Answer: A
The use of psychostimulants, such as methylphenidate, is an effective management for cancer-related fatigue, opioid-induced sedation, and the symptoms of depression in the setting of a limited prognosis. Helping this patient achieve some of his end-of-life wishes is important. Psychostimulants have the benefit of providing more immediate response than conventional therapies. It is improbable that this patient will live long enough to benefit from cognitive behavioral therapy, SSRI, or nutritional support. Starting methylphenidate 2.5 mg PO BID is a reasonable choice when time is limited.

Reference
Li M, Fitzgerald P, Rodin G. Evidence-based treatment of depression in patients with cancer. J Clin Oncol. 2012;30:1187–96.

355. A 67-year-old man is admitted with severe right buttock pain. In the previous year, the patient underwent resection and laminectomy for metastatic renal cell tumor compressing his lower thoracic and upper lumbar spinal cord. The mass is inoperable, and he is receiving palliative chemotherapy. Hospice has not been discussed yet.

During his admission, the pain has been severe and refractory to intravenous opioids. His daily requirement of hydromorphone is 150–175 mg for the past 4 days.

On physical examination, vital signs are stable. He is somnolent, and when he wakes up he is in severe pain. Motor strength assessment is limited by pain.

Which of the following should you recommend now?
    A) Trial of methylphenidate
    B) Placement of an implanted intrathecal drug pump
    C) Optimization of the opioid regimen
    D) A trial of intrathecal analgesia
    E) Lidocaine patch

Answer: D
This patient requires aggressive pain control measures. Changing opioid regimens will probably be of little benefit. Evidence supports the use of intrathecal drug delivery

systems compared with systemic analgesics in opioid-refractory patients. A trial of intrathecal medication is important, to determine the effect, prior to permanent placement of an implanted device.

His previous laminectomy and associated scarring may limit the effect of intrathecal delivery as well as make catheter placement difficult. The use of palliative sedation therapy is indicated in patients with refractory symptoms at the end of life. Although his pain is severe and unresponsive to systemic medications, she is not at the end of life, nor have all interventions been pursued to address her pain.

Reference

Deer TR, Smith HS, Burton AW et al. Comprehensive consensus based guidelines on intrathecal drug delivery systems in the treatment of pain caused by cancer pain. Pain Physician. 2011;14(3):E283–312.

356. A 56-year-old woman has widely metastatic breast cancer. She is admitted for sepsis. The decision has been made to withdraw care and to allow a natural death preferably as an inpatient. The family is at the bedside. Oxygen saturation is 85 % with the patient receiving supplemental oxygen, 2 L/min by nasal cannula.

    On physical examination, she is nonverbal and restless in bed. Her respirations have become more difficult. The family appears fatigued and anxious.

    Which of the following should you do now?
    A) Request a sitter.
    B) Provide 100 % oxygen by face mask.
    C) Administer a dose of parenteral haloperidol.
    D) Administer a dose of parenteral morphine.
    E) Administer a dose of parenteral dexamethasone.

Answer: D

Morphine is the drug of choice with air hunger at the end of life. It is preferred over other sedation. There is no evidence that supplemental oxygen is beneficial at the end of life. In addition, many patients experience increased agitation when a mask is placed over the mouth and nose. Family members may not desire a face mask for the patient as well during this special time.

Reference

Ben-Aharon I, Gafter-Gvili A, Leibovici L, Stemmer SM. Interventions for alleviating cancer-related dyspnea: a systematic review and meta-analysis. Acta Oncol. 2012;51(8):996–1008.

357. A 78-year-old woman who has recurrent breast cancer with metastasis is admitted for decreased appetite. Her last bowel movement was 4 days ago. She is on long-acting morphine with oxycodone for breakthrough pain. Her bowel regimen is docusate, 100 mg twice daily.

On physical examination, her abdomen is distended. A radiograph of the abdomen demonstrates a large amount of stool. She is given three enemas, which produce a small amount of stool.

Which of the following is the most appropriate next step in the management of this patient's constipation?
A) Administer lactulose.
B) Administer methylnaltrexone.
C) Administration of high-dose senna.
D) Placement of a nasogastric tube (NGT) for high-volume laxative.
E) Rotation to another opioid.

Answer: B

Methylnaltrexone is used for severe constipation in opioid-induced ileus. It is well tolerated in most instances. This patient has already shown an intolerance of stimulant laxatives; further measures are unlikely to be successful. An NGT would be uncomfortable.

References

Sawh SB, Selvaraj IP, Danga A et al. Use of methylnaltrexone for the treatment of opioid-induced constipation in critical care patients. Mayo Clin Proc. 2012;87(3):255–9.

Thomas J, Karver S, Cooney GA et al. Methylnaltrexone for opioid-induced constipation in advanced illness. N Engl J Med. 2008;358(22):2332–43.

358. A 68-year-old female is evaluated for preoperative clearance before she goes in for left knee elective surgery. She has a history of chronic hypertension. She has on amlodipine but has been noncompliant with her medicines. Her knee pain limits her activities but she is able to walk up two flights of stairs with minimal difficulty.

    On physical exam her blood pressure is 145/99 mmHg, heart rate is 55 bpm, and respiratory rate is 11 breaths/min. Extremities pulses are 2+ and bilateral. An echo done 7 months ago shows an ejection fraction of 30 %. The patient denies any new complaints.

    What is the next step?
    A) Proceed with surgery without additional preoperative testing.
    B) Control BP to ideal measurement of <130/85.
    C) Delay elective surgery for further evaluation or treatment.
    D) Exercise stress test.
    E) Start metoprolol.

Answer: A

Preoperative hypertension is frequently a hypertensive urgency, not an emergency. In general, patients with chronic hypertension may proceed to low-risk surgery as long as the diastolic BP is <110 mmHg.

There continues to be some debate over the use of beta-blockers preoperatively. Current guidelines state that in patients with no risk factors, starting beta-blockers in the perioperative setting provides unknown benefit.

Reference

Thomas DR, Ritchie CS. Preoperative assessment of older adults. J Am Geriatr Soc. 1995;43(7):811–21.

359. You are asked to admit a 32-year-old female for a 4-day history of lower abdominal pain that she describes as intermittent cramps. She denies nausea or vomiting. She also denies having urinary frequency, dysuria, and flank pain. Her only medication is an oral contraceptive agent.

On physical examination, her temperature is 38.5 °C (101.4 °F), blood pressure is 120/68 mmHg, pulse rate is 100 beats/min, and respiratory rate is 18 breaths/min. Abdominal examination is normal. There is no flank tenderness. Pelvic examination shows cervical motion tenderness. Bilateral adnexal tenderness is appreciated on bimanual examination. She is in minimal distress and is tolerating liquids. The hematologic and serum chemistries are normal. Urine and serum pregnancy tests are negative.

What is the next best step in the management of this patient?
A) Consult for laparoscopic diagnosis and treatment.
B) Admit the patient to the hospital, obtain pelvic ultrasound, and start ceftriaxone.
C) Administer a single-dose IM ceftriaxone and discharge the patient.
D) Administer a single-dose IM ceftriaxone and oral doxycycline for 14 days.
E) Obtain pelvic and abdominal ultrasound and prescribe oral doxycycline with metronidazole.

Answer: D

This patient's clinical findings are compatible with pelvic inflammatory disease (PID). Women with mild to moderate PID may receive outpatient medical treatment without increased risk of long-term sequelae.

Laparoscopy is the criterion standard for the diagnosis of PID, but the diagnosis of PID in emergency departments is often based on clinical criteria, without additional laboratory and imaging evidence.

She should receive intramuscular ceftriaxone and oral doxycycline for 14 days. All women with suspected PID should be tested for infection with gonorrhea and chlamydia. In severe cases, imaging should be performed to exclude a tuboovarian abscess.

Patients with PID should be hospitalized if there is (1) no clinical improvement after 48–72 h of antibiotics, (2) an inability to tolerate food or medicine, (3) severe symptoms, (4) suspected abscess, (4) pregnancy, or (5) predicted noncompliance with therapy.

References
Ness RB, Soper DE, Holley RL, Peipert J, Randall H, Sweet RL et al. Effectiveness of inpatient and outpatient treatment strategies for women with pelvic inflammatory disease: results from the Pelvic Inflammatory Disease Evaluation and Clinical Health (PEACH) Randomized Trial. Am J Obstet Gynecol. 2002;186:929–37.
Paavonen J. *Chlamydia trachomatis* infections of the female genital tract: state of the art. Ann Med. 2012;44(1):18–28.

360. Which of the following is the most common cause of erythema multiforme?
A) *Mycoplasma pneumoniae*
B) *Herpes simplex*
C) Amoxicillin
D) Cytomegalovirus

Answer: B

One of the most common predisposing factors for erythema multiforme is infection with herpes simplex virus, which may or may not be active at the time of the EM eruption. EM is an acute, self-limited, and sometimes recurring skin condition that is considered to be a type IV hypersensitivity reaction. It is associated with infections, medications, and other various triggers. Patients with recurrent EM are typically treated with acyclovir or valacyclovir. Mycoplasma pneumonia, amoxicillin, ibuprofen, and cytomegalovirus may cause EM, but are not as common.

Reference
Aurelian L, Ono F, Burnett J. Herpes simplex virus (HSV)-associated erythema multiforme (HAEM): a viral disease with an autoimmune component. Dermatol Online J. 2003;9:1.

361. A 65-year-old male with a long history of type II diabetes is admitted with the chief complaint of hematuria.

His blood pressure is 130/65 mmHg. Otherwise his physical exam is normal. Urinalysis shows blood 3+ and protein 3+. No casts are seen. A 24-h urinary protein shows 8 g of protein and serum creatinine is normal. Urine microscopy shows isomorphic red blood cells with no casts. Renal and bladder ultrasound are normal. His hematuria is less by day 2 of his admission.

What is the next most appropriate investigation?
A) Renal angiogram
B) Renal biopsy
C) Doppler ultrasound of the kidneys
D) CT scan of the abdomen and thorax alone
E) Cystoscopy
F) Observation alone

Answer: E

This man has hematuria without evidence of dysmorphic red cells or casts in urinary sediment. Macroscopic hematuria in the absence of significant proteinuria or RBC casts is an indication for imaging to exclude malignancy or cystic renal disease. Approximately 80–90 % of patients with bladder cancer present with painless gross hematuria. Urine cytology is extremely valuable but would not eliminate the need for cystoscopy, which is the standard for diagnosing bladder cancer.

Many bleeding urinary tract lesions arise in the bladder and lower urinary tract, and no imaging technique is completely satisfactory for ruling out disease at these sites. Further imaging may be of use but cystoscopy will ultimately be needed.

Reference
Grossfeld GD, Litwin MS, Wolf JS Jr, Hricak H, Shuler CL, Agerter DC et al. Evaluation of asymptomatic microscopic hematuria in adults: the American Urological Association best practice policy – part II: patient evaluation, cytology, voided markers, imaging, cystoscopy, nephrology evaluation, and follow-up. Urology. 2001;57(4):604–10.

362. A 47-year-old woman with a history of ulcerative colitis (UC) is hospitalized for progressive cramping abdominal pain, hematochezia, fever, and up to 15 bloody bowel movements daily. She is resuscitated with IV fluids, and methylprednisolone 60 mg is started. After 5 days of steroids, she continues to have ten bloody bowel movements with persistent abdominal pain.

    Which of the following is NOT an appropriate course of action?
    A) Infectious workup.
    B) Consider starting infliximab.
    C) Surgery consult.
    D) Consider starting cyclosporine.
    E) Increase the dose of steroids.

Answer: E

The American College of Gastroenterology practice guidelines define severe colitis as the passage of six or more stools per day with evidence of systemic toxicity. Intravenous corticosteroids, which are essential in severe cases, are effective in the induction of remission in the majority of cases. A daily intravenous steroid dose of hydrocortisone 300 mg or methylprednisolone 60 mg is suggested. Fortunately, most patients with severe UC respond to intravenous steroid therapy. However, 30 % of patients fail to respond after 5–7 days. These patients are considered to be steroid refractory.

One of the simplest algorithms predicts that at the third day of intravenous steroid therapy, patients with a stool frequency of greater than eight per day or three per day plus a CRP greater than 45 mg/dl have an 85 % likelihood of requiring colectomy.

Medical treatment of steroid-refractory severe UC has expanded with the availability of both cyclosporine and infliximab as rescue agents. The need for colectomy may be reduced with the use of these agents. In addition, stool samples should be collected for culture and toxin analysis to rule out enteric infection.

References
Rosenberg W, Ireland A, Jewell DP. High-dose methylprednisolone in the treatment of active ulcerative colitis. J Clin Gastroenterol. 1990;12(1):40–1.

Travis SP. Predicting outcome in severe ulcerative colitis. Gut. 1996;38(6):905–10.

363. A 67-year-old male is admitted for total knee replacement (TKR). He has a history of severe rheumatoid arthritis (RA) for which he has been on several aggressive medication regimens in the past. In preparation for surgery, he stopped taking ibuprofen a week prior to the surgery.

    On physical exam, he has moderate diffuse joint tenderness which is no different from his baseline. He has some nontender bumps palpated on the forearm bilaterally near to the olecranon process and displacement of metacarpal bones over the proximal phalanges with flexion at proximal joints and with extension of distal interphalangeal joints. Labs are within normal range.

    What is the appropriate recommendation?
    A) CT scan of the neck prior to surgery.
    B) CT scan of the neck prior to surgery.
    C) Avoidance of a paralytic drug during surgery.
    D) Radiograph of the neck in flexion and extension.
    E) Proceed to surgery.

Answer: D

Patients with RA presenting for TKR represent those patients who have failed medical management and are a high-risk group for cervical spine involvement. Radiographic screening of RA patients presenting for joint replacement surgery reveals cervical spine instability in 44 %, which is typically asymptomatic. Lateral flexion/extension views are more sensitive and are recommended. Cervical spine subluxation is less likely in RA patients presenting for general surgery, and there is currently no consensus on who should be screened in this population.

Reference
Neva MH, Hakkinen A, Makinen H et al. High prevalence of asymptomatic cervical spine subluxation in patients with rheumatoid arthritis waiting for orthopaedic surgery. Ann Rheum Dis. 2006;65:884–8.

364. A 33-year-old woman is admitted to the hospital for evaluation of blurry vision and new-onset paraparesis. She has been followed closely by neurology in the past for two recent episodes of optic neuritis in the past 2 years. Her only other history is hypothyroidism. Her only medication is levothyroxine.

On physical examination vital signs are normal. Visual acuity is 20/200 in the right eye and 20/30 in the left. Per ophthalmology consult, optic disks display pallor. Significant spasticity is noted in her legs. The patient requires bilateral assistance to ambulate.

Laboratory studies including a complete blood count, liver chemistry and renal function tests, and erythrocyte sedimentation rate are normal. The antinuclear antibody is positive. Anti-double-stranded DNA and anti-SSA/SSB antibodies are negative. Analysis of the cerebrospinal fluid shows a normal IgG index and no abnormalities in oligoclonal banding.

An MRI of the spinal cord reveals an increased signal extending over five vertebral segments with patchy gadolinium enhancement. An MRI of the brain shows no abnormalities.

Which of the following is the most appropriate next diagnostic test?

A) Electromyography
B) Serum antineutrophil cytoplasmic antibody test
C) Serum neuromyelitis optica (NMO)-IgG autoantibody test
D) Testing of visual evoked potentials
E) Neuromyelitis optica (NMO)-IgG autoantibody test
F) CSF to serum protein ratio

Answer: E

Neuromyelitis optica (NMO), the presentation of myelitis and optic neuritis, may be a variant of multiple sclerosis (MS) or a unique disease. This patient very likely has neuromyelitis optica (NMO). She should be tested for the autoantibody marker NMO-IgG.

Differentiating between NMO and MS early in the disease may be important because the prognosis and treatment of the two diseases are different. NMO is a more severe disease treated with immunosuppressive drugs. MS is often initially treated with immunomodulatory therapies, such as β-interferon and glatiramer acetate.

The MRI is suggested of NMO. In typical MS, lesions are usually less than two segments in length.

The NMO-IgG test is approximately 75 % sensitive and more than 90 % specific for NMO.

References

Lennon VA, Wingerchuk DM, Kryzer TJ, Pittock SJ, Lucchinetti CF, Fujihara K, Nakashima I, Weinshenker BG. A serum autoantibody marker of neuromyelitis optica: distinction from multiple sclerosis. Lancet. 2004;364:2106–12.

Wingerchuk DM, Hogancamp WF, O'Brien PC, Weinshenker BG. The clinical course of neuromyelitis optica (Devic's syndrome). Neurology. 1999;53:1107–14.

Hospital Systems Management

Marianne Maumus and Kevin Conrad

365. As the unit medical director, you are asked by hospital administration to recommend and lead a process that will limit practice variability and better align hospital resuscitation practices with evidence-based guidelines. During codes there is great deal of variability dependent upon the time of day, staff present, and location.

Which of the following would you suggest?
A) Increasing the frequency of advanced cardiovascular life support (ACLS) training to become an annual requirement for all clinical practitioners
B) Interviewing hospital staff using a Delphi method process to enumerate optimal resuscitation practices
C) Implementation of the American Heart Association (AHA) Get with the Guidelines – Resuscitation program
D) Developing resuscitation-specific privileges that are required for all hospital- credentialed

Answer: C
Often the first step in a performance improvement project is to research currently validated programs. According to the American Heart Association (AHA), the Get with the Guidelines program was developed to identify improvement opportunities, allow performance comparison among hospitals, and reduce medical errors through data-driven peer review. The program includes specific up-to-date consensus statements and guidelines for resuscitation, atrial fibrillation, heart failure, and stroke.

Reference
American Heart Association. http://www.heart.org/HEARTORG/HealthcareResearch/GetWithTheGuidelinesHFStroke/GetWithTheGuidelinesStrokeHomePage/Get-With-Guidelines-Stroke-Overview.

366. A 55-year-old male with type 2 diabetes mellitus, hypertension, and hyperlipidemia presents with fever, hypotension, and decreased urine output. He is admitted to the intensive care unit with sepsis due to pyelonephritis. In addition to broad-spectrum antibiotics, the patient has received one liter of fluid resuscitation with 0.9 % saline. Two hours after presentation, the blood pressure is currently 73/42 mmHg. Temperature is 36.8 °C (98.2 °F), pulse rate is 120 beats/minute, and respiratory rate is 24 breaths/minute. Hematocrit is 29 %, blood sugar is 257 mg/dL, and serum lactate is 3.0 mg/dL.

Which of the following is the most likely to improve mortality in this particular patient?
A) Continued fluid resuscitation with colloid added
B) Intensive insulin therapy to maintain euglycemia
C) Vasopressor therapy
D) Bicarbonate infusion
E) Transfusion with PRBC

Answer: C
This patient has not responded to aggressive fluid resuscitation per sepsis guidelines. At this point within 6 h of attempted fluid resuscitation, vasopressor therapy is indicated and has been shown to improve mortality. Intensive insulin therapy and fluid resuscitation with colloid have been recommended for critical illnesses in the past. However, recent trials have failed to show a definitive benefit of these therapies in severe sepsis. Intensive insulin therapy increases

M. Maumus, MD
Department of Hospital Medicine, Ochsner Health Systems, 1521 Jefferson Highway, New Orleans, LA 70121, USA
e-mail: mmaumus@Ochsner.org

K. Conrad, MD, MBA (✉)
Department of Hospital Medicine, Ochsner Health Systems, 1521 Jefferson Highway, New Orleans, LA 70121, USA

Tulane University School of Medicine, New Orleans, LA USA

University of Queensland School of Medicine, New Orleans, LA USA
e-mail: kconrad@ochsner.org

risk of hypoglycemia and has not been shown to improve mortality in an acute setting of sepsis.

Reference

Dellinger RP, Levy MM, Carlet JM, et al. Surviving sepsis campaign: international guidelines for management of severe sepsis and septic shock. Crit Care Med. 2008;36:296–327.

367. Which clinical outcome is reduced with the use of chlorhexidine bathing compared to soap and water bathing in ICU patients?
    A) Global infection rates
    B) Ventilator-associated pneumonia (VAP) rates
    C) Catheter-associated urinary tract infection (CAUTI) rates
    D) All of the above

Answer: D

All of the answers are correct. Bathing with chlorhexidine-impregnated wipes was associated with both global and specific infection rate reduction in a study of >1000 ICU patients when compared to soap and water bathing.

Reference

Michael W. Climo, et al. Effect of daily chlorhexidine bathing on hospital-acquired infection. N Engl J Med. 2013;368:533–42.

368. What is true concerning postoperative cognitive dysfunction (POCD)?
    A) POCD is less likely to occur after operations under regional anesthesia as under general anesthesia.
    B) More likely after major, than minor, operations.
    C) More likely after cardiac surgery than other types of surgery.
    D) More likely in aged than in younger patients.
    E) All of the above.

Answer: E

The risk of POCD increases with age, type, and duration of surgery. There is a very low incidence among all age groups associated with minor surgery. POCD is common in adult patients of all ages at hospital discharge after major noncardiac surgery. The elderly (aged 60 years or older) are at significant risk for long-term cognitive problems, which may last as long as 6 months or become permanent.

Reference

Rasmussen LS. Postoperative cognitive dysfunction: incidence and prevention best practice & research. Clin Anaesthesiol. 2006;20(2):315–30.

369. A 35-year-old female with AIDS is admitted for failure to thrive. She is experiencing chronic diarrhea and anorexia. The family has struggled to get her to eat more than a few bites per day. She has no obvious opportunistic infections. Her family is distressed that the cause of her continued decline appears to be lack of oral intake. They request that home IV nutrition be established.

On physical exam the temperature is 36.2 °C (97.2 °F), heart rate 55 bpm, blood pressure 100/62 mmHg, respiratory rate 12 breaths/min, height 74 in, and weight 45 kg. She appears chronically ill. There is bitemporal wasting, and her hair is thinning.

Which of the following statements regarding home total parenteral nutrition (TPN) is true?
    A) Survival and quality of life are improved in patients with metastatic cancer who are receiving home TPN.
    B) Survival and quality of life are improved in patients with AIDS who are receiving home TPN.
    C) Survival and quality of life are improved in patients with short bowel from Crohn's disease who are receiving home TPN.
    D) No evidence supports the use of home TPN.

Answer: C

Mean survival in AIDS patients or those with metastatic cancer who received home TPN for failure to thrive is about 3 months. There is no evidence that home TPN prolongs life or improves quality of life in these patients. Home TPN is expensive and is indicated in select circumstances. Patients with short bowel resulting from the treatment of Crohn's disease or pseudo-obstruction have a good response to home TPN. In these patients, TPN increases quality-adjusted years of life patients and is cost-effective. There is little evidence to support the use of home TPN, in most chronic diseases resulting in malnutrition.

References

Hoda D, Jatoi A, Burnes J, Loprinzi C, Kelly D. Should patients with advanced, incurable cancers ever be sent home with total parenteral nutrition? Cancer. 2005;103:863–8.

Mullady DK, O'Keefe SJ. Treatment of intestinal failure: home parenteral nutrition. Nat Clin Pract Gastroenterol Hepatol. 2006;3:492–504.

370. A 78-year-old man who has ischemic heart failure, New York Heart Association (NYHA) functional class IV, and severe chronic obstructive pulmonary disease is admitted to the ICU for cardiac decompensation. This is his third admission in the past 2 months, and he is now having difficulty with his activities of daily living. The patient's current medications are carvedilol, lisinopril, spironolactone, furosemide, and beta agonist inhalers. He had previously taken warfarin and aspirin, but had significant bleeding from a gastric ulcer 3 weeks prior to admission, which prompted discontinuation.

Two years ago, an automatic implantable cardioverter defibrillator (AICD) was placed with a transvenous approach for persistent ventricular arrhythmias. In the past 2 weeks, the AICD has fired six times. The patient's daughter reports that since his last hospital discharge, the patient has spent most of his time sleeping in a recliner or in bed and has a poor appetite.

On physical examination, the patient is dyspneic and poorly communicative, but denies current chest pain.

Which of the following is the correct treatment?
A) Initiation of a milrinone infusion
B) Angiography for possi(ble percutaneous intervention
C) Insertion of an intra-aortic balloon pump
D) Deactivation of the AICD
E) AICD recalibration

Answer: D
This patient has multiple indicators for the definition of advanced chronic heart failure, including symptom-based high New York Heart Association (NYHA) classification, severe chronic obstructive pulmonary disease, and left ventricular ejection fraction below 30 %. Palliative care is appropriate and should be offered. The most reasonable intervention at this time is deactivation of the automatic implantable cardioverter defibrillator (AICD). Failure to deactivate the AICD leaves many patients vulnerable to inappropriate device discharge, unnecessary discomfort, and intense anxiety. Other measures, such as infusion of positive inotropes, are used on a temporary basis with a plan for more definitive therapies. The use of intermittent infusions to control symptoms is not recommended by the AHA/ACC guidelines unless the patient is awaiting definitive therapy, such as transplantation.

371. A 64-year-old man has been admitted for a large subarachnoid hemorrhage (SAH) from a ruptured cerebral aneurysm. He has no spontaneous movement for the past week. He remains intubated. There is concern that the patient has brain death.

What test is most commonly used to diagnose brain death in this situation?
A) Cerebral angiography
B) Apnea testing
C) Demonstration of absent cranial nerve reflexes
D) Demonstration of fixed and dilated pupils
E) Performance of transcranial Doppler ultrasonography

Answer: B
Brain death is defined as lack of cerebral function with continued cardiac activity. This state requires support by artificial means. If an individual is determined to have brain death, life-sustaining therapies may be withdrawn. This can occur without the consent of the family. It is important to have

ongoing communication with the family to allow the withdrawal of care without conflict. Most hospitals have developed specific protocols in line with state law to diagnose a patient with brain death.

Three elements should be demonstrated for the diagnosis of brain death. The patient should have widespread cortical damage with the complete absence of response to all external stimuli. Second, the patient should have no evidence of medullary function demonstrated by a lack of oculovestibular and corneal reflexes. A common test is to assess pupillary reaction to light. Finally, there should be no evidence of medullary activity. This is manifested by apnea. Specific protocols have been developed to perform the apnea test.

References
Allen LA, Stevenson LW, Grady KL, et al. AHA scientific statement: decision making in advanced heart failure. Circulation. 2012;125:1928–52.
Wijdicks EFM. The diagnosis of brain death. N Engl J Med. 2001;344:1215–21.

372. A 56-year-old woman is admitted for severe nausea and diarrhea. She complains of nausea and diarrhea that began early that afternoon. She reports that she ate a sandwich from a street vendor for lunch, and she began experiencing symptoms several hours later. She reports no similar experiences in the past; she has no recent travel history, nor has she had any contacts with sick persons. She was treated with a 5-day course of ciprofloxacin for a urinary tract infection 2 months ago and is otherwise healthy.

On physical exam she is heme negative. Abdomen is mildly tender. She is afebrile. Which organism is the most likely cause of this patient's acute diarrheal illness?
A) *Campylobacter jejuni*
B) *Salmonella enteritidis*
C) *Staphylococcus aureus*
D) *C. difficile*
E) *E. coli*

Answer: C
Most acute diarrheas are caused by viral infections, such as adeno, norwalk, and rotavirus. They and are self-limited. Some are caused by bacteria. The most common agents in urban areas are *Campylobacter*, *Salmonella*, *Shigella*, and *Escherichia coli*. Protozoa such as *Giardia lamblia* and *Entamoeba histolytica* account for other common causes.

One mechanism for acute diarrhea is ingestion of a preformed toxin. Several species of bacteria, such as *S. aureus*, *C. perfringens,* and *Bacillus cereus*, can produce toxins that produce syndrome commonly designated as food poisoning. This occurs within 4 h of ingestion. In such cases, the bacteria do not need to establish an intraluminal infection; ingestion of the toxin alone can produce the disease. Symptoms subside after the toxin is cleared, usually by the next day. Symptoms are usually localized and fever is minimal.

Reference

Loir YL, Baron F,Gautier M. Review Staphylococcus aureus and food poisoning. Genet Mol Res. 2003;2(1):63–76.

373. A 52-year-old female with a history of renal transplant 5 years prior presents with headache, fever, and purulent rhinorrhea. This has occurred over the past 5 days. She has been on steroids intermittently over the past 6 months for episodes of acute rejection.

On physical exam, she is lethargic but able to respond to questions appropriately. Her lungs are cleared to auscultation. She has diffuse maxillary tenderness and is noted to have a black nasal discharge.

Which of the following is the likely cause of her illness?

A) *Coccidioides immitis*
B) *Rhizopus* (mucormycosis)
C) *Histoplasmosis capsulatum*
D) *Blastomyces dermatitidis*
E) *Cryptococcus neoformans*

Answer: B

This patient's symptoms are consistent with mucormycosis which is an invasive fungal infection caused by a variety of fungi most commonly rhizopus. This is a rapid opportunistic infection that invades the vascular system. It is a life-threatening condition and urgent consultation with otolaryngology and infectious disease is warranted. Mucormycosis is acquired by inhalation of the spores that are found ubiquitously in soil, decaying fruit, and old bread. Although a black eschar is the classic finding of mucormycosis, it is present in less than half of the patients. The presence of a black eschar indicates vascular invasion and predicts a poor prognosis.

The prognosis of mucormycosis is poor and has varied mortality rates depending on its form and severity. Patients who are immunocompromised have a significantly higher mortality rate from 60 to 80 %. In the rhinocerebral form, the mortality rate is between 30 and 70 %. Disseminated mucormycosis has a very poor prognosis with a mortality rate of up to 90 %

Reference

Roden MM, Zaoutis TE, Buchanan WL, et al. Epidemiology and outcome of Mucormycosis: a review of 929 reported cases. Clin Infect Dis. 2005;41(5):634–53.

374. A 68-year-old male with a past medical history of diabetes mellitus II, hypertension, hypothyroidism, and ESRD on hemodialysis 3 days per week presents with right leg swelling and leg pain.

Imaging confirms lower extremity deep vein thrombosis (DVT). The patient wants to know if there are any other treatment options besides warfarin because he states that grandma "bled too much on that drug."

As the attending physician, you explain to him that his choices are:

A) Rivaroxaban
B) Dabigatran
C) Warfarin (heparin bridge for minimum 5 days)
D) All of the above

Answer: C

There are several alternatives to coumadin in the treatment of DVTs. It is important to know the advantages and disadvantages of each. This patient is on hemodialysis, which limits his medication options for DVT treatment. Rivaroxaban should be avoided once the CrCl <30 mL/min. Dabigatran was not studied in HD patients or in patients with a CrCl <30 mL/min. These populations were excluded from the DVT/PE trials. However, warfarin requires no renal adjustment and is safe to use in HD patients with appropriate monitoring of the INR.

References

Dabigatran Package Insert. http://bidocs.boehringer-ingelheim.com/BIWebAccess/ViewServlet.ser?docBase=renetnt&folderPath=/Prescribing%20Information/PIs/Pradaxa/Pradaxa.pdf. Accessed 6/24/2014. Accessed 25 May 2014.
Rivaroxaban Package Insert. http://www.xareltohcp.com. Accessed 24 May 2014.

375. A 65-year-old female presents with new-onset right hemiplegia. A CT scan is performed and she is found to have had a large left-sided middle cerebral artery stroke. Her past medical history is significant for hypertension and diabetes. Her hospital course is uneventful.

Prior to her transfer to a skilled nursing facility, the patient has initiated physical therapy and is making good progress. She has good family support, and it is anticipated that after her admission to a skilled nursing facility, she will live at home with medical assistance. She has no history of depression or other psychiatric disorder. The patient's family states that she had an extremely active lifestyle before this event and is concerned about the development of depression. They have noticed that she seems a bit down at times and they request that an antidepressant be started for the treatment and prevention of depression.

Which of the following is the most appropriate advice to the family?

A) The incidence of depression is 7 %, and therefore, no therapy is recommended.

B) The incidence of depression poststroke is 29 %, and no therapy is recommended.

C) The incidence of depression is 42 %, and a low-dose selective serotonin reuptake inhibitor would be a reasonable choice.

D) The incidence of depression poststroke is 29 %, and a low-dose selective serotonin reuptake inhibitor would be a reasonable choice.

Answer: B

The incidence of a mild dysthymic state is common after the incidence of stroke. This is due not only to the loss of prior function, but possibly due to chemical changes seen in the cerebral cortex. The duration of this condition may last several weeks.

The lifetime prevalence of depression after stroke is 29 %. The cumulative incidence within 5 years of stroke appears to be 39–52 %. A meta-analysis performed in 2008 revealed no definitive benefit with pharmacological therapy for the prevention of depression after stroke. There was a small but statistically significant benefit of psychotherapy. The most appropriate approach would be to advise the patient and the family to follow for signs of depression and consider treatment when the diagnosis becomes apparent. This patient currently has no signs of depression and has appropriate signs of grieving from the loss of function.

Reference

Mosnik D, Williams LS, Kroenke K, Callahan C. Symptoms of post-stroke depression: a distinct syndrome compared to geriatric depression. Neurology. 2000;54(Suppl 3):A378–9.

376. A 44-year-old female is admitted for community-acquired pneumonia. Her past medical history includes diabetes, hypothyroidism, and vitamin D deficiency. Her clinical course improves with antibiotic therapy and is ready for discharge. She asks you to review her need for lipid-lowering therapy. A lipid panel is not drawn during this admission, and she is currently not taking any lipid-lowering therapy.

Would she benefit from starting a statin and if so, why?

A) Yes, she is diabetic.

B) Yes, she is 44 years old.

C) No, her LDL is unknown.

D) No, need to assess her hemoglobin A1C before deciding to initiate therapy.

Answer: A

Diabetes is one of the four statin benefit groups according to the new lipid guidelines by the American College of Cardiology. Evidence shows that each 39 mg/dL reduction in LDL by statins reduces atherosclerotic cardiovascular disease (ASCVD) risk by about 20 %. The four major statin benefit groups are as follows: clinical ASCVD, LDL $\geq$190, age 40–75 years with diabetes and LDL 70–189 without clinical ASCVD, and age 40–75 years with LDL 70–189 and estimated 10-year ASCVD risk >7.5 % without clinical ASCVD or diabetes. Diabetics (ages 40–75) are further classified according to the patient's 10-year ASCVD risk (<7.5 % = moderate intensity statin or $\geq$7.5 % = high-intensity statin). Initial LDL values are not needed in order to initiate statin therapy in a diabetic patient. In addition, age alone is not a factor, but it helps calculate the 10-year risk. Lastly, hemoglobin A1C does not influence the initiation of statin therapy.

Reference

Stone NJ, Robinson J, Lichtenstein AH, et al. 2013 ACC/AHA guideline on the treatment of blood cholesterol to reduce atherosclerotic cardiovascular risk in adults: a report of the American College of Cardiology/American Heart Association Task Force on Practice Guidelines. J Am Coll Cardiol. 2013;S0735–1097(13):06028–2.

377. Linezolid has the following characteristics as compared to vancomycin:

A) Decreased nephrotoxicity at higher doses

B) Increased intrapulmonary penetration

C) Increased incidence of thrombocytopenia

D) All of the above

E) None of the above

Answer: D

All of the answers are correct. Vancomycin is the current main stay for methicillin-resistant *Staphylococcus aureus* (MRSA) infections, but newer agents will see an increase in use due to better side effect profiles and tissue penetration. Linezolid may be more preferable for treating nosocomial pneumonia due to MRSA.

Reference

Chastre J, et al. European perspective and update on the management of nosocomial pneumonia due to methicillin-resistant Staphylococcus aureus after more than 10 years of experience with linezolid. Clin Microbiol Infect. 2014;20 Suppl 4:19–36.

378. Increasing the dosage of benzodiazepines in cardiac patients admitted to the hospital is associated with:

A) Increased risk of sudden death.

B) Increased heart failure hospitalization.

C) Increased risk of myocardial infarction.

D) Increased risk of dementia.

E) None of the answers is correct.

Answer: A

The adjusted incidence of sudden death was significantly associated with increased benzodiazepine dosage during 4.8 years of follow-up in a 2014 study.

Reference

Wu CK, et al. Anti-anxiety drugs use and cardiovascular outcomes in patients with myocardial infarction: a national wide assessment. Atherosclerosis. 2014;235(2):496–502.

379. A 72- year-old female is admitted with community-acquired pneumonia. On chest X-ray, she is noted to have a marked pleural effusion. You plan to perform a therapeutic thoracentesis of a large right-sided pleural effusion.

　　In addition to confirming the patient's identity verbally and noting the site of the procedure, which of the following has the Joint Commission identified as being a critical component of the time-out in the Universal Protocol for invasive procedures?
A) The patient's admitting diagnosis
B) The patient's date of birth
C) The type of procedure
D) The patient's age and date of admission
E) The follow-up plan after the procedure

Answer: C

The Joint Commission has defined several critical components of the "time-out" in an effort to improve patient safety and reduce medical errors. All components must be performed prior to the procedure. This includes confirming the patient's identity, the site of the procedure, and the type of the procedure.

Reference

A follow-up review of wrong site surgery. Sentinel Event Alert. 2001;24:3.

380. Which of the following statements is false in reference to urinary tract infections?
A) Asymptomatic bacteriuria should be treated when patients are pregnant.
B) Candiduria may represent vaginal flora or colonization.
C) Urine cultures are usually positive in the presence of a Foley catheter and should be treated in the absence of symptoms.
D) A colony count of greater than 100,000 is required to diagnose a UTI.

Answer: C

A common dilemma is the necessity to treat asymptomatic bacteriuria. There are several situations where first-line antibiotics can be avoided in patients who are non-immunocompromised. Positive urine cultures do not necessitate antibiotics in all circumstances. Urine cultures are usually positive in the presence of a Foley catheter and, with the absence of symptoms, should not be treated. If treatment is deemed necessary, remove the Foley catheter and treat for a total of 7 days. Treatment of either bacteriuria or candiduria with a Foley catheter in place is usually ineffective and does nothing more than to increase the resistance for microbes.

Reference

Gould CV, Umscheid CA, Agarwal RK, Kuntz G, Pegues DA. Guideline for prevention of catheter-associated urinary tract infections. Infect Control Hosp Epidemiol. 2010;31(4):319–26.

381. You are preparing to discharge a 77-year-old, retired nurse from your inpatient service after a 4-day hospitalization for heart failure. She has had two admissions this year. The patient has a long history of hypertension and heart failure. Prior to admission, she reported weight gain, peripheral edema, and decreased exercise tolerance for 3 days. While hospitalized, the patient was given intravenous furosemide 40 mg IV BID with a good response. Her admission medications are amlodipine, 5 mg daily; carvedilol, 12.5 mg twice daily; furosemide, 40 mg once daily; and aspirin, 81 mg daily. You suspect that she is compliant with her medications and diet.

　　On day of her discharge, her blood pressure is 125/60 mmHg and heart rate is 60 bpm. Her serum sodium is 134 mEq/L, and serum creatinine is 1.6 mg/dL. A 12-lead electrocardiogram demonstrates normal sinus rhythm, with increased voltages in the precordial leads and left-axis deviation. A transthoracic echocardiogram shows a left ventricular ejection fraction of 60 %, with a mildly thickened left ventricle and an enlarged left atrium.

　　Which of the following should you do next?
A) Increase the amlodipine dosage to 10 mg once daily.
B) Increase the furosemide dosage to 40 mg twice daily.
C) Add digoxin, 0.125 mg daily.
D) Add lisinopril, 2.5 mg daily.
E) Increase carvedilol to 25 mg twice daily.

Answer: D

This patient has responded to diuresis but now may need some intervention to prevent further exacerbations of congestive heart failure. Heart failure with normal left ventricle ejection fraction (HFNEF) is prevalent among older women with a history of hypertension. The mainstays of treatment include blood pressure management, rate control, low-salt diet, weight loss, and exercise that has been attempted here and should be reinforced.

A pair of observational studies demonstrated an association of discharge prescriptions for angiotensin-converting enzyme (ACE) inhibitors and lower overall mortality among patients with HFNEF. In this patient, it would seem reasonable to cautiously add an ACE inhibitor. Increasing her furosemide dosage might further exacerbate her possible volume depletion.

References

Ahmed A, Rich MW, Zile M, et al. Renin-angiotensin inhibition in diastolic heart failure and chronic kidney disease. Am J Med. 2013;126:150–61.

Mujib M, Patel K, Fonarow GC, et al. Angiotensin-converting enzyme inhibitors and outcomes in heart failure and preserved ejection fraction. Am J Med. 2013;126:401–10.

382. A 65-year-old male presents with progressive shortness of breath over the past month. He has a 40 pack-year history of smoking. CT scan of the chest reveals a right middle lobe mass for which he subsequently undergoes biopsy, which reveals adenocarcinoma. Magnetic resonance imaging of the brain reveals a 1 cm tumor in the left cerebral cortex, which is consistent with metastatic disease. The patient has no history of seizures or syncope. The patient is referred to outpatient therapy in the hematology/oncology service as well as follow-up with radiation oncology. The patient is ready for discharge.

    Which of the following would be the most appropriate therapy for primary seizure prevention?
    A) Seizure prophylaxis is not indicated.
    B) Valproate.
    C) Phenytoin.
    D) Phenobarbital.
    E) Oral prednisone 40 mg daily.

Answer: A

There is no indication for antiepileptic therapy for primary prevention in patients who have brain metastasis who have not undergone resection. Past studies have revealed no difference in seizure rates between placebo and antiepileptic therapy in patients who have brain tumors. Antiepileptic therapy has high rates of adverse reactions and caution should be exercised in their use.

Reference

Sirven JI, Wingerchuk DM, Drazkowski JF, Lyons MK, Zimmerman RS. Seizure prophylaxis in patients with brain tumors: a meta-analysis. Mayo Clin Proc. 2004; 79(12):1489–94.

383. An 86-year-old man is admitted to a dedicated geriatric acute care unit from home for treatment of nausea and vomiting related to a urinary tract infection. The unit is staffed by a limited group of trained providers. Outcomes for geriatric patients are assumed to be better on this unit.

    Which of the following statements does not accurately characterize the benefits of a geriatric acute care unit over a general inpatient ward?
    A) The geriatric acute care unit reduces inhospital functional decline.
    B) Patients who receive care in a geriatric acute care unit have improved functional status 3 months after discharge.
    C) The geriatric acute care unit provides patient-centered care that emphasizes independence.
    D) There is an increased likelihood that patients receiving care in a geriatric acute care unit will be able to return home upon discharge.
    E) The geriatric acute care unit provides intensive review of medical care to minimize the adverse effects of medications.

Answer: A

By 90 days after discharge, functional capacity is the same on geriatric units as it is on nonspecialized acute care units.

Geriatric units have specially prepared environments, specific protocols for enhanced discharge planning, and medical care that is designed to minimize the adverse effects of procedures and medications. The geriatric unit is one of several models of comprehensive inpatient geriatric care that have been developed by geriatrician researchers to address the adverse events and functional decline that often accompany hospitalization.

Despite the assumed benefits, studies so far have been mixed. Several short-term favorable outcomes have been recorded. These include reductions in decline of short-term functionality and readmission. Other long-term endpoints have not yet been demonstrated.

Reference

Landefeld CS, Palmer RM, Kresevic DM, Fortinski RH, Kowal J. A randomized trial of care in a hospital medical unit especially designed to improve the functional outcomes of acutely ill older patients. N Engl J Med. 1995;332:1338–44.

384. Which of the following bacteria or virus is the most likely etiology of ventilator-associated pneumonia (VAP) in an 82-year-old nursing home patient who is in the medical ICU for congestive heart failure?
    A) Legionella pneumonia
    B) *E. Coli*
    C) Mycoplasma pneumonia
    D) Respiratory syncytial virus
    E) *Staphylococcus aureus*

Answer: E

Despite geographical variations, *Enterococcus faecium*, *Staphylococcus aureus*, *Klebsiella pneumoniae*, *Acinetobacter baumannii*, *Pseudomonas aeruginosa*, and *Enterobacter* species (ESKAPE) pathogens constitute more than 80 % of ventilator-associated pneumonia (VAP) episodes. The organisms "escape" the biocidal actions of many antibiotics and have developed increasing resistance. As antibiotic development declines and resistance rises, healthcare-associated infections remain a constant threat to patient welfare. The ESKAPE pathogens will be of increasing relevance to antimicrobial chemotherapy in the coming years.

References

Park DR. The microbiology of ventilator-associated pneumonia. Respir Care. 2005;50:742–63.

Sandiumenge A, Rello J. Ventilator-associated pneumonia caused by ESKAPE organisms: cause, clinical features, and management. Curr Opin Pulm Med. 2012;18(3):187–93.

385. Polymerase chain reaction (PCR) bacterial testing has been proven to assist in the diagnosis of what conditions?
     A) Community-acquired pneumonia
     B) Cellulitis
     C) Endocarditis
     D) A and B
     E) A and C

Answer: E

PCR bacterial testing represents a major advance in the rapid diagnosis of infectious diseases. They may be used for blood as well as tissue samples. In a recent study, a broad-range PCR assay diagnosed infective endocarditis with a specificity of 91 %. Sensitivity was 67 %, positive predictive value was 96 %, and negative predictive value was 46 %. In situations where early diagnosis is beneficial or where antibiotics may be given for a long period, it may be cost-effective. So far PCR has shown promise in diagnosing community-acquired pneumonia and endocarditis tissue samples. As costs of PCR testing decrease, further use is anticipated.

References

Barken KB, Haagensen JA, Tolker-Nielsen T. Advances in nucleic acid-based diagnostics of bacterial infections. Clin Chim Acta. 2007;384(1–2):1–11.

Edwards K, Logan J, Langham S, Swift C, Gharbia S. Utility of Real-time amplification of selected 16S rDNA sequences as a tool for detection and identification of microbial signatures directly from clinical samples. J Med Microbiol. 2012;61(5):645–52.

386. Factors not named in the literature as contributing to higher rates of readmission include:
     A) Differences in patient health status
     B) Discharge planning and care coordination
     C) The availability and effectiveness of local primary care

     D) Threshold for admission in the area
     E) Lack of advance directive

Answer: E

Although implementing increased use of advance directives is thought to be an effective tool in decreasing readmissions, so far they have not been demonstrated to be a significant factor in reducing readmissions. Socioeconomic status, comorbidities, and care coordination remain significant factors in determining whether patients are readmitted to the hospital.

Care transitions on discharge should include coordinated with follow-up care and communication as patients transfer between locations of levels of care. This is a time when medical errors and patient harm are known to be more likely.

Due to increasing financial incentives, many studies are currently looking at readmission prevention strategies. As of yet no single factor has been identified as a primary factor in readmission prevention.

Reference

Enguidanos S, Vesper E, Lorenz K. 30-day readmissions among seriously ill older adults, J Palliat Med. 2012;15(12):1356–61. Leonard Davis School of Gerontology. Los Angeles: University of Southern California.

387. Which of the following is a contraindication to the herpes zoster vaccine?
     A) Age younger than 60 years
     B) Chronic post-herpetic neuralgia
     C) History of shingles
     D) Lymphoma
     E) No history of varicella infection

Answer: D

As of 2013 the Advisory Committee on Immunization Practices (ACIP) recommends that herpes zoster vaccine be routinely recommended for adults aged ≥60. The ACIP states that people with primary or acquired immunodeficiency should not receive the vaccine. Immunodeficient states such as lymphoma, AIDS, and leukemia constitute an absolute contraindication to receiving the herpes zoster vaccine.

Both the Centers for Disease Control and Prevention and the ACIP recommend that adults be vaccinated whether or not they report a previous episode of herpes zoster.

There remains a large population of mildly to moderately immunocompromised patients in whom the risk-benefit ratio of vaccination is not well understood.

Reference

Brisson M, Pellissier JM, Camden S, Quach C, De Wals P. The potential cost-effectiveness of vaccination against herpes zoster and post-herpetic neuralgia. Hum Vaccin. 2008;4(3):238–45. Epub 2010 May 25.

388. A 52-year-old man is evaluated in the hospital. The patient was admitted yesterday for treatment of acute pancreatitis secondary to alcohol abuse. He has remained symptomatic for 24 h.

On physical examination, he is lying on his side with his knees drawn to his chest. Vital signs include a temperature of 38.1 °C (100.6 °F), blood pressure is 145/80 mmHg, pulse rate is 106 beats/min, and respiratory rate is 14 breaths/min. Oxygen saturation on ambient air is 94 %. The oral mucosa is dry. Abdominal examination discloses decreased bowel sounds and epigastric tenderness. The remainder of the examination is normal.

Leukocyte count is 12,000/µL, hematocrit is 39 %, blood urea nitrogen is 68 mg/dL, creatinine is 3.4 mg/dL, and amylase is 657 U/L.

Abdominal ultrasonography shows no gallstones or dilatation of the common bile duct.

Which of the following is most predictive of a poor outcome in this patient?
A) Amylase level
B) Anemia
C) Blood urea nitrogen level
D) Leukocytosis
E) Age

Answer: C

Hemoconcentration measurements are the best predictors of higher morbidity and mortality in patients with acute pancreatitis. This includes elevated blood urea nitrogen, serum creatinine, or hematocrit levels. Multiple scoring systems have been devised to measure outcomes in patients with acute pancreatitis. Traditionally utilized, the Ranson criteria rely on parameters that are measured at admission and at 48 h. The Acute Physiology and Chronic Health Evaluation II score is more accurate than the Ranson criteria.

Hemoconcentration may serve as a marker of a capillary leak in acute pancreatitis. This may explain its correlation with mortality. Patients with severe disease tend to have elevated levels of blood urea nitrogen, serum creatinine, and hematocrit. Of these factors, the blood urea nitrogen level is the most accurate for predicting severity. Other factors that predispose patients to a poor prognosis are medical comorbidities, age greater than 70 years, and an increased body-mass index.

There is no correlation between the degree of elevation of the serum amylase level and severity or prognosis of illness in patients with acute pancreatitis. Mild to moderate leukocytosis is common in patients with acute pancreatitis and has no prognostic significance.

Reference

Tenner S, Baillie J, Dewitt J, et al. American College of Gastroenterology guidelines: management of acute pancreatitis. Am J Gastroenterol. 2013;108(9):1400–15.

389. Which of the following therapies for severe acute respiratory distress syndrome (ARDS) has the strongest evidence for improving survival in large randomized studies?
A) Steroids
B) High-frequency oscillation ventilation
C) Prone positioning
D) Nebulized beta-adrenergic agonist therapy
E) Antibiotics

Prone positioning may improve oxygenation in patients who have acute respiratory distress syndrome (ARDS). Several studies have examined strategies to improve outcomes in ARDS with limited positive results. A recent large study of 466 patients found a marked reduction in patients treated with prone positioning. Complications were not different between the two treatments, except for a higher incidence of cardiac arrest in the supine patient group. Another large randomized trial showed potential harm with increased mortality from early use of high-frequency oscillation in ARDS patients. The ARDS network trial of nebulized beta-adrenergic agonist therapy failed to show benefit.

References

Ferguson ND, et al. High-frequency oscillation in early acute respiratory distress syndrome. N Engl J Med. 2013;3368:795–805.

Matthay MA, et al. (ARDSNet). Randomized, placebo-controlled clinical trial of an aerosolized B2-agonist for treatment of acute lung injury. Am J Respir Crit Care Med. 2011;184:561–8.

Soo Hoo GW. In prone ventilation, one good turn deserves another. N Engl J Med. 2013;368(23):2227–8.

390. A 62-year-old white male with a past medical history of diabetes presents to the emergency room for chest pain and is admitted. He rules out for a myocardial infarction and will be scheduled for an outpatient stress test.

His labs are remarkable for increased lipid values, particularly an LDL of 213. On discharge, you inform him that he will be starting a high intensity statin. Which of the following statins, with corresponding dosage regimen, is considered high intensity?
A) Rosuvastatin 10 mg PO QHS
B) Pravastatin 20 mg PO QHS
C) Simvastatin 80 mg PO QHS
D) Atorvastatin 80 mg PO QHS

Answer: D

Atorvastatin 80 mg daily is considered a high-intensity statin according to current guidelines. Rosuvastatin is considered high intensity in doses 20–40 mg daily. Pravastatin 20 mg is considered low intensity. Simvastatin 80 mg daily is not recommended by the FDA due to increased risk of myopathy, including rhabdomyolysis.

Reference

Stone NJ, Robinson J, Lichtenstein AH, et al. 2013 ACC/ AHA guideline on the treatment of blood cholesterol to reduce atherosclerotic cardiovascular risk in adults: a report of the American College of Cardiology/American Heart Association Task Force on Practice Guidelines. J Am Coll Cardiol. 2013;S0735–1097(13):06028–2.

391. A 65-year-old male has been admitted with cellulitis which has developed within the past 2 days. He develops the sudden onset of chest pain 2 h ago. Inspiration and movement exacerbate the pain. The patient has not had hemoptysis. He has no history of recent surgery, prolonged periods of immobility, venous thromboembolism, or cancer.

    Pulse rate is 102 beats/min, respiratory rate is 18 breaths/min, and blood pressure is 185/96 mmHg. Oxygen saturation is 94 % on room air. The patient is anxious; he is alert and oriented to person, place, and time. Physical examination shows no abnormalities of the heart and lungs.

    On laboratory studies, cardiac enzyme levels are within normal limits. Electrocardiography and chest x-ray study show no abnormalities.

    Based on the Wells criteria, which of the following best represents the probability of pulmonary embolism in this patient?
    A) Low
    B) Intermediate
    C) High
    D) None

Answer: A

This patient has a low Wells criteria probability for pulmonary embolism. The Wells criteria are used to determine the pretest probability of pulmonary embolism in patients based on history and physical examination. The Wells criteria allow clinicians to determine which patients need further diagnostic or invasive testing.

    The Wells criteria assign points for presence of signs, symptoms, and historical factors. This includes tachycardia, hemoptysis, and deep venous thrombosis. Additional points are assigned for a history of venous thromboembolism, active malignancy, and recent immobilization and surgery. The Wells criteria assign points if no other alternative diagnosis is likely. This patient has no historical factors or clinical findings suggestive of pulmonary embolism; his Wells score is 1.5/12.5. His symptoms could be related to musculoskeletal pain, pleurisy, or anxiety.

Reference

Wells PS, Anderson DR, Bormanis J, et al. Value of assessment of pretest probability of deep-vein thrombosis in clinical management. Lancet. 1997;350(9094):1795–8.

392. Brain natriuretic factor (BNP) use in the emergency room has resulted in what endpoints?
    A) Decreased admission rates
    B) Decreased all-cause mortality
    C) Decreased length of stay
    D) Decreased readmissions
    E) A and C

Answer: E

Although widely measured, the benefits of BNP measurements on clinical and quality endpoints remain uncertain. A meta-analysis measuring the effects of BNP testing on clinical outcomes of patients presenting to the emergency department with shortness of breath revealed that BNP testing led to a decrease in admission rates and decrease in mean length of stay. No effect on all-cause hospital mortality was seen.

    The BNP test is used as an aid in the diagnosis and assessment of severity of heart failure. The BNP test is also used for the risk stratification of patients with acute coronary syndromes. BNP values may fluctuate due to factors other than heart failure. Lower than predicted levels are often seen in obese patients. Higher levels are seen in those with renal disease, in the absence of heart failure.

    It has been suggested that one of the most important use of natriuretic peptides is in helping to establish the diagnosis of heart failure (HF) when the diagnosis is uncertain. In these patients a value less than 100 makes HF unlikely and a value greater than 400 makes HF likely.

References

Lam LL, Cameron PA, Schneider HG, Abramson MJ, Müller C, Krum H. Meta-analysis: effect of B-type natriuretic peptide testing on clinical outcomes in patients with acute dyspnea in the emergency setting. Ann Intern Med. 2010;153(11):728–35.

Maisel A, Mueller C, Adams K Jr, et al. State of the art: using natriuretic peptide levels in clinical practice. Eur J Heart Fail. 2008;10(9):824–39.

393. An 86-year-old female is admitted from the nursing home with a diagnosis of urinary tract infection and sepsis. She has a history of progressive dementia. She has no known implantable devices or orthopedic, internal hardware.

    Blood cultures are drawn which reveal gram-positive rods. Otherwise, no other source of infection is isolated. Urine cultures are negative. In the first 48 h she clinically improves and is back to her baseline mental status.

    Which of the following explains the positive blood cultures?
    A) Urinary tract infection
    B) Endocarditis
    C) Skin contamination
    D) Chronic wound infection

Answer: C

There are four bacteria that are common contaminants when blood cultures are positive. They are coagulase-negative staph (gram-positive cocci), *Corynebacterium* (gram-positive rods), *Propionibacterium* acnes (anaerobic gram-positive rods), and *Bacillus* species (anaerobic gram-positive rods). These may be considered to be true pathogens when multiple sites are positive, or the patient has prosthetic implants.

Staphylococcus aureus, Streptococcus species, *Enterococcus, Candida, Pseudomonas*, and other gram-negative rods-positive bacillus are usually not a contaminant from the skin. In this particular case, without signs of overwhelming sepsis, the gram-positive rod is almost certainly a contaminant.

Reference

Madeo M, Barlow G. Reducing blood-culture contamination rates by the use of a 2 % chlorhexidine solution applicator in acute admission units. J Hosp Infect. 2008; 69(3):307–9.

394. A 62-year-old Caucasian female with a past medical history of diabetes and osteoarthritis was admitted for right hip total arthroplasty. Perioperatively, she received subcutaneous enoxaparin for anticoagulant therapy. She is on the hip fracture service managed by hospital medicine. You are called to see her on day three for the sudden-onset substernal chest pain. She has minimal response to two doses of sublingual nitroglycerin. Initial 12-lead EKG demonstrates inferior lead ST elevation. Stat labs are drawn and reveal elevated troponins at 45 ng/mL. Complete blood count shows a platelet count of 20,000 cells/mcl which were 238,000 cells/mcl at the time of admission.

Which drug is FDA approved and is indicated for management of acute coronary syndrome of this patient?
A) Oral lepirudin
B) Oral rivaroxaban
C) Intravenous enoxaparin
D) Bivalirudin
E) Fondaparinux

Answer: D

This patient developed heparin-induced thrombocytopenia (HIT) and an acute STEMI. Bivalirudin is a direct thrombin inhibitor that is FDA approved for the management of patients with acute STEMI secondary to or at risk for HIT. Enoxaparin should be avoided in patients with HIT. Although fondaparinux and lepirudin are used in acute coronary syndromes (ACS), they are not indicated in patients who developed ACS with HIT.

Reference

Bittl JA, Chaitman BR, Feit F, et al. Bivalirudin versus heparin during coronary angioplasty for unstable or postinfarction angina: final report reanalysis of the bivalirudin angioplasty study. Am Heart J. 2001;142:952–9.

395. Beta-blockers will provide which of the following benefits in elderly patients with congestive heart failure and preserved ejection fractions?
A) Decreased all-cause mortality
B) Decreased heart failure re-hospitalization
C) All of the above
D) None of the above

Answer: D

Beta-blockers are essential in the treatment of CHF with reduced ejection fraction. However, in patients with CHF with preserved ejection fraction, benefits have not been demonstrated. In a study over 6 years in patients over the age of 65, there was no association with individual endpoints of all-cause mortality or heart failure re-hospitalization, with the use of beta-blockers on discharge.

Reference

Patel K, et al. Beta-blockers in older patients with heart failure and preserved ejection fraction: Class, dosage, and outcomes. Int J Cardiol. 2014;173(3):393–401.

396. Which of the following is the most common type of preventable adverse event in hospitalized patients?
A) Adverse drug events
B) Diagnostic failures
C) Falls
D) Technical complications of procedures
E) Wound infections

Answer: A

The most common adverse event in the hospitalized patient is an adverse drug event (ADE). This occurs in approximately 19 % of hospitalizations. An adverse event is defined as an injury caused by medical management rather than the underlying disease of the patient.

In recent years, there has been increasing focus on the safety of health care provided throughout the world. An Institute of Medicine report identified safety as an essential component of quality in health care. One of the largest studies that has attempted to quantify adverse events in hospitalized patients was the Harvard Medical Practice Study. In that study adverse events included ADE (19 %), wound infections (14 %), technical complications of a procedure (13 %), diagnostic mishaps (15 %), and falls (5 %).

Rounding pharmacists have been shown to greatly reduce preventable adverse drug events. In one study 78 % fewer preventable adverse drug events (ADEs) occurred among patients when a pharmacist participated in weekday medical rounds.

References
Krahenbuhl-Melcher A, Schlienger R, Lampert M, et al. Drug-related problems in hospitals: a review of the recent literature. Drug Saf. 2007;30:397–407.
Kucukarslan SN, Peters M, Mlynarek M, et al. Pharmacists on rounding teams reduce preventable adverse drug events in hospital general medicine units. Arch Intern Med. 2003;163:2014–8.

397. The most common precipitating trigger for type 1 hepatorenal syndrome is:
    A) Sepsis
    B) Large-volume paracentesis
    C) Renal toxic drugs
    D) Increased diuretic dose
    E) Spontaneous bacterial peritonitis
    F) Urinary tract infection

Answer: E
The hepatorenal syndrome (HRS) can develop spontaneously, or it can be triggered by a precipitating event. Type 1 HRS is characterized by rapidly progressive kidney failure, with a doubling of serum creatinine to a level greater than 2.5 mg/dL or a halving of the creatinine clearance to less than 20 mL/min over a period of less than 2 weeks. The most common precipitating trigger for the type 1 hepatorenal (HRS) syndrome is spontaneous bacterial peritonitis, and this should be considered in any end-stage liver disease (ESLD) patient with hepatorenal syndrome. It is important that this is considered even in the absence of symptoms.

Type 1 HRS occurs in approximately 25 % of patients with SBP, despite rapid resolution of the infection with antibiotics.

Hepatorenal syndrome is primarily induced by renal arterial vasoconstriction. Several conditions that decrease renal blood flow can also induce type 1 hepatorenal syndrome. This includes sepsis, volume depletion, and volume shifts. This may occur when a large-volume paracentesis is undertaken. Adequate plasma expansion should be undertaken when a large-volume paracentesis occurs.

Reference
Betrosian AP, Agarwal B, Douzinas EE. Acute renal dysfunction in liver diseases. World J Gastroenterol. 2007;13(42):5552–9.

398. A 47-year-old female is admitted to the hospital medicine service for possible osteomyelitis. Past medical history includes hypertension, diabetes mellitus type 2, depression, and hyperlipidemia.

Labs are within normal limits except for an elevated WBC count. As her medication admission orders are being completed, the emergency room physician orders pantoprazole 40 mg PO daily for stress ulcer prophylaxis. Is the pantoprazole indicated in this patient?
    A) Yes
    B) No

Answer: B
Prophylactic proton pump inhibitor therapy is recommended for any of the following major risk factors: respiratory failure requiring mechanical ventilation (likely for greater than 48 h) or coagulopathy defined as platelet count <50,000, INR >1.5, or a PTT >2× the control (prophylactic or treatment doses of anticoagulants do not constitute a coagulopathy). Additional risk factors warranting stress ulcer prophylaxis are as follows: head or spinal cord injury, severe burn (more than 35 % BSA), acute organ dysfunction, history of GI ulcer/bleeding within 1 year, high doses of corticosteroids, liver failure with associated coagulopathy, postoperative transplantation, acute kidney injury, major surgery, and multiple trauma.

Suppressing the acid production of the stomach may lead to adverse side effects, such as an increased risk of aspiration pneumonia.

References
ASHP Commission on Therapeutics. ASHP Therapeutic Guidelines on Stress Ulcer Prophylaxis. Am J Health Syst Pharm. 1999;56:347–79.
Sessler JM. Stress-related mucosal disease in the intensive care unit: an update on prophylaxis. AACN. Adv Crit Care. 2007;18:199–206.

399. As the unit medical director, you are asked by the hospital administration to align the current cardiac code policies with evidence-based guidelines. In particular you are asked to reduce the variability that currently occurs.
    Which of the following would you suggest?
    A) Increasing the frequency of advanced cardiovascular life support (ACLS) training to become an annual requirement for all clinical practitioners
    B) Interviewing hospital staff using a Delphi method process to enumerate optimal resuscitation practices
    C) Developing resuscitation-specific privileges that are required for all hospital credentialed
    D) Implementation of the American Heart Association (AHA) Get with the Guidelines – Resuscitation program

Answer: D
The American Heart Association (AHA) has put a great deal of effort and expertise into developing evidence-based guidelines for cardiac resuscitation.

The AHA "Get with the Guidelines" program was developed to identify improvement opportunities, allow performance comparison among hospitals, and reduce medical errors through data-driven peer review. The AHA has reviewed the most up-to-date research and scientific publications in developing this program. The program includes guidelines for resuscitation, atrial fibrillation, heart failure, and stroke.

Reference

American Heart Association (AHA) Get with the Guidelines – Resuscitation program 2012. http://www.heart.org/HEARTORG/HealthcareResearch/GetWithTheGuidelinesHFStroke/GetWithTheGuidelinesStrokeHomePage/Get-With-Guidelines-Stroke-Overview. Accessed 12 Dec 2014.

400. The US government's National Quality Forum-approved methodology for calculating excess 30-day readmission rates includes all of the following except:
A) Adjustment for clinically relevant patient comorbidities
B) The patient's socioeconomic status, specifically federally defined income level below the poverty line
C) Established 3-year period for which discharges are calculated
D) Readmissions from all causes to the same or another hospital for patients with specified diagnoses
E) Minimum number of cases (25) annually for the hospital for each listed

Answer: B

Thirty-day hospital readmissions are common and costly and because they may signal an unnecessary use of resources have been the focus of US health policy interventions to reduce cost.

In March 2010, the comprehensive health reform act, the Patient Protection and Affordable Care Act, went into law. The law established a program to encourage reduction in hospital readmissions, which requires the US Centers for Medicare and Medicaid Services to reduce payments to hospitals with excess readmissions.

Thirty-day hospital readmission calculations do not consider socioeconomic status, race or ethnicity, or English language proficiency in the risk adjustments. These are strong risk factors for readmission. Some hospital advocates feel these are factors that clinicians have no control over and should not be considered in penalty determinations.

Reference

CMS.gov. Readmissions reduction program 2013. www.cms.gov/Medicare/Medicare-Feefor-Service-Payment/AcuteInpatientPPS/Readmissions-Reduction-Program.html. Accessed 14 Nov 2014.

401. Which of the following statements is true comparing dopamine with norepinephrine as a first-line vasotherapy for septic shock?
A) Increased 28-day overall death rate
B) Increased death rate among the septic shock group
C) Increased arrhythmias
D) Increased use of additional vasopressors

Answer: C

Although there has been a long-standing debate, no single vasopressor has been definitively shown to have a mortality benefit over another in patients with septic shock. To help better answer the question of whether there is a mortality benefit from the initial vasopressor used, the Sepsis Occurrence in Acutely Ill Patients II (SOAP II) study randomized 1679 patients with shock to norepinephrine or dopamine as the initial vasopressor. The study found no difference between the two groups in 28-day mortality, although there were significantly more cardiac arrhythmias in the dopamine group.

References

Havel C, Arrich J, Losert H, Gamper G, Müllner M, Herkner H. Vasopressors for hypotensive shock. Cochrane Database Syst Rev. 2011;5:CD003709.

Marik PE, Mohedin M. The contrasting effects of dopamine and norepinephrine on systemic and splanchnic oxygen utilization in hyperdynamic sepsis. JAMA. 1994;272(17):1354–57.

402. A 92-year-old female presents with confusion, diaphoresis, and mild shortness of breath. A rapidly performed EKG reveals possible ischemia.

The most common symptom of acute myocardial infarction in patients older than 85 years old is:
A) Chest pain
B) Altered mental status
C) Syncope
D) Dyspnea
E) Fever

Answer: D

In patients older than 85 years of age, shortness of breath is the most common symptom during a myocardial infarction. This may be due acute congestive heart failure or anxiety. Elderly, diabetic, and female patients often have atypical anginal symptoms. The initial evaluation of an elderly patient with suspected myocardial ischemia should begin with a high index of suspicion for atypical symptoms.

References

Aronow WS, Epstein S. Usefulness of silent ischemia, ventricular tachycardia, and complex ventricular arrhythmias in predicting new coronary events in elderly patients with coronary artery disease or systemic hypertension. Am J Cardiol. 1990;65:511–2.

Siegel R, Clements T, Wingo M, et al. Acute heart failure in elderly: another manifestation of unstable "angina." J Am Coll Cardiol. 1991;17:149A.

403. Which antibiotic may be associated with the greatest odds for ventricular arrhythmia and cardiovascular death in adult patients?
    A) Levofloxacin
    B) Azithromycin
    C) Moxifloxacin
    D) Clarithromycin
    E) Clindamycin

Answer: B
There has been concern that azithromycin may increase the risk of ventricular arrhythmias in susceptible adults. A database analysis found increased arrhythmias and cardiovascular events in patients treated with azithromycin and found no association between clarithromycin or ciprofloxacin and adverse cardiac outcomes.

Many authorities suggest that older individuals and those at high risk for cardiovascular disease may be more vulnerable to adverse effects and should use extra caution when taking this antibiotic.

It has also been suggested that inappropriate use has led to widespread antibiotic resistance and is contributing to the emergence of resistant bacteria.

Azithromycin was developed in 1980 and has been marketed in the United States since 1991. As of 2011, it was the most commonly prescribed antibiotic.

References
Bril F, Gonzalez CD, Di Girolamo G. Antimicrobial agents-associated with QT interval prolongation. Curr Drug Saf. 2010;5(1):85–92.
Ray WA, Murray KT, Hall K, Arbogast PG, Stein CM. Azithromycin and the risk of cardiovascular death. N Engl J Med. 2012;366(20):1881–90.

404. A 45-year-old male was admitted the prior morning with suspected meningitis. Blood cultures done in the emergency room now reveal *Neisseria meningitidis*. The patient was started 12 h ago with vancomycin and ceftriaxone. The patient is currently afebrile. Neck stiffness and photophobia have decreased.

    When is the appropriate time to remove the patient from isolation?
    A) Discontinuation now
    B) 48 h following admission
    C) 24 h after antibiotics have been started
    D) Upon complete resolution of clinical symptoms
    E) Upon discharge

Answer: C
For most cases of bacterial meningitis, isolation can be discontinued 24 h after the initiation of antibiotics. It is important to remove isolation when it can be safely done to reduce the psychological stress placed on the patient, improve patient care, and facilitate discharge planning.

Reference
Chaudhuri A, Martinez–Martin P, Martin PM et al. EFNS guideline on the management of community-acquired bacterial meningitis: report of an EFNS Task Force on acute bacterial meningitis in older children and adults. Eur J Neurol. 2008;15(7):649–59.

405. A pharmaceutical company does not publish inconclusive results of new drug that it is marketing. This is an example of:
    A) Reporting bias
    B) Underestimation
    C) Cofounding
    D) None of the above

Answer: A
Reporting bias continues to be a major problem in the assessment of health-care interventions. Several prominent cases of reporting or publication bias have been described in the literature. These have included trials reporting the effectiveness of antidepressants, class I anti-arrhythmic drugs, and selective COX-2 inhibitors. Studies in which drugs are shown to be ineffective are often not published, delayed, or modified to emphasize the positive results suggested.

In addition, trials with statistically significant findings were generally published in academic journals with higher circulation more often than trials with nonsignificant findings. In general, published evidence tends to overestimate efficacy and underestimate safety risks. The extent of this is often unknown.

References
MacAuley D. READER: an acronym to aid critical reading by general practitioners. Br J Gen Pract. 1994;44:83–5.
Sterne J, Egger M, Moher D. Addressing reporting biases. In: Higgins JPT, Green S, editors. Cochrane handbook for systematic reviews of interventions. Chichester: Wiley; 2008. p. 297–334.

406. Compared with central venous catheters (CVCs), peripherally inserted central catheters (PICCs) are associated with which of the following?
    A) Lower patient satisfaction
    B) Lower cost-effectiveness
    C) Greater risk of bloodstream infection
    D) Greater risk of deep vein thrombosis

Answer: D

PICCs have many advantages over central venous catheters. PICCs are a reliable alternative to short-term central venous catheters, with a lower risk of complications. PICCs have higher patient satisfaction and lower infection rates and are more cost-effective than other CVCs.

However, PICCs are associated with a higher risk of deep vein thrombosis than are central venous catheters (CVCs). This risk is increased in patients who are critically ill or those with a malignancy. Also, to meet the definition of a PICC, the distal tip of the catheter must terminate in the superior vena cava, the inferior vena cava, or the proximal right atrium. Thrombosis may be a result of PICCs being inserted into peripheral veins that are narrower and more likely to occlude in the presence of a catheter than the large veins used for CVCs.

Reference

Chopra V, Anand S, Hickner A, et al. Risk of venous thromboembolism associated with peripherally inserted central catheters: a systematic review and meta-analysis. Lancet. 2013;382:311–25.

407. What is the 30-day hospital readmission rate for patients in the United States?
   A) 20 % of all Medicare discharges
   B) 10 % of all Medicare discharges
   C) 12 % of hospitalized patients covered by commercial payers
   D) 20 % of Medicare and commercial payers
   E) None of the above

Answer: A

19.6 % of 11,855,702 Medicare beneficiaries who had been discharged from a hospital in 2003 and 2004 were rehospitalized within 30 days, and 34 % were rehospitalized within 90 days. Since that time small reductions in readmissions have occurred.

Reducing readmission rates is a major priority for hospitals given that the Affordable Care Act (ACA) established a Hospital Readmissions Reduction Program that requires the Centers for Medicare and Medicaid Services (CMS) to reduce payments to hospitals with excessive readmissions.

Not all readmissions are avoidable. But unplanned readmissions frequently suggest breakdowns in continuity of care and unsuccessful transitions of care between settings. Studies suggest that readmissions are not usually tied to medical errors committed during the hospital stay, but rather to social issues, poor follow-up, or the patient's lack of understanding of post-hospital care.

Reducing readmissions has proven to be difficult. No simple fix has been found. Most gains are seen in institutions that employed a multifactorial approach.

Reference

Jencks SF, Williams MV, Coleman EA. Rehospitalizations among patients in the Medicare fee-for-service program. N Engl J Med. 2009;360:1418–28.

408. A 27-year-old man presents painful swelling of the right knee and swelling of several fingers. He is otherwise healthy but does recall a severe bout of diarrheal illness about 3–4 weeks prior that spontaneously resolved. He takes no medications and reports rare marijuana use.

   On physical exam he has limited motion and swelling of the right knee. You suspect reactive arthritis due to a diarrheal illness.

   Which of the following is the most likely etiologic agent of his diarrhea?
   A) *Campylobacter jejuni*
   B) *Clostridium difficile*
   C) *Escherichia coli*
   D) *Helicobacter pylori*
   E) *Shigella flexneri*

Answer: E

The most common organism associated with reactive arthritis in diarrheal illness is the *Shigella* species. Reactive arthritis refers to an acute, nonpurulent arthritis that occurs after an infection elsewhere in the body. In shigella infections, it often presents with lower joint inflammatory arthritis occurring 1–4 weeks after a diarrheal episode. Reactive arthritis may also include uveitis or conjunctivitis, dactylitis, and urogenital lesions. It can occur with yersinia, chlamydia, and, to a much lesser extent, salmonella and campylobacter.

Reference

Hannu T, Mattila L, Siitonen A, Leirisalo-Repo M. Reactive arthritis attributable to Shigella infection: a clinical and epidemiological nationwide study. Ann Rheum Dis. 2005;64(4):594–8.

409. An 82-year-old nursing home resident has been admitted for melena. You are called to see him the first night because he was found unresponsive in his bed immersed in black stool. His past medical history is remarkable for Alzheimer's dementia.

   On physical his pressure is 85/50 mmHg and heart rate is 130 beats/min. He is transferred to the ICU and a central venous catheter is placed that reveals CVP less than 5 mmHg. Catheterization of the bladder yields no urine. Anesthesiology has been called to the bedside and is assessing the patient's airway.

In the patient described, which of the following is true regarding his clinical condition?

A) Loss of 20–40 % of the blood volume leads to shock physiology.
B) Loss of less than 20 % of the blood volume will manifest as orthostasis.
C) Oliguria is a prognostic sign of impending vascular collapse.
D) Symptoms of hypovolemic shock differ from those of hemorrhagic shock.
E) The first sign of hypovolemic shock is mental obtundation.

Answer: C

Oliguria is a very important clinical parameter that should help guide volume resuscitation. Volume resuscitation should be initiated with rapid IV infusion of isotonic saline or Ringer's lactate. After assessing for an adequate airway and spontaneous breathing, initial resuscitation aims at reexpanding the intravascular volume and controlling ongoing losses. Transfusion with packed red blood cells (PRBC) should be considered with hemorrhagic shock, continued blood losses, and a hemoglobin of less than 10 g/dL

Symptoms of hemorrhagic and nonhemorrhagic shock are indistinguishable. Up to 20 % of the blood volume can be lost with few clinical symptoms except mild tachycardia. Orthostasis is seen with a loss of 20–40 % of the blood volume. Shock occurs with loss of more than 40 % of the blood volume. This results in marked tachycardia, hypotension, oliguria, and finally obtundation. Central nervous system perfusion is maintained until shock becomes severe.

Once hemorrhage is controlled, transfusion of PRBCs should be performed only for hemoglobin of 7 g/dL or less. Patients who remain hypotensive after volume resuscitation have a poor prognosis. Inotropic support and intensive monitoring should be initiated in these patients.

Reference

Stainsby D, MacLennan S, Thomas D, Isaac J, Hamilton PJ. Guidelines on the management of massive blood loss. Br J Haematol. 2006;135(5):634–41.

410. In which of the following circumstances would albumin infusion be most beneficial?
A) A patient with the end-stage liver disease and ascites requiring paracentesis
B) A patient with hypotension and a serum albumin of 1.8 g/dL
C) A patient with acute blood loss awaiting type and match for packed red blood cell infusion
D) A patient who is hypotensive with sepsis syndrome and a serum albumin of 2.0 g/dL

Answer: A

The role of albumin infusion remains uncertain in many clinical situations. Albumin composes 50–60 % of blood plasma proteins. It is effective in preventing the complications of high-volume paracentesis in patients with cirrhosis and ascites undergoing paracentesis. Indications and the use of albumin administration in critically ill patients are uncertain. In general, albumin is not given specifically to treat hypoalbuminemia, which is a marker for serious disease.

Reference

McGibbon A, Chen GI, Peltekian KM, van Zanten SV. An evidence-based manual for abdominal paracentesis. Dig Dis Sci. 2007;52(12):3307–15.

411. For patients greater than 65 years of age and hospitalized with heart failure and preserved ejection fraction, discharging with a new prescription for calcium channel blockers (CCBs) provides what benefit?
A) Decreased mortality
B) Decreased 30-day heart failure admissions
C) Decreased 90-day incidence of myocardial infarction
D) None of the above

Answer: D

New discharge prescriptions for CCBs have no correlation with improved endpoints in older patients hospitalized with HF and ejection fraction ≥40 %. This is according to 2014 study.

Reference

Patel K, et al. Calcium-channel blockers and outcomes in older patients with heart failure and preserved ejection fraction. Circ Heart Fail. 2014;7(6):945–52.

412. A 62-year-old white female presents with confusion. She has a known history of alcoholism, ascites, and hepatic encephalopathy. Ammonia upon admission is elevated. Her husband claims she has not being taking her lactulose as often as prescribed. He also reports that she is having about 1–2 bowel movements per day. Upon admission, her lactulose is restarted at 30 g PO TID. By day 3 in the hospital, the patient is more alert and closer to baseline per her husband. The nurses have charted the following bowel movements: day 1, 2; day 2, 4; and day 3 so far, 2.

How does lactulose work in the setting of hepatic encephalopathy?
A) Decreases the amount of ammonia-producing bacteria in the gut
B) Creates an acidic ph in the gut, which in turn causes NH3 to become NH4+ resulting in an osmotic effect in the gut due to the nonabsorbable ammonium ion

C) Creates a resin in which ammonia can bind and then be excreted fecally

D) Works as a stimulant laxative

Answer: B

Option A describes the mechanism of action of rifaximin. Option C is incorrect as there is no resin that forms from lactulose. Option D is incorrect because lactulose works as an osmotic rather than a stimulant.

Reference

Als-Nielsen B, Gluud LL, Gluud C. Non-absorbable disaccharides for hepatic encephalopathy: systematic review of randomised trials. BMJ. 2004;328(7447):1046.

413. A 61-year-old man is admitted for cellulitis. He has responded to antibiotics and is ready for discharge. He would like to get off warfarin, which was started six months ago for atrial fibrillation. He underwent ablation 6 months ago for long-standing atrial fibrillation. He has had no symptoms of palpitations since. He has hypertension and type 2 diabetes mellitus. Medications are lisinopril, atenolol, insulin, and warfarin.

Blood pressure is 124/82 mmHg and pulse rate is 72 beats/min. Cardiac examination and EKG disclose regular rate and rhythm. The rest of the physical examination is normal.

Which of the following is the most appropriate treatment?

A) Continue warfarin.

B) Switch to aspirin.

C) Switch to clopidogrel.

D) Switch to aspirin and clopidogrel.

E) 24 h halter monitor.

Answer: A

Warfarin should be continued indefinitely in this patient. All patients after an atrial fibrillation ablation should take warfarin for 2–3 months. The best management strategy after that is to provide anticoagulation as if the ablation did not occur. Tools such as the CHADS2 score are commonly used to guide therapy options. Although the patient has had no symptoms of atrial fibrillation since his ablation procedure, warfarin is still indicated.

Hypertension and diabetes mellitus give this patient a CHADS2 score of two. He has a 4.0 % risk of stroke per year. If the CHADS2 score is zero, aspirin alone is the preferred agent. New agents such as dabigatran and rivaroxaban may be an option. These agents have not been studied in the post-atrial fibrillation ablation setting.

Reference

Ouyang F, Tilz R, Chun J, Schmidt B, Wissner E, Zerm T, Neven K, Köktürk B, Konstantinidou M, Metzner A, Fuernkranz A, Kuck KH. Long-term results of catheter ablation in paroxysmal atrial fibrillation: lessons from a 5-year follow-up. Circulation. 2010;122:2368–77.

414. A 35-year-old woman presents to the emergency room with complaints of fever, diarrhea, nausea, and vomiting. She recently returned from Africa after spending 6 months there on a medical mission. Emergency isolation procedures are activated. She remains ill and develops worsening symptoms of odynophagia, sore throat, and conjunctivitis. She is diagnosed with Ebola virus. Finally, she develops disseminated intravascular coagulation, mucosal bleeding, altered mental status, and anuria, and she dies 9 days later. An emergency room nurse may have been exposed to the patient's bodily fluids.

How long should the nurse be followed for signs of Ebola infection?

A) 10 days

B) 21 days

C) 36 days

D) 48 days

Answer: B

The Centers for Disease Control and Prevention recommends that people with possible Ebola exposure should receive medical evaluation and close follow-up care including fever monitoring twice daily for 21 days after the last known exposure.

Contact tracing has been shown to be effective if cases are followed for 21 days after exposure and has been effective in limiting outbreaks worldwide. In rural areas, moving exposed patients with symptoms from the home or community to designated area of isolation has also proven to be successful in control efforts. It has been suggested that exposed health care personnel be medically followed for 21 days for signs and symptoms of Ebola virus.

References

West TE, von Saint André-von Arnim A. Clinical presentation and management of severe Ebola virus disease. Ann Am Thorac Soc. 2014;11:1341–1350.

World Health Organization Ebola response team. Ebola virus disease in West Africa—the first 9 months of the epidemic and forward projections. N Engl J Med. 2014;371:1481–95.

415. Patients who are admitted with community-acquired pneumonia who have been on statins have the following characteristics?

A) Decreased inhospital death

B) Decreased need for mechanical ventilation

C) Decreased acute respiratory failure

D) Decrease ICU admission

E) All of the above

Answer: E

Regular statin use may be significantly associated with favorable outcomes during admission for community-acquired pneumonia. In addition, statins may have beneficial effects on the clinical course of several infectious diseases, including bacterial sepsis in animals and humans. The protective benefits of statins are presumably related to their anti-inflammatory and immunomodulatory activities. Investigators have even suggested that statins might be useful in the treatment and prophylaxis of pandemic influenza.

References

Chung SD, et al. Statin use and clinical outcomes among pneumonia patients. Clin Microbiol Infect. 2014;20(9):879–85.
Fedson DS. Pandemic influenza: a potential role for statins in treatment and prophylaxis. Clin Infect Dis. 2006;43(2): 199–205.

416. According to a review of available studies, what are the effects of starting alpha blockers prior to the removal of a urinary catheter in order to prevent retention?
    A) Reduces urinary retention
    B) Increased side effects compared to placebo
    C) Increase success rate of catheter removal
    D) Prevents long-term urinary retention
    E) No better than placebo in catheter removal success rate

Answer: C
The limited available evidence suggests that alpha blockers increase success rates of catheter removal in high-risk patients. Fortunately, alpha blocker side effects are low and comparable to placebo. It is uncertain whether alpha blockers reduce the risk of recurrent urinary retention. The cost-effectiveness and recommended duration of alpha blocker treatment remain unknown. Alpha blockers prior to removal of a catheter for acute urinary retention in adult men caused few vasodilatation-related side effects.

Reference

Zeif H-J, Subramonian K. Alpha blockers prior to removal of a catheter for acute urinary retention in adult men. Cochrane Database Syst Rev. 2009;(4):CD006744.

417. Which of the following patient groups would be adequately treated for pneumonia utilizing ceftriaxone and azithromycin therapy upon presentation to the emergency department?
    A) A 77-year-old female who attends dialysis on Tuesday, Thursday, and Saturday
    B) A 22-year-old male undergoing chemotherapy for acute leukemia
    C) An 82-year-old female with a history of hypertension and glaucoma which has never been hospitalized
    D) A 54-year-old male who resides in a nursing home due to early-onset dementia

Answer: C
The majority of hospitalized patients with community-acquired pneumonia can be treated with either a respiratory fluoroquinolone or a combination or cephalosporin and a macrolide. Currently, duration of treatment is recommended between 7- and 10-day total therapy course. It is important for physicians to assess patients who are at increased risk for bacterial resistance to this empirical antibiotic regimen. Patients that meet criteria for health-care-associated pneumonia should be identified as their antibiotic regimens may need to include coverage for methicillin-resistant *Staphylococcus aureus* (MRSA) and multidrug-resistant (MDR) gram-negative pathogens.

Criteria for Health-Care-Associated Pneumonia:

Hospitalization for ≥2 days during the previous 90 days

Development of pneumonia greater than 48–72 h post-admission to hospital

Residence in a nursing home or extended-care facility

Long-term use of infusion therapy at home, including antibiotics

Hemodialysis during the previous 30 days

Home wound care

Family member with multidrug-resistant pathogen

Immunosuppressive disease or therapy such as organ transplantation or active chemotherapy

Reference

Solomon C. Community-acquired pneumonia. N Engl J Med. 2014;270:543–51.

418. What is the most commonly used illegal substance in an urban setting?
    A) Cocaine
    B) Marijuana
    C) Prescription opioids
    D) Nonpresription opioids
    E) Amphetamines

Answer: B
Marijuana is the most commonly used illegal substance followed by cocaine, opioids, and prescription opioids. Marijuana use remained stable in 2014, even though the percentage of people describing the drug as harmful went down. All illicit drug use has generally declined over the past two decades.

Marijuana was legal in the United States until 1937, when Congress passed the Marijuana Tax Act, effectively making the drug illegal.

Reference

Wilkinson ST, D'Souza DC. Problems with the medicalization of marijuana. JAMA. 2014;311:2377–8.

419. A 77-year-old man is admitted to a nursing home after having a stroke 2 weeks ago. The patient has residual right-sided paralysis, aphasia, and urinary incontinence. He can respond to verbal commands but cannot speak well enough to make his needs known. He spends most of the day in bed or in a chair. His expected physical progress will be slow. He needs assistance with all activities of daily living. The patient has a poor appetite, cannot use his right arm to feed himself, and is eating only half his meals. He also has intermittent urinary incontinence. He currently has no skin breakdown.

Which of the following is the most appropriate intervention for preventing pressure ulcers in this patient?
A) An air-fluidized bed
B) A doughnut cushion when seated
C) A foam mattress overlay
D) Bladder catheterization
E) Massage of skin over pressure

Answer: C

This patient has many risk factors for pressure ulcers. This includes advanced age, reduced mobility, poor nutrition, and urinary incontinence. The most appropriate cost-effective preventive measure for this patient is a foam mattress overlay. A systematic review concluded that specialized foam mattresses overlays and specialized sheepskin overlays reduce the incidence of pressure ulcers compared with standard mattresses.

Since a limited preventive approach to pressure ulcers is less costly than one focused on treating established ulcers, patients should be identified as quickly as possible.

Whether there is any additional advantage for ulcer prevention by using a more expensive air-fluidized bed is unclear. These beds make nursing care more difficult and are usually reserved for treating patients with established extensive ulcers.

The preferred seat cushion is one that distributes pressure uniformly over the weight-bearing body surface. Doughnut cushions do not do this and should not be used as a preventive measure.

An indwelling or condom catheter is sometimes needed when treating a stage IV ulcer, but should be used with caution.

Reference

Pham B, Teague L, Mahoney J, Goodman L, Paulden M, Poss J, et al. Early prevention of pressure ulcers among elderly patients admitted through emergency departments: a cost-effectiveness analysis. Ann Emerg Med. 2011;58(5):468–78.e3.

420. You are asked to see a 72-year-old male in the emergency department with a 3-day history of cough and increasing shortness of breath. He has enjoyed good health and is on no medications.

On physical examination, his temperature is 38 °C (101.5 °F) and blood pressure is 150/80. There are crackles noted in his right lower lung field. The remainder of his physical examination is normal.

Laboratory data reveals a hemoglobin of 13.4 and a leukocyte count of 10,500 µ/L. Blood urea nitrogen is 24 mg/dL and creatinine is 1 mg/dL. Glucose is 110. Chest X-ray reveals a right lower lobe infiltrate. Blood cultures and sputum gram stain are pending.

Which of the following is the most appropriate management of this patient?
A) Begin empiric antibiotics and admit him to the intensive care unit.
B) Begin empiric antibiotics and admit him to the medical ward.
C) Discharge on oral antibiotic therapy.
D) Administer a single dose of empiric antibiotic and discharge on oral antibiotic therapy.

Answer: B

The correct level of care for this patient includes admitting to the medical ward with intravenous antibiotics. The CURB-65 score estimates mortality risk based upon the following indicators: confusion, blood urea nitrogen level >19.6, respiratory rate ≥30 per minute, systolic blood pressure <90, diastolic pressure ≤60, and age 65 years or older. One point is scored for each positive indicator. Patients with a score of 0–1 have a low mortality risk and can be considered for outpatient treatment. Those with a CURB-65 score of 2 or more should be hospitalized. Patients with a score of 3 or more should be considered for admission to the intensive care unit. This patient's CURB-65 score is 2, and his predicted mortality risk is 17 %. Hospitalization is recommended for patients with a score of 2 or higher.

The CURB-65 has been compared to the more complicated pneumonia severity index (PSI) in predicting mortality from pneumonia. It has been shown that the PSI is a better predictor for short-term mortality.

Reference

Howell MD, Donnino MW, Talmor D, Clardy P, Ngo L, Shapiro NI. Performance of severity of illness scoring systems in emergency department patients with infection. Acad Emerg Med. 2007;14(8):709–14.

421. Your hospital is initiating a performance improvement plan to decrease the rate of catheter-associated urinary tract infections. Which of the following patients currently meet indications for indwelling urinary catheter usage?
A) A 49-year-old male with prostate cancer who has not urinated for 2 days and had 850 cc of urine present on bladder scan

B) A 62-year-old female who is unable use the bedside commode and is requesting a Foley catheter
while in the hospital

C) An 85-year-old man with urinary incontinence
who has a stage 4 sacral ulcer

D) All of the above

E) A and C

F) B and C

Answer: E

Some acceptable indications for an indwelling urinary catheter include the following:

1) Clinically significant urinary retention for temporary
relief

2) For comfort in a terminally ill patient

3) Accurate urine output monitoring in the critically ill
patient

4) During prolonged surgical procedures with general or
spinal anesthesia

5) To aid in healing stage 4 sacral decubitus ulcer that has failed
treatment and is worsened due to urinary incontinence

Patient preference, urinary incontinence, and monitoring
urinary output in the stable patient are not indications for
indwelling urinary catheters and should be avoided.

Reference

Hooton TM, Bradley SF, Cardenas DD, Colgan R, Geerlings
SE, Rice JC, Saint S, Schaeffer AJ, Tambayh PA, Tenke P,
Nicolle LE; Infectious Diseases Society of America.
Diagnosis, prevention, and treatment of catheter-associated
urinary tract infection in adults: 2009 International Clinical
Practice Guidelines from the Infectious Diseases Society
of America. Clin Infect Dis. 2010;50:625–63.

422. A 48-year-old woman is admitted to the stroke unit for
new-onset left hemiparesis and left-sided neglect. A
CT scan of the head shows a right middle cerebral
artery infarction. An MRI done 2 h after presentation
shows an intraluminal thrombus consistent with internal carotid artery dissection.

On physical examination 2 days after admission,
temperature is normal, blood pressure is 140/78 mmHg,
pulse rate is 68 beats/min, and respiratory rate is 12
breaths/min. The cardiopulmonary examination is normal. She is lethargic. Family reports that she is
depressed. She has dysarthria and left arm and leg
weakness. Some upper airway congestion is noted. On
bedside dysphagia screening, she is unable to safely
swallow water and has a mild cough.

Which of the following is the most appropriate next
step in management?

A) Early rehabilitation

B) Amoxicillin

C) Modafinil

D) Stenting of the internal carotid

E) Paroxetine

Answer: A

Rehabilitation should be initiated in this patient as soon as she is
medically stable. She has had an acute ischemic stroke with an
identified cause that resulted in significant motor dysfunction.

Early rehabilitation can have multiple beneficial effects on
stroke recovery. Physical therapy may prevent risk for deep
venous thrombosis, atelectasis, contractures, and skin breakdown. She should be evaluated by speech and swallow therapists
for the ability to swallow liquids safely.. Other steps to improve
stroke recovery include screening for and treating poststroke
depression and minimizing the occurrence of poststroke medical
complications, such as pneumonia and urinary tract infections.

Prophylactic antibiotics in stroke patients who are at risk
for aspiration have not been shown to be effective in reducing the incidence of pneumonia.

The central nervous system stimulant modafinil is unlikely
to help this patient early in her recovery . In general, pharmacological agents, including amphetamines, and antidepressants are not indicated in the acute phase. They have not yet
to be shown to improve stroke recovery.

Stenting of the internal carotid artery is not indicated in
this patient who has not experienced recurrent symptoms.
The indications for stenting in the setting of carotid artery
dissection are not known.

References

Jauch EC, Saver JL, Adams HP Jr, Bruno A, Connors JJ,
Demaerschalk BM, Khatri P, McMullan PW Jr, Qureshi AI,
Rosenfield K, Scott PA, Summers DR, Wang DZ,
Wintermark M, Yonas H; American Heart Association
Stroke Council; Council on Cardiovascular Nursing;
Council on Peripheral Vascular Disease; Council on Clinical
Cardiology. Guidelines for the early management of patients
with acute ischemic stroke: a guideline for healthcare pro-
fessionals from the American Heart Association/American
Stroke Association. Stroke. 2013;44(3):870–947.

423. Which of the following best describes the Plan-Do-
Study-Act (PDSA) cycle for quality improvement in
health care?

A) PDSA obviates the need for performance
measurement.

B) PDSA activities require approval by the institutional review board.

C) Randomized, controlled trials have greater validity.

D) PDSA describes a process for measuring the effect
of changes.

Answer: D

PDSA cycles form part of the improvement guide, which
provides a framework for developing, testing, and implementing changes leading to improvement. It is commonly

used in the health-care setting. It emphasizes measurement taken after the implement of change and calls for these measurements to be built into the process. It discourages change without measurement.

The model is based in scientific method and moderates the desire to take immediate action by insisting on careful study. Most quality improvement activities do not require approval from the institutional review board.

References
Curtis JR, Levy MM. Improving the science and politics of quality improvement. JAMA. 2011;305(4):406–7.
Fan E, Laupacis A, Pronovost PJ, et al. How to use an article about quality improvement. JAMA. 2010;304(20):2279–87.

424. Which of the following is the leading cause of preventable hospital deaths?
    A) Falls with resulting trauma
    B) Central line-associated bloodstream infections
    C) Surgical errors
    D) Venous thromboembolism
    E) Medical errors

Answer: D
This is according to the US Department of Health and Human Services for Healthcare Research and Quality.

Despite an overall decline in thrombotic events due to increase use of prevention prophylaxis, pulmonary embolism resulting from deep vein thrombosis thromboembolism remains the most common preventable cause of hospital death.

There is some debate over which event is defined as a preventable death and some suggest that there is an overestimate in number of pulmonary embolisms cases classified as a preventable hospital death.

References
Cohen AT, Tapson VF, Bergmann JF, et al. Venous thromboembolism risk and prophylaxis in the acute hospital care setting (ENDORSE study): a multinational cross-sectional study. Lancet. 2008;371(9610):387–94E.
Kopcke D, Harryman O, Benbow EW, Hay C, Chalmers N. Mortality from pulmonary embolism is decreasing in hospital patients. J Roy Soc Med. 2011;104(8):327–31.

425. When is *Pneumocystis carinii* (PcP) pneumonia most likely to present?
    A) Winter
    B) Fall
    C) Summer
    D) Spring

Answer: C
There can be seasonal variations in disease presentations. This may be due to a variety of environmental factors.

Increased levels of air pollutants, including carbon monoxide, nitrogen dioxide, ozone, sulfur dioxide, and particulate matter, are well-known risk factors for the development of pneumonia, asthma, COPD, and other pulmonary diseases

In a study of 457 patients with HIV and microscopically confirmed PcP, hospital admissions were significantly higher in the summer than in other seasons. Increases in temperature and sulfur dioxide levels were independently associated with hospital admissions for PcP.

Reference
Dyawe K, et al. Environmental risk factors for Pneumocystis pneumonia hospitalizations in HIV patients. Clin Infect Dis. 2013;56(1):74–81.

426. A 35-year-old man is admitted to the hospital with acute pancreatitis. In order to determine the severity of disease and risk of mortality, the Bedside Index of Severity in Acute Pancreatitis is calculated. All of the following variables are used to calculate this score except:
    A) Age greater than 60 years
    B) BUN greater than 35
    C) Impaired mental status
    D) Pleural effusion
    E) White blood cell count greater than 12,000 leukocytes/µL

Answer: E
Most patients with acute pancreatitis recover without complications, the overall mortality rate of this illness is between 2 and 5 %. Several tools have been developed to predict outcomes in pancreatitis. The Bedside Index of Severity in Acute Pancreatitis (BISAP) score may replace the Ranson criteria and APACHE II severity scores as the modality to assess the severity of pancreatitis. It has been validated in studies as an accurate measure of severity in pancreatitis.

It is easier to calculate and is a better predicted of outcomes. The Bedside Index of Severity in Acute Pancreatitis score incorporates five variables in determining severity: BUN greater than 35 mg/dL, impaired mental status, presence of SIRS, age above 60 years, and pleural effusion on radiography. The presence of three or more of these factors is associated with an increased risk for inhospital mortality.

Reference
Papachristou GI, Muddana V, Yadav D, O'Connell M, Sanders MK, Slivka A, Whitcomb DC. Comparison of BISAP, the Ranson, APACHE II, and CTSI scores in predicting organ failure, complications, and mortality in acute pancreatitis. Am J Gastroenterol. 2010;105(2):435–41.305.

427. According to a 2012 Minneapolis Heart Institute study, what were the outcomes of cardiologist as compared to

hospitalists in the management of congestive heart failure?

A) Cardiology-treated patients had fewer 30-day readmissions.
B) Hospitalist-treated patients had fewer 30-day readmissions.
C) Costs were the same.
D) Readmission rates were the same.

Answer: A

Care must be taken in interpreting studies that look at quality endpoints among different hospital services. Studies often show conflicting results as to what specialty service provides better quality and most cost-efficient care. This may depend on resources allocated, patient selection, and who is conducting the study.

The research conducted at the Minneapolis Heart Institute tracked readmission rates for patients admitted with heart failure from 2009 to 2011. The 30-day readmission rate for cardiologists was 16 % vs. 27.1 % of patients discharged by hospitalists, even though cardiologists treated patients with more severe disease.

Researchers found that the cardiologists did a better job than hospitalists of calling patients after discharge, making sure patients had outpatient appointments and ensuring follow-up with a nurse practitioner. The length of stay was similar for both specialties. Cardiologists utilized more resources and delivered more expensive care. Their cost per case was $9850 for cardiologists vs. $7741 for hospitalists.

Reference

Minneapolis Heart Institute Foundation. Heart failure patients treated by a cardiologist, rather than hospitalist, have fewer readmissions. American Heart Association's scientific sessions in Los Angeles, November 2012.

428. Which of the following has been shown to be effective in improving sleep and reducing delirium in patients in the ICU?
A) Back massages
B) Ear plugs
C) Eye shades
D) Lorazepam
E) Midazolam

Answer: B

Preventing delirium in the hospital and, in particular, the ICU continues to be a challenge. Simple measures seem to work best. Ear plugs may provide some filtering of the almost constant auditory stimulation which occurs in the hospital. This has been validated by recent studies. Ear plugs may facilitate normal sleep patterns.

Medicines should be limited and may contribute to delirium. Multiple studies have shown an association between

sedative drugs and delirium, with benzodiazepines being the most strongly associated. Orientation to place and time may be accomplished by promoting visual clues. It is important to not underestimate the disruptive nature of the hospital environment and its effect on the cognitive function of frail patients.

Reference

Jones SF, Pisani MA. ICU delirium: an update. Curr Opin Crit Care. 2012;18(2):146–51.

429. A 55-year-old male is admitted with pyelonephritis. Urinalyses on admission is performed and showed 10 RBCs/hpf and 20 WBC/hpf. Nitrite and leukocyte esterase are positive. Urine culture grows *E. coli*. The patient is treated with antibiotics for urinary tract infection and is ready for discharge.
What should be the next step?
A) Repeat urine culture to confirm eradication of the organism.
B) Renal ultrasound.
C) Cystoscopy.
D) Repeat the urinalysis in 2 weeks.

Answer: D

The American Urological Association recommends urine testing, imaging, computed tomography scans, or intravenous pyelogram plus renal ultrasound and cystoscopy for patients aged 35 years or older with 3 or more red blood cells per high power field on two of three properly collected urinalyses. This patient has a classic UTI, which may account for the RBCs seen. It would be reasonable to repeat the urinalysis in 2 weeks.

He is also a smoker and therefore at risk for uroepithelial malignancies. Follow-up with urology as well may be appropriate in this case.

Reference

Khadra MH, Pickard RS, Charlton M, Powell PH, Neal DE. A prospective analysis of 1,930 patients with hematuria to evaluate current diagnostic practice. J Urol. 2000;163:524–7.

430. The use of diuretics in the treatment of acute kidney injury (AKI) in critically ill patients is most likely to result in which of the following?
A) Reduction in mortality
B) Improvement in renal recovery
C) Shortening of the duration of acute kidney illness
D) Reduction of the need for renal replacement therapy
E) Increase in urine output and sodium excretion

Answer: E

Although it is tempting to use diuretics in anuric and oliguria renal failure, there is no data to support their use. Diuretics may increase urine output and sodium excretion but are ineffective and even detrimental in the prevention and treatment of AKI. They neither shorten the duration of AKI nor reduce the need for renal replacement therapy.

Reference
Dennen P, Douglas IS, Anderson R. Acute kidney injury in the intensive care unit: an update and primer for the intensivist. Crit Care Med. 2010;38:261–75.

431. Cardiovascular events contribute to what percentage of deaths at long-term follow-up in patients with community-acquired pneumonia (CAP)?
    A) 37 %
    B) 30 %
    C) 15 %
    D) 10 %
    E) Less than 5 %

Answer: B
CAP increases the risk for cardiovascular events in the 90 days after discharge. Both plaque-related and plaque-unrelated cardiovascular events are increased. The 90-day incidence of cardiovascular events in discharged community-acquired pneumonia patients was 1.5 % for myocardial infarction, 10.2 % for congestive heart failure, 9.5 % for arrhythmia, 0.8 % for unstable angina, and 0.2 % for stroke. Overall 30 % of patients who died in long term did so from cardiovascular events.

Reference
Soto-Gomez N, et al. Pneumonia: an arrhythmogenic Disease? Am J Med. 2013;126(1):43–8.

432. A 63-year-old male is admitted with a diagnosis of urosepsis. On his admission, his hemoglobin is noted to be 9.3 g/dL. The patient has clinical improvement. On the third day of his admission, his hemoglobin is noted to be 6.1 g/Dl. Hemoccult studies are negative. Fecal hemoccult is negative. A peripheral smear reveals schistocytes on the blood smear.
    What is the most likely cause of this patient's drug-induced hemolytic anemia (DIHA)?
    A) Piperacillin/tazobactam
    B) Haloperidol
    C) Fentanyl
    D) Metformin

Answer: A
A variety of drugs can cause drug-induced hemolysis. Of the drugs listed, piperacillin/tazobactam has the highest risk, followed by metformin. In the 30-year experience of a reference laboratory, cefotetan, ceftriaxone, and piperacillin were responsible for 76 % of all cases of DIHA, with cefotetan accounting for the majority of cases.

References
Garratty G. Drug-induced immune hemolytic anemia. Hematology Am Soc Hematol Educ Program. 2009;73–79.
Mayer B, Yürek S, Salama A. Piperacillin-induced immune hemolysis: new cases and a concise review of the literature. Transfusion. 2010;50:1135–8.

433. A 67-year-old man is admitted to the medical intensive care unit with sepsis associated with pneumococcal pneumonia. He required mechanical ventilation as well as vasopressors while in the ICU.
    On the third hospital day, he is transferred to your service. His urine output drops and his creatinine increases to 4.0 mg/dL. Acute tubular injury is suspected. For the next 3 days, the creatinine continues to rise slowly to 5.4 mg/dL, but then stabilizes. Potassium remains below 5 meq/L. The patient is oliguric, but urine output continues to increase. He has recovered well from the pneumonia and is eating well and participating with physical therapy.
    Which of the following would improve renal recovery?
    A) Furosemide
    B) Bosentan
    C) Low-dose dopamine
    D) Continuous renal replacement therapy (CRRT)
    E) Hemodialysis
    F) None of the above

Answer: F
There is no clear consensus on when or how often to perform hemodialysis in the setting of acute kidney injury (AKI). Some studies have suggested that early initiation may be beneficial. In one prospective trial, aggressive dialysis did not improve recovery or survival rates. Many authorities suggest that hemodialysis may delay the recovery of patients with AKI. In addition there seems to be no difference in outcome between the use of intermittent hemodialysis and continuous renal replacement therapy (CRRT). In severe AKI hemodialysis is still considered standard therapy.

Once dialysis is started, the ability to measure recovery is limited. In this patient urine output is increasing, creatinine has stabilized, and sepsis has resolved. All of these point toward recovery of renal function.

Indications for dialysis in AKI include hyperkalemia refractory to medical therapy, correction of severe acid-based disturbances that are refractory to medical therapy, and severe azotemia (BUN >80–100).

Most clinical studies have failed to establish this beneficial role of low-dose dopamine infusion.

References
Macedo E, Mehta RL. When should renal replacement therapy be initiated for acute kidney injury? Semin Dial. 2011;24(2):132–7.
Palevsky PM, Zhang JH, O'Connor TZ, Chertow GM, Crowley ST, Choudhury D, et al. Intensity of renal support in critically ill patients with acute kidney injury. N Engl J Med. 2008;359(1):7–20.

434. Compared to middle age and younger adults, elderly patients have an increase in 30-day readmission rates for which of the following conditions:
    A) Heart failure.
    B) Pneumonia.
    C) Acute MI.
    D) All of the answers are correct.
    E) None of the above.

Answer: E
Despite social situations that often differ, young and middle-aged adults have 30-day readmission rates that are similar for most conditions.

References
Jencks SF, Williams MV, Coleman EA. Rehospitalizations among patients in the medicare fee-for-service program. New Eng J Med. 2009;360:1418–28.
Ranasinghe I, et al. Readmissions after hospitalization for heart failure, acute myocardial infarction, or pneumonia among young and middle-aged adults: a retrospective observational cohort study. PLoS Med. 2014;11(9):e1001737.

435. A 68-year-old man who has severe coronary artery disease is admitted to the ICU with respiratory failure and shock. The source of the shock is uncertain. A procalcitonin level is ordered.
    Which of the following is true concerning procalcitonin levels?
    A) An elevated procalcitonin level mitigates against myocardial infarction.
    B) A procalcitonin-guided strategy will decrease the patient's mortality risk.
    C) A low procalcitonin level excludes bacterial infection.
    D) A high procalcitonin level is specific for bacterial infections.
    E) A low procalcitonin level makes septic shock less likely.

Answer: E
A low procalcitonin level is primarily predictive of a decrease incidence of septic shock. Procalcitonin (PCT) is a biomarker that exhibits greater specificity than other markers in identifying patients with sepsis. It can aid in the diagnosis of bacterial infections.

Levels of procalcitonin increase in sepsis in proportion to the severity of the infection. PCT levels are highest in patients who have a bacterial infection, but these levels have also high in patients who have viral and fungal infections. Bacteremia is usually associated with high procalcitonin levels, but low levels do not exclude this diagnosis. Procalcitonin levels have been reported to be increased in myocardial infarction and pancreatitis.

Its exact clinical use is yet to be determined, and its use in studies has not resulted in decreased mortality yet. Procalcitonin levels predictably decline if successful source control, which may be the best use of this marker. One use may be in the de-escalation of antibiotics. Procalcitonin is a prohormone of calcitonin.

References
Heyland D. Procalcitonin for reduced antibiotic exposure in the critical care setting. Crit Care Med. 2011;39: 1792–9.194.
Reinhart K, Meisner M. Biomarkers in the critically ill patient: procalcitonin. Crit Care Clin. 2011;7:253–63.

436. A healthy 45-year-old hospice nurse has been caring for a patient who is terminally ill with AIDS. She accidentally stuck herself with a needle that was used to draw his blood. The needle that pricked her skin drew a barely noticeable amount of blood. The nurse is very upset and calls you immediately regarding her risk of exposure to the HIV virus and postexposure treatment.
    What is the most appropriate action?
    A) Reassurance.
    B) Treat only if she tests positive.
    C) Start three-drug antiretroviral therapy and continue for 28 days.
    D) Start antiretroviral therapy with zidovudine and continue for 6 months.

Answer: C
This nurse should immediately be treated with three-drug antiviral therapy. The nurses' risk of infection is based on the source and type of exposure. For HIV, the circulating viral burden is highest at the initial stage of infection and in the preterminal advanced stage, which is the case here.

Hollow needles used for drawing blood are associated with higher viral inoculum than solid needles. An expanded regimen of three drugs for 28 days is advocated by the Centers for Disease Control and Prevention. HIV postexposure prophylaxis should be initiated, ideally within 1 h of the injury.

Hospitalists and nursing staff should be aware of current protocols and how they are activated in a timely manner.

References

Cardo DM, Culver KH, Ciesielski C, Srivastava PU, Marcus R, Abiteboul D, et al, A case–control study of HIV sero-conversion in health-care workers after percutaneous exposure. N Engl J Med. 1997;337:1485–90.

Diprose P, Deakin CD, Smedley J. Ignorance of post-exposure prophylaxis guidelines following HIV needle-stick injury may increase the risk of seroconversion. Br J Anaesth. 2000;84 (6):767–70.

437. A 67-year-old man with ETOH-related cirrhosis is admitted with hematemesis. He has been taking twice daily propranolol for 4 months for esophageal varices. He has not had prior bleeding before this. He has been abstinent from alcohol for 3 years. He is stabilized and given 4 units of fresh frozen plasma and 2 units of packed red blood cells. His INR on admission is 1.6.

An octreotide infusion is started. An esophagogastroduodenoscopy shows three columns of grade 3 esophageal varices. An active bleeding source is found. Hemostasis is achieved with band ligation of several esophageal varices.

His vital signs remain stable post procedure and he is transferred back to the floor.

Which of the following should be done to increase this patient's survival?

A) Packed red blood cells to achieve a target hematocrit of greater than 30 %
B) Continued octreotide infusion for 5 days total
C) Intravenous ceftriaxone now and daily for 5 days
D) Fresh frozen plasma to correct coagulopathy to an INR of less than 1.5
E) Intravenous pantoprazole now and twice daily for 2 days

Answer: C

Intravenous antibiotics such as ceftriaxone or ciprofloxacin have a proven survival benefit in patients who have cirrhosis with portal hypertensive bleeding. It is recommended that it be administered early in the course and continued for 5–7 days.

A target hematocrit of 30 % risks increasing portal pressure. Excessive fresh frozen plasma administration increases portal pressure and the risk for transfusion-associated lung injury. There is no clear survival benefit from intravenous pantoprazole in the setting of variceal bleeding, even after band ligation. Octreotide infusion can lower portal pressures, but are usually emergency and recommended for 72 h.

Reference

Garcia-Tsao G, Sanyal AJ, Grace ND, Carey W; Practice Guidelines Committee of the American Association for the Study of Liver Diseases; Practice Parameters Committee of the American College of Gastroenterology. Prevention and management of gastroesophageal varices and variceal hemorrhage in cirrhosis. Hepatology. 2007;46(3):922–38.

438. Which percentage of C. difficile infections are community acquired?
A) 5 %
B) 10 %
C) 15 %
D) 35 %
E) 50 %

Answer: D

C. difficile infection is now recognized as a common cause of community-acquired diarrhea. 22–44 % of cases are thought to occur within the community. Many patients lack the typical risk factors associated with an acquisition. Community-acquired patients tend to be younger and more likely to be female than hospital-acquired C. difficile-infected patients.

Reference

Sahil Khanna MBBS; Darrell S Pardi MD; MS; FACG; Scott L Aronson MD; Patricia P Kammer CCRP; Robert Orenstein DO; Jennifer L St Sauver PhD; W Scott Harmsen MS; Alan R Zinsmeister PhD Am J Gastroenterol. 2012;107(1):89–95.

439. In patients with chronic liver disease, which hemoglobin threshold for transfusion of red cells in patients with acute gastrointestinal bleeding is associated with significantly improved outcomes?
A) Below 10 g/dL (aggressive)
B) Below 9 g/dL (liberal strategy)
C) Below 7 g/dL (restrictive strategy)
D) No threshold

Answer: C

The restrictive strategy below 7 g/dL improved probability of survival and decreased further bleeding in a recent study. Within the first 5 days, the portal-pressure gradient increased significantly in patients assigned to the liberal strategy but not in those assigned to the restrictive strategy. It was significantly higher in the subgroup of patients with cirrhosis and Child-Pugh class A, B, or C disease., possibly due to an increase in portal pressures seen in that group.

Mortality at 45 days was significantly lower in the group with fewer transfusions. In addition, patients with a lower transfusion goal were less likely to rebleed and were discharged from the hospital sooner.

Patients in hypovolemic shock, and those with cardiovascular disease, might still benefit from higher transfusion thresholds.

Reference

Villanueva C, Colomo A, et al. Transfusion Strategies for acute upper gastrointestinal bleeding. N Engl J Med. 2013;368:11–21.

440. Most high-risk peptic ulcer rebleeding after successful endoscopic hemostasis occurs within how many days?
    A) 3
    B) 4–7
    C) 15–30
    D) 8–14

Answer: A

Most patients with high-risk peptic ulcers rebleed within the first 72 h. Major clinical parameters for predicting rebleeding after receiving endoscopic treatment are hemodynamic instability at admission and hemoglobin value. Major endoscopic predictors for rebleeding are active bleeding at endoscopy, large ulcer size, and ulcer location.

Reference

El Ouali S, et al. Timing of rebleeding in high-risk peptic ulcer bleeding after successful hemostasis: a systematic review. Can J Gastroenterol Hepatol. 2014;28(10):543–8.

441. The 2013 American Heart Association Guidelines for reducing heart failure readmissions include all of the following except:
    A) Identifying patients suitable for guideline-directed medical therapy
    B) Developing patient education programs that emphasize discharge care
    C) Developing home electronic monitoring systems
    D) Utilizing nursing staff for disease management
    E) Conducting patient follow-ups at 3 days and 2 weeks post-discharge

Answer: C

Interventions that were relatively inexpensive and available to all hospitals were chosen. They include four simple, low-tech interventions. Identify heart failure patients appropriate for goal-directed therapy, developing transitional care, and discharge planning that emphasizes patient education to increase treatment compliance, manage comorbid conditions effectively, and tackle psychosocial barriers to care.

Readmissions will continue to be a significant reform topic because they are seen as maker of overall system quality and can be objectively measured.

References

Dellinger RP, Levy MM, Carlet JM, et al. Surviving sepsis campaign: international guidelines for management of severe sepsis and septic shock: 2008. Crit Care Med. 2008;36:296–327.

Roger VL, Lloyd-Jones D, Emelia J, et al. Heart disease and stroke statistics— 2012 update: a report from the American Heart Association. Circulation. 2012;125:e2–e220.

442. What is the approximate percentage of patients being treated for a deep vein thrombosis (DVT) who have a silent pulmonary embolism (PE)?
    A) 13%
    B) 40 %
    C) 22 %
    D) 4 %

Answer: B

Silent PE is common in patients with a DVT. Estimates on the frequency of a silent PE are as high as 50 %, based on several study results, though identification of the PE would have little impact on treatment.

Investigation of a silent pulmonary embolism in patients with deep vein thrombosis may be of some benefit. Those who have suffered a pulmonary embolism are at increased risk of embolic recurrence, especially in the first 15 days. There is also the concern that if PE is found during follow-up, it may be incorrectly diagnosed as a new PE. This may lead to the false assumption that anticoagulation failed in this patient. Despite these factors guidelines do not currently recommend PE screening in patients with DVT.

References

Meignan M, et al. Systematic lung scans reveal a high frequency of silent pulmonary embolism in patients with proximal deep venous thrombosis. Arch Intern Med. 2000;160(2):159–64.

Tzoran I, et al. Silent pulmonary embolism in patients with proximal deep vein thrombosis in the lower limbs. J Thromb Haemost. 2012;10(4):564–71.

443. A 75-year-old male was admitted with a diagnosis of COPD exacerbation 3 days ago. He developed acute respiratory distress with elevated carbon dioxide so the patient was intubated and placed on invasive mechanical ventilation. He has improved with the treatment including methylprednisolone, albuterol, and levofloxacin. He tolerates a weaning trial well, and the decision is made to extubate. He does well but remains hypercapnic. He is transferred to the floor.

On physical examination, he is alert and awake. Blood pressure is 128/63 mmHg and pulse rate is 80 beats per minute. Pulmonary examination reveals normal breath sounds with mild wheezes.

Which of the following interventions will decrease patient's risk for reintubation?
    A) Incentive spirometry every 2 h
    B) Noninvasive positive pressure ventilation
    C) Nebulized N-acetylcysteine
    D) Inhaled helium-oxygen mixture

Answer: B

Noninvasive positive pressure ventilation (NPPV) in the 24 h after extubation may reduce the need for reintubation. As a method of weaning critically ill adults from invasive ventilation, NPPV was significantly associated with reduced mortality and ventilator-associated pneumonia. In many circumstances, NPPV is not tolerated.

The use of incentive spirometry reduces the risk of postoperative pulmonary complications but has a limited role in the routine management of nonsurgical patients following extubation. N-acetylcysteine is a mucolytic agent. In this particular patient, secretions do not seem to be a confounding factor. In addition, N-acetylcysteine may trigger bronchospasm and would not be recommended here.

Reference

Ferrer M, Sellares J, Valencia M, et al. Non-invasive ventilation after extubation in hypercapnic patients with chronic respiratory disorders: randomised controlled trial. Lancet. 2009;374(9695):1082–8.

444. Which of the following drugs is not listed on the 2012 Beers criteria for potentially inappropriate sue?
    A) Hydroxyzine
    B) Promethazine
    C) Nitrofurantoin
    D) Methyldopa
    E) E) None of the above

Answer: E

Mark H. Beers, MD, a geriatrician, first created the Beers criteria in 1991. The criteria were developed utilizing a field of experts and statistical modeling. He and his colleagues published criteria listing potentially inappriate medications for older patients. Updates to these criteria have subsequently been published on a regular basis.

Drugs listed on the Beers list are categorized according to stratified risks. The tables include medications that have relative and absolute contraindications. The list emphasizes stopping medications that are unnecessary and have a high risk-benefit ratio.

The criteria are used in clinical care, training, research, and health-care policy to develop performance measures and document outcomes. The "Beers criteria" apply to people 65 and older. As this age group grows, the delivery of safe and effective health care has become increasingly important.

Reference

Fick DM, Cooper JW, Wade WE, et al. Updating the Beers criteria for potentially inappropriate medication use in older adults: results of a US consensus panel of experts. Arch Intern Med. 2003;163(22):2716–24.

445. A 78-year-old man who has coronary artery disease and heart failure is admitted to the hospital because of worsening shortness of breath. His outpatient medications are an ACE inhibitor, aspirin, and a beta-adrenergic blocking agent. He has no underlying pulmonary disease.

On physical exam, the temperature is 37.0 °C (98.6 °F), pulse rate is 117 beats per minute, respiratory rate is 33 breaths per minute, and blood pressure is 112/63 mmHg. Arterial PO2 is 56 mmHg, PCO2 is 57 mmHg, and pH is 7.32 on 100 % oxygen by nonbreathing mask. Radiograph of the chest reveals diffuse opacities consistent with pulmonary edema. He is started on continuous positive airway pressure ventilation (CPAP).

Which of the following is decreased with the use of CPAP in acute cardiogenic edema?
    A) Stroke
    B) Intra-aortic balloon pump support
    C) Need for revascularization surgery
    D) New myocardial infarction
    E) Worse outcomes than BIPAP
    F) Death

Answer: F

Respiratory compromise may develop in patients with cardiogenic pulmonary edema, and these patients may require respiratory support. Continuous positive airway pressure (CPAP) is effective for acute cardiogenic pulmonary edema. A meta-analysis has demonstrated that CPAP reduces the risk of intubation and death. It does not protect against a new myocardial infarction, need for revascularization, stroke, or use of balloon pump.

Positive airway pressure has been well used for acute exacerbations of chronic obstructive pulmonary disease. It can also be used effectively for cardiogenic edema well.

Currently, the data are insufficient to compare the efficacy and safety of BiPAP with those of CPAP.

References

Peter JV, Moran JL, Phillips-Hughes J, et al. Effect of noninvasive positive pressure ventilation (NIPPV) on mortality in patients with acute cardiogenic pulmonary edema: a meta-analysis. Lancet. 2006;367:1155–63. 1661655.

Weng CL, Zhao YT, Liu QH, et al. Meta-analysis: noninvasive ventilation in acute cardiogenic pulmonary edema. Ann Intern Med. 2010;152(9):590–600.

446. In 2013, what specialty among the choices had the lowest rate of malpractice claims per practicing physician?
    A) Neurosurgery
    B) Hospitalists
    C) Gastroenterology
    D) Cardiology
    E) Neurology

Answer: B

Because the hospitalist field is relatively new, there has been little formal research as to how malpractice claims against hospitalists compare against other specialists and internists for liability risk. Overall malpractice claims against hospitalists appear to be low. Although malpractice claims against hospitalist are low compared to other specialties, in some areas hospitalists have seen an increase in claims. This has probably occurred as hospitalists continue to expand their scope of practice, particularly in the areas of comanagement with neurosurgical patients.

A study of closed claims by The Doctors Company found that the most common allegations involving hospitalists are improper management of treatment course, delay in treatment, failure to treat, diagnosis-related error improper medication management, and failure to monitor the physiologic status of the patient.

Reference

Hospital Medicine 2013: Society of Hospital Medicine (SHM) Annual Meeting. Presented on May 18, 2013.

447. The most common cause of acute mesenteric ischemia is:
    A) Superior mesenteric artery embolism
    B) Mesenteric vein thrombosis
    C) Noninclusive mesenteric vascular disease
    D) Thrombosis of the superior mesenteric artery
    E) Abdominal aortic aneurysm involving the superior mesenteric artery

Answer: A

Fifty percent of the cases of acute mesenteric ischemia (AMI) are caused by an embolism. Emboli usually originate in the left atrium or ventricle. Often a source is found such as atrial fibrillation or recent myocardial infarction. Most emboli lodge distal to a major branch point.

Abdominal distention and gastrointestinal bleeding are the primary presenting symptoms in as many as 25 % of patients. Pain may be abrupt, severe, and unresponsive to opioids. As the bowel becomes gangrenous, rectal bleeding and signs of sepsis develop.

If not rapidly recognized and treated, AMI has a poor outcome. It should be considered in any patient with abdominal pain disproportionate to physical findings and the presence of risk factors, especially age older than 60 years.

Because of the high mortality and the difficulty of diagnosis, mesenteric ischemia poses a substantial legal risk. Legal risk is reduced with early surgical consultation and prompt imaging.

Reference

Sachs SM, Morton JH, Schwartz SI. Acute mesenteric ischemia. Surgery. 1982;92(4):646–53.

448. What is the most common missed diagnosis found on autopsy among hospitalized patients?
    A) Pulmonary embolism
    B) Myocardial infarction
    C) Aortic aneurysm
    D) Infection
    E) Malignancy

Answer: A

Due to its frequency and variety of presentations, pulmonary embolism remains the most common missed diagnosis found on autopsy. This has been true both with past and current studies. Studies of patients who died unexpectedly from pulmonary embolism both in the hospital and outside have revealed that the patients complained of a variety of vague symptoms, often for weeks. Forty percent of these patients had been seen by a physician in the weeks prior to their death.

In high-risk patients, the diagnosis of pulmonary embolism should be sought actively in patients with respiratory symptoms unexplained by an alternative diagnosis.,

References

Aalten CM, Samson MM, Jansen PA. Diagnostic errors: the need to have autopsies. Neth J Med. 2006;64(6):164–5.
Al-Saidi F, Diaz-Granados N, Messner H, Herridge MS. Relationship between premortem and postmortem diagnoses in critically ill bone marrow transplantation patients. Crit Care Med. 2002;30:570–3.
Barendregt WB, de Boer HHM, Kubat K. Quality control in fatally injured patients: the value of the necropsy. Eur J Surg. 1993;159:9–13.

449. A 78-year-old male with severe chronic obstructive pulmonary disease was admitted the ICU. He develops acute delirium post-extubation for 36 h. He gradually improves with supportive care and is transferred to the medicine service. He is being prepared for discharge to a skilled nursing facility. He is debilitated but his cognitive abilities seem to be near baseline. Prior to this episode, he was living by himself. The family is concerned about any further cognitive decline which would impact his ability to live independently.

Which of the following statements is correct?
    A) Patients with the same admitting diagnosis, who develop delirium in the hospital, have the same neurological outcome as those who do not.
    B) Long-term cognitive impairment in patients with delirium is not seen in younger patients.
    C) The use of antipsychotics in the hospital correlates with the level of cognitive impairment.
    D) Patients who develop delirium after critical illness are at risk of developing persistent cognitive impairment after 1 year.

Answer: D

Development of delirium is predictive of cognitive impairment 1 year after a critical illness. In this case, there may be some permanent cognitive decline. The duration of delirium is an independent predictor of long-term cognitive impairment. This is noted in patients under the age of 40 as well. The development of delirium may be a predictor of underlying cognitive impairment, such as dementia.

References

Bergeron N, Dubois MJ, Dumont M et al. Intensive care delirium screening checklist: evaluation of a new screening tool. Intensive Care Med. 2001;27:859–64.

Jackson JC, Gordon SM, Girard TD et al. Delirium as a risk factor for long-term cognitive impairment in mechanically ventilated ICU survivors. Am J Respir Crit Care Med. 2007;175:A22.

450. On your first day as a hospitalist, you are called to the emergency room to admit a case of abdominal pain due to pancreatitis. The ED physician starts his presentation by stating the patient is an alcoholic. On your questioning, the patient reports that he has a history of alcoholism, but denies any recent alcohol intake in the past several years. You suspect that he still drinks. Amylase and lipase are normal. ETOH is not detected. You admit him with the diagnosis of pancreatitis. He is started in IV fluids and pain control.

    Several days later with no resolution of symptoms, gastroenterology is consulted. They conclude that pancreatitis is unlikely and he undergoes an EGD. The diagnoses of severe gastritis are made.

    Which of the following is the type of medical error made?
    A) Anchoring
    B) Heuristic
    C) Cultural bias
    D) Framing

Answer: A

Anchoring errors occur when clinicians cling to an initial impression even as conflicting and contradictory data accumulate. There is a tendency to frame a clinical problem around the first piece of information we receive. There is often a sense of reward and confidence in going with your first instinct. In addition, the hierarchical nature of medicine often places greater emphasis on the opinions of certain staff.

    In this case, pancreatitis is certainly possible, but the data points otherwise. There is a tendency to stick with the original diagnosis and not consider other options even in the face of conflicting evidence.

Reference

Furnham A, Boo, Hua CH. A literature review of the anchoring effect. J Soc Econ. 2011;40(1):35–42.

451. A 57-year-old male was hospitalized for the treatment of osteomyelitis of her left foot. This has resulted from a chronic diabetic ulcer. Medical history is significant for type 1 diabetes mellitus, hypertension, and chronic kidney disease. His baseline serum creatinine is 3.7 mg/dL. There was creatinine change this admission. She is currently followed by the renal service. The patient was initiated on broad-spectrum antibiotics. Subsequent, cultures grew *Klebsiella*. He will be discharged to a long-term care facility for physical therapy and to complete a 4-week course of intravenous antibiotics.

    Which of the following is the most appropriate route of access for antibiotics in this patient?
    A) Left subclavian catheter
    B) Left internal jugular catheter
    C) Peripheral intravenous access
    D) Right peripherally inserted central catheter

Answer: C

Every attempt should be made to continue the use of peripheral intravenous access in this patient. This patient has chronic kidney disease and will eventually require hemodialysis. A central catheter may interfere with the placement of the future graft. It should only be placed after a discussion with the nephrology and vascular service.

Reference

Trainor D, Borthwick E, Ferguson A. Perioperative management of the hemodialysis patient. Semin Dial. 2011;24(3):314–26.

452. A 72-year-old female is admitted to the hospital with congestive heart failure. You are the attending physician. She has a history of New York Heart Association class III ischemic cardiomyopathy. Her past medical history is significant for congestive heart failure as well as syncope due to recurrent ventricular tachycardia.

    On the third day of her hospitalization, patient is found to be nonresponsive. The cardiac arrest team is called. You arrive at the same time as the cardiac arrest team. The patient is pulseless and chest compression have begun. The family is in the room. The family requests to stay present during the resuscitation efforts.

    Which of the following is true concerning outcomes when family members are present during cardiac resuscitation?
    A) Lower rates of post-traumatic stress disorder are seen in family members.
    B) Longer duration of cardiac resuscitation.
    C) Increased rates of stress noted by team members.
    D) Improved outcomes.
    E) Worse outcomes.

Answer: A

Several studies have looked at the presence of family members during cardiac resuscitation. Most have shown positive outcomes in many parameters. Most who were offered elected to remain present. Significant findings have demonstrated a lower risk of post-traumatic stress disorder in family members 90 days after the event. Clinical outcomes, as well as duration of resuscitation, were found to be equal. It is suggested that the duration of codes may actually be shorter when family members are present.

Several current guidelines now suggest that family members be offered the opportunity to be present during cardiac resuscitative measures, if space allows. Hospital staff may feel uncomfortable with this arrangement and should be provided training prior to establishing this protocol.

Reference

Meyers TA, Eichhorn DJ, Guzzetta CE, et al. Family presence during invasive procedures and resuscitation: the experience of family members, nurses, and physicians. Am J Nurs. 2000;100:32–41.

453. Which device has been shown to be the most effective in preventing decubitus ulcers?
    A) Air mattress.
    B) Water flotation systems.
    C) Egg crate mattress.
    D) Foam mattress.
    E) None are effective.
    F) All are equal.

Answer: F

Clinical trials suggest that devices that reduced pressure are superior to standard mattresses. There is no clear advantage of one device over another. The goal is to maintain tissue pressures less than 32 mmHg. In theory, reduction of tissue pressures below capillary filling pressures should allow adequate tissue perfusion.

Any individual thought to be at risk for developing pressure ulcers should be placed on a pressure-reducing device.

Several trials compared different devices: dynamic air mattresses, water flotation systems, and static support overlay, in terms of the incidence and severity of pressure ulcers that occurred with their use. In these studies, no device was more effective than any other in preventing pressure ulcers.

References

Daechsel D, Connine TA. Special mattresses: effectiveness in preventing decubitus ulcers in chronic neurologic patients. Arch Phys Med Rehabil. 1985;66:246–48. Vilter RW.

Whitney JD, Fellows BJ, Larson E. Do mattresses make a difference? J Gerontol Nurs. 1984;10:20–5.

454. What percent of patients experiencing refractory recurrent *Clostridium difficile* infections (CDI) is cured via intestinal microbiota transplantation (IMT)?
    A) 80 %
    B) 25 %
    C) 50 %
    D) 100 %

Answer: A

A small study of 14 patients with severe and refractory CDI found that 79 % were cured after IMT was delivered via a nasogastric tube. There were no CDI recurrences in the IMT group.

Currently, there are several other randomized controlled studies recruiting patients with recurrent CDI. Evidence continues to increase that donor feces infusion may be superior to antibiotics in patients with recurrent CDI.

Reference

Van Nood E, Vrieze A, Nieuwdorp M, Fuentes S, Zoetendal EG, de Vos WM, Visser CE, Kuijper EJ, Bartelsman JF, Tijssen JG, Speelman P, Dijkgraaf MG, Keller JJ. Duodenal Infusion of Donor Feces for Recurrent Clostridium difficile. N Engl J Med. 2013;368(5):407–15.

455. A 60-year-old female presents to the emergency room due to confusion and headache for the past 8 h. She has a history of hypertension that is often uncontrolled and is treated with hydrochlorothiazide and clonidine. As reported by family, her blood pressure is often above 190 systolic.

    On physical exam, the patient is noted to be diaphoretic and confused. Her heart rate is 120 beats per minute, and her blood pressure is 220/130 mmHg. She is tachycardic and has 1+ edema noted. No focal neurological deficits are noted.

    Laboratory studies are significant for a creatinine of 2.5 mg/dL with a baseline of 1.8 mg/dL. The rest of her chemistries are within normal limits.

    Which of the following is the most appropriate blood pressure goal during the first hour of treatment?
    A) 200/100 mmHg
    B) 180/100 mmHg
    C) 160/9 mmHg
    D) 140/90 mmHg
    E) 130/80 mmHg

Answer: B

This patient has a hypertensive emergency. A hypertensive emergency, formerly called malignant hypertension, is hypertension with acute impairment of one or more organ systems. It is defined as a blood pressure greater than 180/120 with progressive target organ dysfunction, encephalopathy, intracerebral hemorrhage, myocardial infarction, acute left ventricular failure, unstable angina, dissecting aortic aneurysm, or eclampsia. Hypertensive emergency differs from hypertensive crisis in that, in the former, there is evidence of acute organ damage.

The goal of therapy is to reduce blood pressure by 25 % within the first hour and then to 160/100 within the next 2–6 h. Further reductions can then occur over the next 24–48 h, except in the management of acute cerebrovascular accidents. Excessive reduction in blood pressure can precipitate coronary, cerebral, or renal ischemia and, possibly, infarction.

No trials exist comparing the efficacy of various agents in the treatment of hypertensive emergencies. Drugs are chosen based on their onset of action, ease of use, predictability, and convention.

Reference
Thomas L. Managing hypertensive emergencies in the ED. Can Fam Physician. 2011;57(10):1137–97.

456. Which of the following increases with age?
    A) Plasma D-dimer concentrations
    B) Positive antinuclear antibodies
    C) Erythrocyte sedimentation rate
    D) All of the above

Answer: D
Erythrocyte sedimentation rate, plasma D-dimer concentrations, and positivity of antinuclear antibodies increase in the elderly. Electrolytes are remarkably stable and deviate from the values in the young adults only in the very old (>90 years). As a result, traditional thresholds may result in more false positives. It has been suggested that the D-dimer traditional cutoff of 500 mcg/L be adjusted in the elderly population to 750 mcg/L.

Reference
Spring JL, Winkler A, Levy JH. The influence of various patient characteristics on d-dimer concentration in critically ill patients and its role as a prognostic indicator in the intensive care unit setting. Clin Lab Med. 2014;34(3):675–68.

457. Which of the following is true concerning significant lower gastrointestinal bleeding (LGIB)?
    A) Diverticulosis is the most common etiology.
    B) Colonic angiodysplasia is the most common etiology.
    C) Hemorrhoids are the most common etiology.
    D) Malignancy is the most common etiology.
    E) The upper gastrointestinal tract is responsible for 30 % of cases.

Answer: A
Lower gastrointestinal bleeding (LGIB) is a frequent cause of hospital admission and is a factor in hospital morbidity and mortality. The most common etiologies for LGIB are diverticulosis (33.5 %), hemorrhoids (22.5 %), and carcinoma (12.7 %)

Diverticulosis is the dominant etiology for massive LGIB in most publications. Most diverticular bleeding occurs without concomitant diverticulitis. Risk factors for diverticular bleeding include lack of dietary fiber, constipation, advanced age, and use of nonsteroidal anti-inflammatory drugs (NSAIDs) and aspirin. In about 10 % of patients presenting with LGIB, the source of bleeding is from the upper gastrointestinal (GI) tract.

Reference
Gayer C, Chino A, Lucas C, Tokioka S, Yamasaki T, Edelman DA, et al. Acute lower gastrointestinal bleeding in 1,112 patients admitted to an urban emergency medical center. Surgery. 2009;146(4):600–6; discussion 606–7.

458. Which of the following is a not a predictor of a cardiac etiology for chest pain?
    A) Nonresponse to GI cocktail
    B) Duration of pain
    C) Location of pain
    D) None of the above

Answer: A
Approximately 5 million patients per year present to the emergency department with chest pain. In adults the most common causes of chest pain include gastrointestinal (42 %), coronary artery disease (31 %), musculoskeletal (28 %), pericarditis (4 %), and pulmonary embolism (2 %)

A recent review found that for patients with chest pain and suspected acute coronary syndrome (ACS), use of GI cocktails did not improve accuracy of diagnosis compared with standard diagnostic protocols for ACS.

Reference
Chan S, Maurice AP, Davies SR, Walters DL. The use of gastrointestinal cocktail for differentiating gastro-oesophageal reflux disease and acute coronary syndrome in the emergency setting: a systematic review. Lung Circ. 2014;(10):913–23.

459. Which of the following scenarios is it appropriate to allow outpatient treatment for community acquired pneumonia (CAP)?
    A) 65-year-old male with CAP and confusion
    B) 66-year-old male with CAP and respiratory rate of 18/min
    C) 72-year-old female with CAP and creatinine of 2.2 mg/dL
    D) 45-year-old female with CAP, low blood pressure, and some confusion
    E) 28-year-old female with CAP, altered mental status, respiratory rate 35/min, and blood pressure of 90/50 mmHg

Answer: B

Some cases of CAP can be safely treated as an outpatient. CURB-65 guidelines have been developed to assist in appropriate level of care in treating CAP. The CURB-65 acronym stands for C, confusion; U, uremia; R, respiratory rate greater than 30/min; B, blood pressure that is low, less than 90 mmHg systolic or less than 60 mmHg diastolic; and 65, age 65 years or greater. Each category is assigned 1 point; 0–1 point total means the patient can be treated as an outpatient, 2 points total requires treatment in the medical ward, and 3 or more points total requires ICU admission

The 66-year-old male with CAP and respiratory rate of 18/min can be treated as an outpatient. This patient only has one point, age greater than 65 years of age. The CURB score simply serves a guideline. Other factors such as home situation, comorbidities, and access to health care must be considered.

References

Aujesky D, Auble TE, Yealy DM, et al. Prospective comparison of three validated prediction rules for prognosis in community-acquired pneumonia. Am J Med. 2005;118(4): 384–92.

Howell MD, Donnino MW, Talmor D, Clardy P, Ngo L, Shapiro NI. The performance of severity of illness scoring systems in emergency department patients with infection. Acad Emerg Med. 2007;14(8):709–14.

460. A 75-year-old female presents with sepsis due to pneumonia. She is admitted to the intensive care unit and is intubated and started on broad-spectrum antibiotics. She has a history of vitamin D deficiency. She has been prescribed replacement therapy but she has noted been taking them.

    She is found to have marked vitamin D deficiency.

    Which is true concerning high-dose vitamin D replacement?
    A) Length or stay will be improved.
    B) Six-month mortality will be improved.
    C) Functional status will be improved.
    D) All of the above.
    E) None of the above.

Answer: E

Low vitamin D status is linked to increased mortality and morbidity in patients who are critically ill. The mechanism through which vitamin D deficiency is associated with increased mortality in patients with sepsis may be related to its immunological effects.

It is unknown if replacement therapy improves outcome. Critically ill patients with vitamin D deficiency did not benefit from D3 replacement as compared with placebo. No reductions in length of stay, hospital mortality, or 6-month mortality were noted in a 2014 study.

Reference

Amrein K, Schnedl C, Holl A, et al. Effect of high-dose vitamin D3 on hospital length of stay in critically ill patients with vitamin D deficiency: the VITdAL-ICU randomized clinical trial. JAMA. 2014;312(15):1520–30.

461. An 89-year-old female is admitted for UTI. According to previous cultures, patient was positive for a pansensitive *Escherichia coli*. Ciprofloxacin will be started empirically until new cultures return. In deciding on which dosage regimen to start for this patient, which renal dosage adjustment equation should be utilized?
    A) Cockcroft-Gault (CG)
    B) The modification of diet in renal disease (MDRD)
    C) The Chronic Kidney Disease Epidemiology Collaboration (CKD-EPI)
    D) Schwartz

Answer: A

The Cockcroft-Gault (CG) equation provides an estimate of creatinine clearance and is the equation most commonly used to determine drug dosages in patients with impaired kidney function. Currently the MDRD or the CKD-EPI equations are not recommended in drug dosage adjustment. Further studies need to be conducted. Also, keep in mind the package insert for medications bases the recommendations for renal dosage adjustment on the CG equation, which are FDA labeled. Lastly, the Schwartz equation is used for the pediatric population.

Reference

National Kidney patients with renal insufficiency. Can Med Assoc J 200 Foundation. KDOQI. Clinical Practice Guidelines and Clinical Practice Recommendations for Chronic Kidney Disease. Am J Kidney Dis. 2007;49:1–180.

462. Which of the following are not measurements in the Crohn's Disease Activity Index?
    A) Number of stools
    B) Endoscopic grade of inflammation
    C) Hematocrit
    D) Abdominal pain
    E) Taking Lomotil for diarrhea

Answer: B

The Crohn's Disease Activity Index or CDAI is a clinical tool used to quantify the symptoms of patients with Crohn's disease. Most major studies on newer medications use the CDAI in order to standardize a define response or remission of disease. The CDAI does not incorporate a subjective assessment of quality of life, endoscopic factors, or systemic features.

While the CDAI is considered to be the standard for assessing disease activity in Crohn's disease, validation of the index has been varied.

The Inflammatory Bowel Disease Questionnaire (IBDQ) was developed to incorporate subjective elements pertaining to quality of life as well as bowel-related symptoms into an activity index.

Reference

Best WR, Becktel JM, Singleton JW, Kern F Jr. Development of a Crohn's disease activity index. National Cooperative Crohn's Disease Study. Gastroenterology. 1976;70(3):439–44.

463. An internal medicine resident sustains a needlestick injury while attempting to insert a central line on a patient on your service. The resident contacts you. She is in severe emotional distress due to the possibility of HIV transmission.

The source patient, who is competent, is informed of the injury but refuses to provide consent for human immunodeficiency virus (HIV) testing. A year ago, this same resident became ill after taking postexposure prophylaxis (PEP) for a similar exposure. She asks you if she can use blood for complete blood count already taken from the source patient for other reasons and test it for HIV.

Which of the following are true statements?

A) HIV testing of source patients is permitted in all states without consent.

B) HIV testing of source patient is not allowed without consent in any states.

C) HIV testing of source patient is only allowed without consent by court order.

D) HIV testing of source patient without consent is allowed in some states.

Answer: D

State laws regulate HIV source patient testing practices in the United States. The controversy over HIV testing in cases of occupational exposure is reflected in variations in state laws and policies. As of 2011, 36 states have laws that allow unconsented HIV testing of source patients in cases of occupational exposure. Each state has its own requirements for unconsented HIV testing. Variations exist in numerous procedures, including who can authorize an unconsented test, how the test is documented in the medical record, and who is informed of the test results.

In this particular case prompt postexposure treatment may be needed. It is important that state policy be understood to allow or a rapid decision-making process to occur.

Reference

Henderson DK. Management of needlestick injuries: a house officer who has a needlestick. JAMA. 2012;307(1):75–84.

464. Which of the following symptoms is inconsistent with a diagnosis of Guillain-Barré syndrome (GBS)?

A) A 5-day history of bilateral weakness with abdominal and thigh pain

B) Bilateral lower extremity weakness and a normal magnetic resonance imaging of the head and spine

C) A patient with bilateral lower extremity weakness and paresthesia who has markedly decreased reflexes in his lower extremities

D) A patient who presents with symmetrical sensory loss but on physical examination has no motor weakness

E) Facial droop and dysarthria

Answer: D

On presentation the classic symptoms of Guillain-Barré are often not present. Patients with atypical presentation often have a delayed diagnosis. They are often diagnosed as having a psychological reaction. They are frequently sent home from the emergency department and then return with persistent or progressive symptoms hours to days later.

A hallmark of Guillain-Barré is ascending motor weakness. Sensory loss may be present, but motor weakness is the predominant consistent finding. Universal are flexia is usually present with Guillain-Barré syndrome, although some patients only have distal areflexia. Pain-related symptoms occur in more than half.

Urinary retention is rarely persistent. Anal sphincter muscles are rarely affected as well. The classic cerebrospinal spinal finding, an elevated protein with a normal white blood cell count, is present 50 % of the time within the first week. By the second week, 80 % of patients will have an elevated CSF protein level. EMG often do not show the typical pattern on presentation and may evolve with time.

Cranial nerve involvement is observed in 45–75 % of patients with GBS. Cranial nerves III–VII and IX–XII may be affected.

The mean time from presentation to the clinical function nadir is 12 days. 98 % of patients reaching a nadir by 4 weeks. Progression of symptoms beyond 4 weeks brings the diagnosis under question. Recovery usually begins 2–4 weeks after all progression ceases. The mean time to clinical recovery is 200 days.

References

Hughes RA, Rees JH. Clinical and epidemiologic features of Guillain-Barré syndrome. J Infect Dis. 1997;176(Suppl 2):S92–8.

Rinaldi S. Update on Guillain-Barré syndrome. J Peripher Nerv Syst. 2013;18(2):99–112.

465. You are an attending hospital physician on the day shift, while checking out to your nighttime colleague, you notice slightly slurred speech and alcohol on her breath.

Otherwise, she seems functional and is able to comprehend the patients presented. As far as you know, she has not had trouble with substance abuse in the past.

The appropriate action should be:

A) Notify hospital administration.
B) Advise colleague to seek care, respecting her right to privacy.
C) Inform the colleague that she must remove herself from the practice area immediately.
D) Inform the chief of hospital medicine.

Answer: C

In this circumstance, you are the hospital's advocate and are responsible for managing the situation until handed off to the appropriate treatment team. You are secondarily responsible to the colleague as a patient. Immediate and definitive action is required.

In the setting of suspected acute intoxication of a physician or health-care provider who provides patient care or who might be reasonably expected to provide care in the near future, immediate removal from the practice setting is essential. In such cases, an intervention may include accompanying the suspected physician to an established health care environment, such as the emergency department. Security if needed may be involved.

Reference

Baldisseri M. Impaired healthcare professional. Crit Care Med. 2007;35(2):106–16.

466. Which of the following oral anticoagulants affects prothrombin time, partial thromboplastin time, and thrombin time coagulation assays?
    A) Apixaban
    B) Dabigatran
    C) Rivaroxaban
    D) Warfarin

Answer: B

Warfarin has been the standard therapy for oral anticoagulation for decades. Its side effects and efficacy profile are well known. It is used for atrial fibrillation, venous thromboembolism (VTE) prophylaxis, VTE treatment, and valvular heart disease.

Newer agents have been developed in an effort to improve upon warfarin's deficiencies. The entire side affect the profile of the newer agents is not yet known. Of the drugs listed, only dabigatran causes alteration in all of the coagulation assays.

Reference

Eriksson BI, et al. Comparative pharmacodynamics and pharmacokinetics of oral direct thrombin and factor Xa inhibitors in development. Clin Pharmacokin. 2009; 48(1):1–22.

467. According to the 2013 INTERACT 2 trial, improved outcomes were seen in patients with intracerebral hemorrhage whose blood pressure was aggressively lowered to what level?
    A) 140 mmHg
    B) 180 mmHg
    C) 160 mmHg
    D) 120 mmHg

Answer: A

Rapid intensive blood pressure lowering in patients with intracerebral hemorrhage (ICH) appears to be related to less long-term disability, according to the results of the INTERACT 2 (Intensive Blood Pressure Reduction in Acute Cerebral Hemorrhage Trial 2) trial. The Chinese trial compared lowering blood pressure to a target of less than 140 mmHg systolic within 1 h with the guideline-recommended approach of lowering pressure to less than 180 mmHg. The drug most commonly used was urapidil, a popular drug in China but not used extensively in the United States.

Quality-of-life assessment suggested that patients in the intensive treatment group had fewer problems and had a significantly better overall health-related quality of life at 90 days than the standard treatment group. In a subgroup who underwent brain imaging, there was a small reduction in hematoma growth in the intensive treatment group, but this finding was not significant.

References

Honner SK, Singh A, Cheung PT, Alter HJ, Dutaret CG, Patel AK, et al. Emergency department control of blood pressure in intracerebral hemorrhage. J Emerg Med. 2011;41(4):355–61.

Qureshi AI, Palesch YY, Martin R, Novitzke J, Cruz-Flores S, Ehtisham A. Effect of systolic blood pressure reduction on hematoma expansion, perihematomal edema, and 3-month outcome among patients with intracerebral hemorrhage: results from the antihypertensive treatment of acute cerebral hemorrhage study. Arch Neurol. 2010;67(5):570–6.

468. What is true concerning Cochrane reviews?
    A) It was founded in the United States.
    B) It has an official partnership with the World Health Organization.
    C) It is a for-profit organization.
    D) The group conducts randomized controlled trials.

Answer: B

Systematic reviews are important in practicing evidence-based health care. One of the largest organizations doing them is the Cochrane collaboration. The Cochrane collaboration is an independent, nonprofit, non-governmental organization. It consists primarily of more than 31,000 volunteers in more than 120 countries.

The group conducts systematic reviews of randomized controlled trials of medical and non medical interventions. It does not undertake prospective trials. The Cochrane collaboration is split into smaller divisions composed of centers, review groups, methods groups, and fields.

On average a Cochrane systematic review takes 23 months from protocol to publication. Some have criticized this time frame. Although Cochrane reviews are done with much diligence, some reviews have come under scrutiny for their overreaching conclusions.

Reference
Hill GB. Archie Cochrane and his legacy. An internal challenge to physicians' autonomy? J Clin Epidemiol. 2000;53(12):1189–92.

469. Hospitalist often have schedules that result in patients seeing several attendings during one hospital stay.
     What is the reported impact of this fragmented hospitalist care on the length of stay?
     A) Increased length of stay
     B) Decreased length of stay
     C) Decreased patient satisfaction
     D) No change

Answer: A
Several studies have shown that fragmented care causes an increase in length of stay (LOS). One study published in the 2010 Journal of Hospital Medicine revealed that a 10 % increase in fragmentation was associated with an increase of 0.39 days for pneumonia and an increase of 0.30 days in LOS for heart failure. Fragmentation was defined as the percentage the patient was seen by physicians other than the physician providing the majority of care.

Reference
Epstein K, Juarez E, Epstein A, Loya K, Singer A. The impact of fragmentation of hospitalist care on length of stay. J Hosp Med. 2010;5:335–8.

470. A 82-year-old woman is brought to the emergency department because she has had a progressive cough, fevers, and confusion for the past 3 days. She has moderate Alzheimer's disease that has been progressing slowly. She is cared for at home by her daughter. She was treated for a urinary tract infection 1 year ago. Six months ago a mammogram showed suspicious microcalcifications, but the patient and her family decided not to pursue additional evaluation.
     The patient is oriented only to person. Temperature is 38.9 °C (102.0 °F), pulse rate is 110 beats per min-

ute, respiratory rate is 28 per minute, and blood pressure is 152/96 mmHg. Oxygen saturation is 84 %. Crackles are heard in the lower lung fields.
     Which of the following is the most important piece of information that you should obtain before you treat this patient?
     A) Influenza occurrence in the local area
     B) Pneumococcal vaccination status of the patient
     C) Methicillin-resistant *Staphylococcus aureus* prevalence of her care facility
     D) Prior urine cultures
     E) Advance directives

Answer: E
A significant number of patients admitted to the hospital do not want aggressive life-prolonging care. It is important to recognize what hospice, palliative care, and advance directives have to offer to individuals and families who face serious, life-threatening advanced illness issues.

Protocol-driven admission processes can make it easy to overlook the fundamental right of patient autonomy. Goals of care in this situation should be determined before any significant effort is undertaken.

Reference
Celso B, Meenrajan, S. The triad that matters: palliative medicine, code status, and health care costs. Am J Hosp Palliat Med. 2010;27(6):398–401.

471. Which of the following factors increases the risk of a falsely low B-type natriuretic peptide level?
     A) Female sex
     B) Kidney failure
     C) Obesity
     D) Older age
     E) Pulmonary embolism

Answer: C
Obesity increases the risk of a falsely low B-type natriuretic peptide (BNP) level. BNP is especially helpful in differentiating dyspnea as a result of heart failure versus dyspnea as a result of pulmonary disease. BNP has a good negative predictive value. Among patients presenting to the emergency department with dyspnea of undetermined cause, a BNP level of less than 100 pg/mL accurately excludes decompensated heart failure as a cause.

The clinical use in the ambulatory setting is uncertain. Among ambulatory patients with established heart failure, normal ranges for BNP during periods of clinical stability may be as high as 500 pg/mL. Factors other than heart failure that affect BNP levels include kidney failure, older age, and female sex. These increase BNP level.

The BNP level may also be elevated with many causes of ventricular strain. These include pulmonary embolism, acute myocardial infarction, and acute tachycardia.

Reference

Daniels LB, Clopton P, Bhalla V, Krishnaswamy P, Nowak RM, McCord J, et al. How obesity affects the cut-points for B-type natriuretic peptide in the diagnosis of acute heart failure. Results from the Breathing Not Properly Multinational Study. Am Heart J. 2006;151(5):999–1005.

472. What are the established benefits of inferior vena cava (IVC) filters?
    A) Reduction in mortality
    B) Reduction in recurrent pulmonary embolism
    C) Reduction in deep vein thrombosis (DVT)
    D) Prevent the need for anticoagulation

Answer: B

Inferior vena cava filters have been widely used with little evidence to support their use. Inferior vena cava filters have been compared to no filters in only two studies. These studies showed reduced recurrent PE but an increased risk of DVT with IVC filters. There was not an associated reduction in mortality with filter use.

IVC filters have been commonly used for prophylaxis in high-risk patients including trauma patients, neurosurgical patients, patients with malignancy, and super-obese patients undergoing surgery; whether or not their use leads to a net benefit is not known.

With IVC placement, it is recommended that anticoagulation be resumed as soon as possible after filter insertion because the filter alone is not an effective treatment of venous thromboembolism (VTE).

Retrievable filters may offer some benefit without the long-term complications of IVC filters.

References

Ghanim AJ, Daskalakis C, Eschelman DJ, Kraft WK. A five-year, retrospective, comparison review of survival in neurosurgical patients diagnosed with venous thromboembolism and treated with either inferior vena cava filters or anticoagulants. J Thromb Thrombolysis. 2007;24(3):247–254.

Kim HS, Young MJ, Narayan AK, Hong K, Liddell RP, Streiff MB. A comparison of clinical outcomes with retrievable and permanent inferior vena cava filters. J Vasc Interv Radiol. 2008;19(3):393–9.

473. What are the characteristics of patients who are rate physicians highest in patient satisfaction scores?
    A) Lower mortality
    B) Decreased health-care expenditures
    C) Decreased prescription drug use
    D) All of the above
    E) None of the above

Answer: E

Patient satisfaction has become a common metric for hospital medicine physicians. The balance between providing quality care and meeting the expectations of the patient can be challenging.

Satisfied patients are not necessarily healthy patients. In a paper published in 2012, researchers at the University of California, Davis, using data from nearly 52,000 adults, found that the most satisfied patients spent the most on health-care and prescription drugs. They were 12 % more likely to be admitted to the hospital and accounted for 9 % more in total health-care costs. Their mortality was also increased.

Although this study does not prove a causal effect, it does question the relationship between patient satisfaction and quality.

Reference

Friedberg MW, Gelb Safran D, Schneider EC. Satisfied to death: a spurious result? Arch Intern Med. 2012;172:1112–3.

474. A 47-year-old man is admitted for a 3-week history of cough and dyspnea and hemoptysis. He also has had fevers, night sweats, and a 30-lb weight loss over the last 3 months. He has no significant medical history and does not smoke, use alcohol, or take drugs. He is married and employed as an accountant. He takes no medications.

On physical examination, he appears thin and coughs frequently. Temperature is 38.3 °C (101.0 °F), blood pressure is 100/60 mmHg, pulse rate is 101 beats/min, and respiratory rate is 30/min. Pulmonary examination shows crackles over the right upper lung field.

Which of the following are the most appropriate infectious precautions to order for this patient?
    A) Airborne
    B) Contact
    C) Droplet
    D) Standard

Answer: A

Not all patients with pneumonia can or should be isolated. Although this patient apparently has no risk factors, *Mycobacterium tuberculosis* (TB) should be in the differential in any patient with cough for greater than 3 weeks, loss of appetite, unexplained weight loss, night sweats, hoarseness, fever, fatigue, or chest pain. The index of suspicion should be substantially higher in high-risk groups where it is most often seen.

Airborne precautions are recommended for patients infected with microorganisms such as avian influenza, varicella, disseminated zoster, severe acute respiratory syndrome, or smallpox and the agents of viral hemorrhagic fever. Airborne precautions, which may be dependent on local regulations, include placing the patient in an isolation room with high-efficiency particulate air filtration and negative pressure. Anyone entering the room should wear a fit-tested N-95 or higher disposable respirator. The patient should also wear one during transport out of the room. Goggles, gowns, and gloves should be worn if contact with respiratory secretions is anticipated.

Contact precautions are indicated for patients with known or suspected infections that are transmitted by direct contact, such as vancomycin-resistant enterococci and methicillin-resistant *Staphylococcus aureus*.

Droplet precautions are used for protection against microorganisms transmitted by respiratory droplets larger than 5 μm. These droplets can usually be transmitted over distances of less than 3–10 ft. Examples of pathogens and diseases that require the institution of droplet isolation precautions include *Neisseria meningitidis*, pneumonic plague, diphtheria, *Haemophilus influenzae* type b, *Bordetella pertussis*, influenza, mumps, rubella, and parvovirus B19. Droplet precautions include placing the patient in an isolation room, wearing a face or surgical mask when in the room, and wearing goggles, gowns, and gloves. Standard precautions are used with all patients.

475. A 78-year-old female who has mild dementia and chronic kidney disease stage 3 was admitted to the hospital for pyelonephritis and acute or chronic renal failure. Since the admission 2 days ago, she has improved clinically. Her laboratory parameters have been improving, with a decrease in leukocytosis, repeat negative blood cultures, and slight decrease in his serum creatinine.

Despite having mild dementia, at baseline the patient recognized her family, could express her needs, and participate in daily activities. Current medications are ceftriaxone, aspirin, and acetaminophen.

On hospital day 2, she develops mild delirium which is worse at night. Last evening, she repeatedly tried to climb out of bed. Today, she pulled out her intravenous line again even though nursing staff had her under close observation.

On physical examination, the temperature is 38.0 °C (100.1 °F), heart rate is 90 beats per minute, and blood pressure is 146/75 mmHg. The patient appears restless and is oriented only to person. Her speech is mildly distorted, and she cannot repeat three numbers.

Which of the following should you recommend?
A) Keeping the television on for distraction
B) Initiating a bedside sitter
C) Placing bilateral wrist restraints
D) Administration of quetiapine, 25 mg once mg/dL
E) Lorazepam 2 mg nightly

Answer: B
Current evidence supports a role for a sitter as part of the management of patients with delirium. Although once only used for observation of high-risk psychiatric patients, the use of sitters is now most commonly employed as part of the cost-effective management for delirious patients. Of the choices here it is the only option with proven benefits.

A limiting factor in utilizing sitters is obviously their cost. It is uncertain in what circumstances sitters are cost-effective. In studies utilizing sitters, length of stay and duration of delirium were not significantly reduced; however, falls were. To help with identification of patients who would benefit from sitter use and improve the process of sitter requests, an assessment tool, the 'Patient Attendant Assessment Tool, (PAAT), was created. In addition the use of trained volunteers has been suggested as a method to increase sitter use.

476. A 82-year-old man is admitted for a hemorrhagic stroke. No deep venous thrombosis prophylaxis is administered because of his central nervous system bleeding. His outpatient medications included aspirin, and this was withheld as well.

Recovery is good and the patient will be transferred to acute rehabilitation 72 h after his admission.

On physical examination, the patient cannot raise his affected arm or leg off the bed. Since having her stroke, he is incapable of walking without assistance.

What is the value in ordering intermittent pneumatic compression (IPC) device for this patient?
A) Reduced risk of deep venous thrombosis
B) Reduced mortality risk
C) Increased risk of falls
D) Increased risk of lower leg ischemia or amputation

Answer: A
IPC devices prevent VTE after stroke. Thromboembolism is a common complication of stroke and can have lethal consequences, but DVT prophylaxis can be risky. The Clots in Legs Or Stockings after Stroke (CLOTS 3) trial studied the efficacy and adverse effects of IPC devices in a stroke population At 30 days, patients receiving IPCs had a significant reduction in any DVT compared to those who had none. This protective effect was persistent through 6 months. The effect was similar whether anticoagulants were used or not. There was also benefit to IPCs whether the stroke was hemorrhagic or not. Falls which may be increased with devices that limit movement were not different between the groups. There was a slight increase in skin breaks in the IPC group compared to those who had no IPC with 20 skin breaks. The IPC group did not have a higher incidence of ischemia or limb amputation.

Reference
Dennis M, Sandercock P, Reid J, et al. Effectiveness of intermittent pneumatic compression in reduction of risk of

deep vein thrombosis in patients who have had a stroke (CLOTS 3): a multicentre randomised controlled trial. Lancet. 2013;382(9891):516–24.

477. A 77-year-old woman who had been admitted for pneumonia is ready for discharge. The patient has responded well to therapy. On admission, she was noticed to be disheveled, and there is some concern about her living arrangements. Her BMI is currently 26. The patient lives alone and reports no difficulty with daily living. Her daughter has been hard to contact. A friend reports that the patient's home is cluttered and dirty. A nursing home is offered but the patient insists that her goal is to return home. The patient is competent to make decisions.

Which of the following may best assist in improving the safety at home?
A) Ethics consultation
B) Performing a home visit
C) Insisting on a higher standard for safety in the home
D) Avoiding negotiation that allows the patient to choose her living arrangements
E) Avoiding worst-case scenario discussions

Answer: B
Self-neglect is common in geriatric practice and family support is increasingly absent. Hospitalists are under increasing pressure to reduce readmissions, and self-neglect is associated with readmissions.

A review article by Smith et al. suggests four practical approaches to managing self-neglecting patients and a discussion of tactics that generally do not work. A home visit by the care provider team can be the means of allowing others to support the patient in the home. It can also introduce members of the home care team to the reluctant patient. Although self-neglecting patients often lack resources, there is no ethical justification to insist a higher standard for safety. Ageism is to be avoided. Negotiation is generally only useful in trying to help the patient with shared goals. An uncompromising approach should be avoided. Worst-case scenarios will occur and plans should be developed to address these situations.

Reference
Smith AK, Lo B, Aronson L. Elder self-neglect—how can a physician help? N Engl J Med. 2013;369:2476–9.

478. What is true concerning the use of flumazenil in treating benzodiazepine (BZD) overdose?
A) It can be used in patients with an increased risk of seizures.
B) Its best use may be isolated iatrogenic benzodiazepine overdose.
C) It can be used with tricyclic antidepressant overdose.
D) It will consistently reverse benzodiazepine-induced respiratory depression.

Answer: B
Flumazenil is a competitive BZD receptor antagonist. It is the only available specific antidote for BZDs. Its beneficial use in acute BZD is not well established. Flumazenil does not consistently reverse central respiratory depression due to BZDs. Re-sedation occurs in over half the patients, and they should be followed closely.

In long-term BZD users, flumazenil may precipitate withdrawal and seizures. Flumazenil should not be used in any patient at an increased risk of having a seizure, such as head injury and co-ingestion of BZD and tricyclic antidepressant or other agents which may lower the seizure threshold. The ideal use for flumazenil may be isolated iatrogenic BZD overdose in BZD-naive patients

Reference
Marraffa JM, Cohen V, Howland MA. Antidotes for toxicological emergencies: a practical review. Am J Health Syst Pharm. 2012;69(3):199–212.

479. A 72-year-old male is admitted for ETOH withdrawal. Mild delirium develops, and the patient becomes agitated and combative. He is transferred to the ICU. The nurse requests an order for physical restraints. You suggest a sitter but none are available. Physical restraints are applied to the patient.

Compared with nonrestrained patients, which of the following is this patient at risk for?
A) Increased use of sedation
B) Increased patient safety
C) Decreased days of intensive care
D) Decreased incidence of adverse events

Answer: A
It is important to recognize potential negative physical and psychological consequences of restraints. The use of physical restraints is often necessary for the protection of staff and of patients and should be continued to be used judiciously. Attacks on nurses can be sudden, serious, and life threatening. The trend in health-care literature is that violence against nurses appears to be a growing problem globally.

Physical restraints placed have been shown to require higher doses of benzodiazepines, opioids, and antipsychotic medications. Patients have prolonged length of stay in the intensive care unit (ICU). Patients have higher rates of self-extubation and accidental removal of intravenous catheters, urinary catheters, and feeding tubes. After discharge, elderly patients who have undergone physical restraint have higher levels of post-traumatic stress disorder. All of these factors make physical restraints one of the least preferred options.

References
Chang LY, Wang KW, Chao YE. Influence of physical restraint on unplanned extubation of adult intensive care patients: a case–control study. Am J Crit Care. 2008;17:408–15.

Happ MB, Kagan SH, Strumpf NE, et al. Elderly patients' memories of physical restraint use in the intensive care unit (ICU). Am J Crit Care. 2001;10:367–9.

Lepping P, Lanka S, Turner J, Stanaway SE, Krishna M. Percentage prevalence of patient and visitor violence against staff in high-risk UK medical wards. Clin Med. 2013;13:543–6.

Swickhamer C, Colvig C, Chan SB. Restraint use in the elderly emergency department patient. J Emerg Med. 2013;44(4):869–74.

480. A 68-year-old female who has been admitted for pneumonia experiences cardiac arrest with pulseless electrical activity. You are first to arrive. The peripheral intravenous catheter becomes dislodged. Rapid review of past medical history reveals marked dehydration. During the first moments of the code, the nurses report that she has poor peripheral veins, and they are having difficulty achieving venous access. You request an intraosseous (IO) cannula to be placed in the patient's right medial malleolus.

Which of the following additional information is true concerning an IO cannula?
A) Intraosseous cannulation may put this patient at greater risk for cerebral fat emboli or bone-marrow emboli.
B) Epinephrine administration by intraosseous injection is acceptable.
C) Administration of medications by the intraosseous route is at the same dose.
D) Infusion rates achieved through an intraosseous cannula are comparable to rates achieved through a 21-gauge peripheral intravenous catheter.
E) All of the above.

Answer: E
IO administration of emergency medications has been proven to be effective in patients needing resuscitation in whom establishing intravenous (IV) access is difficult.

Medications, such as antibiotics, epinephrine, blood products, or neuromuscular-blocking agents, can be delivered through an intraosseous cannula. There is no requirement for dose adjustment. Infusion rates are similar to those achieved with a 21-gauge peripheral intravenous catheter. IO techniques have fewer serious complications than central lines and may be performed much faster than central or peripheral lines when vascular access is difficult.

Patients who have a right-to-left shunt are at higher risk for fat emboli or bone-marrow components migrating to the cerebral circulation, and intraosseous cannulation should be avoided in these patients if at all possible.

Reference
Ngo AS, Oh JJ, Chen Y, Yong D, Ong ME. Intraosseous vascular access in adults using the EZ-IO in an emergency department. Int J Emerg Med. 2009;2(3):155–60.

481. In the treatment of hyperkalemia, one dose of calcium gluconate provides cardioprotection for what time period?
A) 15–30 min
B) 30–60 min
C) 2–3 h
D) 4–6 h

Answer: B
Calcium gluconate increases the threshold potential which is abnormally elevated in hyperkalemia. The onset of action is rapid within 5 min, and duration of action is about 30–60 min. It is recommended to repeat the dose if ECG changes do not normalize within 3–5 min.

Calcium agents are the first-line treatment for severe hyperkalemia greater than >7 mEq/L or when the electrocardiogram (ECG) shows significant abnormalities.

Administration of calcium should be accompanied by other therapies that help lower serum potassium levels.

Reference
Fordjour KN, Walton T, Doran JJ. Management of hyperkalemia in hospitalized patients. Am J Med Sci. 2012;347(2):93–100.

482. What percentage of patients who die of pulmonary embolism (PE) do so within the first hour?
A) 10 %
B) 30 %
C) 50 %
D) 70 %

Answer: D
70 % of patients who die of a pulmonary embolus do so within the 1st hour after onset of symptoms. This fact demonstrates the need for early treatment without the delay of imaging in suspected cases PE.

Reference
Aklog L, Williams CS, Byrne JG, Goldhaber SZ. Acute pulmonary embolectomy: a contemporary approach. Circulation. 2002;105(414):1416–9.

483. Which of the following anticoagulants has genotype dosing shown to be effective in achieving target dose?
A) Warfarin
B) Heparin
C) Low-molecular-weight heparin
D) Rivaroxaban

Answer: A
Anticoagulant therapy with warfarin is characterized by a wide variation among individuals in dose requirements. Its narrow therapeutic index and constant need for monitoring have made its use challenging.

There has been investigation into the genetic influences on warfarin dose requirements. Three single-nucleotide polymorphisms (SNPs) have been found to play key roles in determining the effect of warfarin therapy on coagulation. Studies have shown that achieving a target INR occurs more rapidly after patients have undergone genetic testing. Whether this is clinically significant or cost-effective is uncertain.

Reference
Caraco Y, Blotnick S, Muszkat M. CYP2C9 genotype-guided warfarin prescribing enhances the efficacy and safety of anticoagulation: a prospective randomized controlled study. Clin Pharmacol Ther. 2008;83(3):460–70.

484. You are urgently contacted by your resident who has had an exposure to blood from an HIV-positive patient. While placing a central line, her glove was ripped by the suture needle. When she removed the glove, she noticed blood on her hands and a small scratch mark. She is not sure where the scratch came from.
     Which of the following is the best postexposure management strategy for the resident?
     A) Tenofovir and emtricitabine
     B) Tenofovir, emtricitabine, and raltegravir
     C) Tenofovir, emtricitabine, and nevirapine
     D) No postexposure prophylaxis
     E) An immediate pregnancy test before prescription

Answer: B
The US Public Health Service now recommends that three drugs be used in all postexposure prophylaxis regimens regardless of exposure type. Previous guidelines offered only two drug regimens for exposures that were considered to be associated with a lower level of transmission. A three-drug combination of tenofovir, emtricitabine, and raltegravir is the current recommendation and should be given as soon as possible. It is well tolerated and has relative safety in pregnancy.

Reference
Kuhar DT, Henderson DK, Struble KA, et al. Updated U.S. Public Health Service guidelines for the management of occupational exposures to human immunodeficiency virus and recommendations for postexposure prophylaxis. Infect Control Hosp Epidemiol. 2013;34(9):875–92.

485. What is the impact of having advanced residents in training cover patients in the ICU that they are not following during the day?
     A) Higher mortality, no difference in interventions
     B) No difference in mortality or interventions
     C) Higher patient mortality and fewer interventions
     D) Lower patient mortality and more interventions

Answer: D
Transferring care does not necessarily increase complications. Interestingly in one study comparing patient outcomes when critical care fellows were assigned to cover patients overnight in an ICU, mortality actually decreased but interventions increased. This effect could possibly be explained by the impact of having a new review of existing data or the increased diligence, which may occur when dealing with new patients.

Reference
Amaral ACK-B, Barros BS, Barros CCPP, et al. Nighttime cross-coverage is associated with decreased intensive care unit mortality. Am J Respir Crit Care Med. 2014;189(11):1395–401.

486. How does propofol compare to benzodiazepines for sedation in the ICU?
     A) Propofol and benzodiazepine usage have similar ICU outcomes.
     B) Benzodiazepine usage has better outcomes.
     C) Propofol usage has better outcomes.

Answer: C
Propofol as opposed to benzodiazepines usage appears to be associated with better outcomes in the ICU. Benzodiazepines have been shown to induce delirium and oversedation and are difficult to titrate. Some believe that inappropriate dosing of benzodiazepines is unavoidable given their unpredictable pharmacokinetics. Benzodiazepines may lead to prolonged ICU stays and increased mortality. A recent large study with more than 3300 patients examined associations between sedative use and ICU outcomes. Propofol use was associated with a reduction in clinically important outcomes, including ICU mortality, hospital mortality, ICU length of stay, ventilator removal, and sedation days. Propofol use is expensive and not without complications. Further studies may be needed to establish that reductions in complications offset this expense.

Reference
Ferrell BA, Girard TD. Sedative choice: a critical decision. Am J Respir Crit Care Med. 2014;189(11):1295–7.

487. Which of the following infections is the leading cause of death among HIV-infected patients worldwide?
     A) *Cytomegalovirus*
     B) *Escherichia coli*
     C) *Mycobacterium tuberculosis*
     D) *Pneumocystis jiroveci*
     E) *Staphylococcus aureus*

Answer: C
Tuberculosis (TB) remains one of the most important infectious complications of HIV. It is the leading cause of death among

HIV-infected persons worldwide. In developed countries, malignancy, cardiovascular disease, and complications from antiviral agents have emerged as causes of HIV-related mortality.

Reference

Nahid P, Menzies D. Update in tuberculosis and nontuberculous mycobacterial disease 2011. Am J Respir Crit Care Med. 2012;185:1266–70.

488. A 27-year-old female presents with acute ingestion of acetaminophen. She reports that she took approximately fifteen 650 mg tablets 4 h ago. A family member is with her and confirms the amount and time of ingestion.

    Which of the following is the lowest acute toxicity ingested to require an acetylcysteine in the adult patient?
    A) 25 g
    B) 20 g
    C) 15 g
    D) 7.5 g
    E) 5 g

Answer: D
A single dose of 7.5 g of acetaminophen is enough to warrant acetylcysteine administration. In this case 9.75 g has been ingested and N-acetylcysteine therapy should be initiated.

Patients presenting less than 8 h after acetaminophen overdose have a significantly reduced risk of hepatotoxicity with acetylcysteine use. Although acetylcysteine is most effective if given within 8 h of ingestion, it still has beneficial effects if given as late as 48 h after ingestion. The mortality rate from acetaminophen overdose increases 2 days after the ingestion, reaches a maximum on day four, and then gradually decreases.

Acetylcysteine is usually well tolerated and should be considered when the total amount of ingestion is uncertain. The most common adverse reaction to acetylcysteine treatment is an anaphylactoid reaction, manifested by rash, wheeze, or mild hypotension.

Reference

Heard KJ. Acetylcysteine for acetaminophen poisoning. N Engl J Med 2008;359(3):285–92.

489. An 80-year-old woman with advanced dementia is hospitalized with pneumonia. The family is actively discussing the goals of care. Before a final decision is made however, the patient's respiratory failure worsens that evening when the patient is intubated and given ventilator support. The family decides on comfort care. However, they request that the patient remain in the hospital with the best medical care. They believe that the patient will have the best care if she remains in the ICU.

Which of the following choices would most likely promote well-being in the patient and family?
A) Allow the patient to die with ventilatory support in the ICU without further escalation of heroic measures.
B) Allow the patient to die with ventilatory support in the ICU.
C) Extubate and allow the patient to die in the ICU.
D) Transfer the patient out of the ICU.

Answer: D
At this point transfer out of the ICU is the most appropriate. Death in the ICU may lead to increased interventions, increased suffering for the patient, and an increase in post-traumatic stress disorder (PTSD) among family members. Studies have demonstrated that stress for family members can often be less on the floor which is less hectic, more quiet, and often more convenient as opposed to the ICU.

References

Mularski RA, Heine CE, Osborne ML, et al. Quality of dying in the ICU: ratings by family members. Chest. 2005;128:280–7.
Wright AA, Keating NL, Balboni TA, et al. Place of death: correlations with quality of life of patients with cancer and predictors of bereaved caregivers' mental health. J Clin Oncol. 2010;28:4457–64.
Wunsch H, Linde-Zwirble WT, Harrison DA, et al. Use of intensive care services during terminal hospitalizations in England and the United States. Am J Respir Crit Care Med. 2009;180:875–80.

490. Spironolactone has a black box warning for patients with:
    A) Family history of breast cancer
    B) Family history of thyroid cancer
    C) Family history of bladder cancer
    D) Personal history of colon cancer
    E) Personal history of rectal cancer

Answer: A
The strongest warning that the US Federal Drug Administration (FDA) requires is the boxed warning. It signifies that medical studies indicate that the drug carries a significant risk of serious or is even life threatening. Black box warnings have had significant effects on drug use.

Spironolactone is an antiandrogenic potassium-sparing diuretic. It can be used for women for adult acne that is recalcitrant to treatment. Although it is not first line, it helps to block androgens that cause acne in the jawline. Spironolactone has a black box warning against patient with a personal history of breast cancer or family history of breast cancer.

Reference
Shah ND, Montori VM, Krumholz HM, Tu K, Alexander
  GC, Jackevicius CA. Geographic variation in the response
  to FDA boxed warnings for rosiglitazone. N Engl J Med.
  2010;22(455):2081–4.

491. Which of the following statements regarding the diag-
  nosis of community-acquired pneumonia is true?
  A) Directed therapy specific to the suspected caus-
     ative organism is more effective than empirical
     therapy in hospitalized patients.
  B) Ten percent of patients hospitalized with
     community-acquired pneumonia will have positive
     blood cultures.
  C) In patients who have bacteremia caused by
     Streptococcus pneumoniae, sputum cultures are
     positive in more than 70 % of cases.
  D) Polymerase chain reaction tests are widely avail-
     able and should be utilized for diagnosis in patients
     hospitalized with community-acquired pneumonia.
  E) In 40 % of all case of pneumonia, the specific
     infectious agent will be identified.

Answer: B
It can be a challenge to find the specific etiology of community-
acquired pneumonia. Overall a cause is found approximately
in only 15 % of cases. Generally, the yield from sputum culture, even in cases of fulminant bacteremic pneumococcal
pneumonia the yield from sputum is no greater than 50 % .
The yield from blood cultures is also low at 5–14 %.

  Empirical broad-spectrum therapy remains the standard
therapy. Expanded polymerase chain reaction assays show
promise as a means to target more specific bacterial etiologies. As availability and cost of these tests continue to
decline, expect more widespread use.

Reference
Hoare Z, Lim WS. Pneumonia: update on diagnosis and
  management (PDF). BMJ. 2006;332(7549):1077–9.
  doi:10.1136/bmj.332.7549.
  1077. PMC 1458569. PMID 16675815301).

492. Which one of the following factors suggests that a non-
  purulent, para-pneumonic effusion should be drained
  by a chest tube?
  A) The presence of pneumococcal pneumonia
  B) A pleural fluid pH <7.20
  C) A temperature of 104 °F
  D) A pleural fluid nucleated cell count of 30,000/mL

Answer: B
Pleural effusions are a common finding in patients with pneumonia. More than 40 % of patients with bacterial pneumonia
develop para-pneumonic effusions. Several studies have

documented that in a nonpurulent, para-pneumonic effusion,
a low pleural pH of less than 7.20 has the highest predictive
value for the need for pleural space drainage. Although any
organism causing pneumonia can be associated with a pleural
effusion, anaerobic organisms, Streptococcus pyogenes,
Staphylococcus aureus, and gram-negative bacilli tend to
have a higher frequency based on the number of cases.

Reference
Sahn SA. Diagnosis and management of parapneumonic
  effusions and empyema. Clin Infect Dis.
  2007;45(11):1480–6.

493. What is the most common cause of nursing homeac-
  quired pneumonia (NHAP)?
  A) Streptococcus pneumoniae
  B) Branhamella catarrhalis
  C) Haemophilus influenzae
  D) Legionella
  E) Staphylococcus aureus

Answer: A
NHAP more closely resembles community-acquired pneumonia (CAP) than nosocomial pneumonia with the usual
pathogens being the most common. Streptococcus pneumoniae is still the most common. In severe cases of NHAP
requiring mechanical ventilation, the rates of infection with
Staphylococcus aureus and enteric gram-negative organisms
appear to exceed those of S. pneumoniae.

References
El-Solh AA, et al. Etiology of severe pneumonia in the very
  elderly. Am J Respir Crit Care Med. 2001;163(3 pt
  1):645–51.
Mills K, Graham AC, Winslow BT, Springer KL. Treatment
  of nursing home-acquired pneumonia. Am Fam Physician.
  2009;79(11):976–82.

494. A 25-year-old nurse picked up the urine sample from
  the patient infected with HIV and while leaving the
  room slipped and fell down spilling the urine on her
  hands and clothes. After thorough washing of her
  hands with soap and water and changing her clothes,
  she asks you for advice. She understands that time is an
  important factor in HIV prophylaxis exposure. She has
  no cuts, abrasions, or dermatitis. The source patient is
  HIV positive.
     What is the appropriate management for this health-
  care worker?
  A) Efavirenz and lamivudine
  B) Efavirenz, lamivudine, and zidovudine
  C) Kaletra, lamivudine, and zidovudine
  D) Abacavir, lamivudine, and zidovudine
  E) Observation

Answer: E
Treatment with antiretroviral therapy is reserved for high-risk exposure such needlestick and exposure to bloody fluids and is not necessary in this case. In the absence of blood, saliva, sputum, sweat, tears, feces, nasal secretions, urine, and vomitus carry a very low risk of transmission of HCV and HIV.

Reference
Henderson DK, Fahey BJ, Willy M, Schmitt JM, Carey K, Koziol DE. Risk for occupational transmission of human immunodeficiency virus type 1 (HIV-1) associated with clinical exposures. A prospective evaluation. Ann Intern Med. 1990;113(10):740–6.

495. A 52-year-old man is admitted for dysarthria and right and lower extremity weakness of 20 min duration. He has a history of diabetes, hypercholesterolemia, and hypertension. He takes aspirin, hydrochlorothiazide, metformin, and simvastatin daily. A CT of head without contrast showed no acute abnormalities. tPA was administered in the radiology interventional lab. Subsequent CT scan 2 days later of head demonstrated ischemic stroke involving right parietal area. Echocardiography of the heart was normal.

     What other intervention should be done to reduce recurrence of the stroke?
     A) Add clopidogrel at discharge.
     B) Aspirin and warfarin on discharge.
     C) Discontinue aspirin and start warfarin.
     D) Add dipyridamole at discharge.
     E) Nothing else as she is on optimal treatment.

Answer: D
Starting clopidogrel alone and adding dipyridamole to his aspirin are reasonable options. Guidelines from the Seventh American College of Chest Physicians (ACCP) Conference on Antithrombotic and Thrombolytic Therapy suggest that the combination of extended-release dipyridamole and aspirin is more efficacious than clopidogrel.

     The patient was already on aspirin and addition of dipyridamole has shown to reduce risk of stroke recurrence in ESPRIT and PRoFESS trials. The addition of clopidogrel to aspirin has increased risk of cerebral and GI bleeds and there is no substantial increase in benefit. Anticoagulants are not used to reduce stroke recurrence.

References
Albers GW, Amarenco P, Easton JD, Sacco RL, Teal P. Antithrombotic and thrombolytic therapy for ischemic stroke: the Seventh ACCP Conference on Antithrombotic and Thrombolytic Therapy. Chest. 2004;126(3 Suppl):483S–512S.
Meschia JF, Bushnell C, Boden-Albala B, Braun LT, Bravata DM, Chaturvedi S, et al. Guidelines for the primary prevention of stroke: a Statement for healthcare professionals from the American Heart Association/American Stroke Association. Stroke. 2014;45(12):3754–832.

496. A 55-year-old woman with insulin-dependent diabetes is admitted for epigastric pain. Esophagogastroduodenoscopy (EGD) is performed and reveals mild gastric mucosal erythema but no additional abnormalities. She is started on metoclopramide for presume diabetic gastroparesis.

     Which of the following is true regarding metoclopramide?
     A) It has a 10 % risk of tardive dyskinesia.
     B) Long-term efficacy has been proven.
     C) It improves symptoms of tachygastria, not bradygastria.
     D) It improves survival in gastoparetics.
     E) Patients should be on the shortest course and at the minimal dose required, with every effort made to avoid chronic use of metoclopramide.

Answer: E
Metoclopramide is approved for short-term use in diabetic gastroparesis. It is one of the few options available. Five controlled trials have evaluated the efficacy of metoclopramide in the treatment of diabetic gastroparesis. Benefits have been limited. Metoclopramide has been demonstrated to be effective for the short-term treatment of gastroparesis for up to several weeks, but long-term efficacy has not been proven. In one study, no consistent benefit was observed from the use of metoclopramide for more than 1 month. Survival in diabetics with gastroparesis is not impacted by metoclopramide use. While symptoms of bradygastria are improved, diabetics may also have tachygastric symptoms which would be worsened, not improved with metoclopramide.

     National guidelines estimate the risk of developing tardive dyskinesia (TD) from metoclopramide to be 1–15 %. Chronic use of metoclopramide appears to increase the risk of developing TD. Prior to initiating treatment with metoclopramide, it may be reasonable to obtain informed consent with the physician, patient, and family members. This should also be documented in the medical chart for medicolegal reasons.

References
Hasler WL. Gastroparesis: symptoms, evaluation, and treatment. Gastroenterol Clin North Am. 2007;36:619–47.
Shaffer D, Butterfield M, Pamer C, Mackey AC. Tardive dyskinesia risks and metoclopramide use before and after U.S. market withdrawal of cisapride. J Am Pharm Assoc. 2003;44(6):661–5.

497. A 88-year-old white female presenting from her nursing home with watery diarrhea × 4 days. She is found to be positive for *Clostridium difficile*. This is her first occurrence, and she is started on metronidazole 500 mg PO TID.

Which of the following medications should not be on her inpatient profile?

A) Polyethylene glycol
B) Loperamide
C) Both A and B
D) Cholestyramine

Answer: C

Polyethylene glycol is an osmotic agent that would increase bowel movements. Loperamide acts on opioid intestinal muscle receptors to inhibit peristalsis and prolong transit time in the GI tract. Neither would be appropriate in an acute *Clostridium difficile* infection. Loperamide would potentially inhibit the excretion of toxins, leading to toxic megacolon. On the other hand, polyethylene glycol would cause more cramping and discomfort for the patient who is already experiencing frequency in bowel movements.

Cholestyramine has shown only modest activity in reducing stool frequency and is not recommended for use in patients with severe cases of *C. difficile* colitis. Cholestyramine binds to vancomycin and must be dosed separately if it is used in combination with this antibiotic.

Reference
Cohen SH, et al. Clinical practice guidelines for clostridium difficile infection in adults : 2010 Update by the Society for Healthcare Epidemiology of America (SHEA) and IDSA. Infect Cont Hosp Epidemiol. 2010;31:431–55.

498. Approximately what percent of empirical antimicrobial regimens remain unchanged after 5 days of hospitalization?

A) 25 %
B) 45 %
C) 65 %
D) 85 %
E) 3 %

Answer: C

Broad-spectrum empirical therapy is common, and in many cases it is protocol driven. This is beneficial in many instances, and certainly many antibiotic guidelines have improved mortality. However, there is often a reluctance to deescalate a regimen that has been working even when clinical signs of infection are no longer present.

Deescalation of antibiotics when indicated is associated with a lower mortality. At 48–72 h, it is suggested to review microbiologic data, and if the patient is improving, deescalate from broad-spectrum antibiotics to a more narrow spectrum. Procalcitonin levels are also being utilized to guide therapy. Many health-care systems are developing antibiotic stewardship programs to address these issues.

References
Dellit TH, et al. Infectious Diseases Society of America and the Society for Healthcare Epidemiology of America guidelines for developing an institutional program to enhance antimicrobial stewardship. Clin Infect Dis. 2007;44:159–77.

Garnacho-Montero J, Gutierrez-Pizarraya A, Escoresca-Ortega A, et al. De-escalation of empirical therapy is associated with lower mortality in patients with severe sepsis and septic shock. Intensive Care Med. 2014;40(1):32–40.

499. Which of the following in acute exacerbations of COPD is not predicted by a BAP-65 score?

A) Inhospital mortality
B) The risk of mechanical ventilation
C) Length of stay
D) Long-term mortality
E) None of the above

Answer: D

The BAP-65 system represents a simple tool to categorize patients with acute exacerbation of COPD. It is calculated by measuring B blood urea nitrogen, A altered mental status, P pulse, and age. Patients ≤ 65 years of age are class 1. For patients older than 65 years of age, the score is stratified based upon a number of risk factors: class 3 has one risk factor, class 4 has two risk factors, and class 5 has three risk factors.

BAP-65 is primarily used to predict the inhospital severity and possible need for intubation. It does not predict out-of-hospital mortality.

The BODE index is utilized to predict long-term outcome for patients with COPD. It is composed of body-mass index, airflow obstruction, dyspnea, and exercise.

References
Celli BR, Cote CG, Marin JM, et al. The body-mass index, airflow obstruction, dyspnea and exercise capacity index in chronic obstructive pulmonary disease. N Engl J Med. 2004;350(10):1005–12.

Shorr AF, Sun X, Johannes RS, Yaitanes A, Tabak YP. Validation of a novel risk score for severity of illness in acute exacerbations of COPD. Chest. 2011;140(5): 1177–83.

500. In alcohol withdrawal, when does a seizure usually occur?

A) 6–8 h after the cessation of drinking
B) 8–12 h after the cessation of drinking
C) 6–48 h after the cessation of drinking
D) 72 h after the cessation of drinking
E) 1 week after the cessation of drinking

Answer: C

Withdrawal seizures occur within 6–48 h of alcohol cessation. Alcohol withdrawal may present with a seizure as the first sign. No other symptoms of withdrawal may occur after the seizure abates. About 30–40 % of patients with alcohol withdrawal seizures progress to delirium tremens. Alcohol withdrawal seizures usually occur only once or recur only once or twice, and they generally resolve spontaneously. Withdrawal generally occurs 10–72 h after the last drink.

Reference

Eyer F, Schuster T, Felgenhauer N, Pfab R, Strubel T, Saugel B. Risk assessment of moderate to severe alcohol withdrawal – predictors for seizures and delirium tremens in the course of withdrawal. Alcohol Alcohol. 2011;46(4):427–33.

501. How do academic versus nonacademic hospitalists' services compare in the following parameters?
  A) Increased length of stay (LOS).
  B) Increased all-cause inhospital mortality.
  C) Decreased all-cause mortality.
  D) No changes were observed.

Answer: A

In studies that compared a teaching hospitalist service with a staff-only hospitalist service, LOS was significantly shorter in the staff-only hospitalist group. Other factors remained the same.

Reference

Everett GD, Anton MP, Jackson BK, Swigert C, Uddin N. Comparison of hospital costs and length of stay associated with general internists and hospitalist physicians at a community hospital. Am J Manag Care. 2004;10(9): 626–30.

502. In which of the following situations do patients warrant stress ulcer prophylaxis?
  A) Platelet count = 37,000 with an INR = 1.9
  B) Patients in the ICU on a ventilator (>48 h)
  C) High-dose corticosteroid use
  D) All the above

Answer: D

Stress ulcer prophylaxis is recommended for any of the following major risk factors: respiratory failure requiring mechanical ventilation (likely for greater than 48 h) or coagulopathy defined as platelet count <50,000, INR >1.5, or a PTT >2× the control (prophylactic or treatment doses of anticoagulants do not constitute a coagulopathy). Additional risk factors warranting stress ulcer prophylaxis are as follows: head or spinal cord injury, severe burn (more than 35 % BSA), hypoperfusion, acute organ dysfunction, history of GI ulcer/bleeding within 1 year, high doses of corticosteroids, liver failure with associated coagulopathy, postoperative transplantation, acute kidney injury, major surgery, and multiple trauma.

References

ASHP Commission on Therapeutics. ASHP Therapeutic Guidelines on Stress Ulcer Prophylaxis. Am J Health Syst Pharm. 1999;56:347–79.

Sessler JM. Stress-related mucosal disease in the intensive care unit: an update on prophylaxis. AACN Adv Crit Care. 2007;18:199–206.

Index

A

Abdominal compartment syndrome
  physical examination, 65
  surgical depression, 66
Academic *vs.* nonacademic hospitalists, 193
Acetaminophen, 72, 189
Acetylcysteine, 189
Acid-fast bacilli (AFB), 57
Acute coronary syndrome (ACS), 53, 159, 179
Acute kidney injury (AKI)
  cause, 90–91
  urine output and sodium excretion, 170–171
Acute mesenteric ischemia (AMI)
  abdominal distention and gastrointestinal bleeding, 176
  classification, 24
  legal risk, 176
  superior mesenteric artery embolism, 176
Acute respiratory distress syndrome (ARDS), 8, 142, 157
Acute tubular necrosis (ATN), 64
Acyclovir
  Bell's palsy, 4
  therapy, 62–63
Adenocarcinoma, 6, 14, 85, 115, 155
Adjuvant albumin treatment, 48
Adrenal adenomas, 25
Adrenal insufficiency, 53
Adult-onset Still disease (AOSD), 9–10
Adult Still's disease, 46
Adverse drug event (ADE), 159–160
Advisory Committee on Immunization Practices (ACIP), 156
Affordable Care Act (ACA), 163
Aggressive fluid resuscitation
  blood transfusion, 26
  fluid requirements, 26
  sepsis from pyelonephritis, 61
  vasopressor therapy and, 149
Aggressive hydration, 29, 56, 133
Agitation, psychosocial support, 30
Airborne precautions, 184–185
Air trapping, COPD, 99
Albumin infusion, 164
Alcoholic hepatitis, 39–40, 50
Alcohol withdrawal
  diagnosis, 24
  pharmacologic treatment, 25
  seizures, 32, 192
Alkalosis, 75
Alpha blockers, 166
Amebic liver abscess, metronidazole treatment, 74–75
American Academy of Neurology (AAN), 2
American Association of Clinical Endocrinology, 34

American College of Cardiology (ACC)
  amiodarone, class IIa recommendation, 55
  guidelines, 96
American College of Cardiology/American Heart Association
  (ACC/AHA) guidelines, 53
American College of Chest Physicians, 62, 109, 123
American College of Emergency Physicians (ACEP)
  Clinical Policy, 18
American College of Gastroenterologists (ACG), 103
American College of Gastroenterology, 147
American Diabetes Association (ADA), 34
American Heart Association (AHA), 8, 97–98, 149, 160–161
American Heart Association/American Stroke Association, 68
American Urological Association, 170
AMI. *See* Acute mesenteric ischemia (AMI)
Aminoglycoside toxicity, 23
Amiodarone, 55
Amniotic fluid embolism, 110
Amphotericin B, 37
Ampicillin, 10–11
Analgesia in cirrhotic patients, 72
Anchoring errors, 177
Anemia
  blood loss source, 101
  mean corpuscular volume (MCV), 42
  oxygen carrying capacity, 101
Anorexia and gastrointestinal symptoms, 133
Anterior myocardial infarction, 42
Anthrax, 100
Antibiotics, deescalation, 192
Anticoagulant therapy, 86, 159, 187–188
Antidopaminergic medicines, 114
Antiepileptic therapy, 155
Antileukocyte antibodies, 112
Antineutrophil cytoplasmic antibodies (pANCA), 87
Antinuclear antibodies (ANA), 20
Antipsychotics
  atypical, 22, 81
  frontotemporal dementia (FTD), 83
  medications, 5
  neuroleptic medications, 11
Antiretroviral therapy, 172, 190
Anti-*Saccharomyces cerevisiae* antibodies (ASCA), 87
Antituberculous therapy, 57
Aortic abdominal aneurysm, ruptured, 79
Aortic stenosis, 25
Aortic valve replacement, 25, 97
Aplastic crisis
  erythema infectiosum, 29
  parvovirus B19, 29
Appendicitis, 131

Printed in the United States
By Bookmasters